Pain Relief
With Trigger Point
Self-Help

Valerie DeLaune, LAc

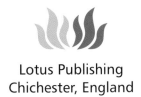

Lotus Publishing
Chichester, England

North Atlantic Books
Berkeley, California

First published in 2011 by
Lotus Publishing
Apple Tree Cottage, Inlands Road, Nutbourne, Chichester, PO18 8RJ and
North Atlantic Books
P O Box 12327
Berkeley, California 94712

Drawings Amanda Williams
Photographs Skip Gray, Don Douglas
Pain Relief Guides SarahGraphics
Text and Cover Design Wendy Craig
Printed and Bound in the UK by Scotprint

Pain Relief With Trigger Point Self-Help is sponsored by the Society for the Study of Native Arts and Sciences, a nonprofit educational corporation whose goals are to develop an educational and crosscultural perspective linking various scientific, social, and artistic fields; to nurture a holistic view of arts, sciences, humanities, and healing; and to publish and distribute literature on the relationship of mind, body, and nature.

MEDICAL DISCLAIMER: The following information is intended for general information purposes only. Individuals should always see their health care provider before administering any suggestions made in this book. Any application of the material set forth in the following pages is at the reader's discretion and is his or her sole responsibility.

British Library Cataloguing-in-Publication Data
A CIP record for this book is available from the British Library
ISBN 978 1 905367 25 2 (Lotus Publishing)
ISBN 978 1 58394 400 4 (North Atlantic Books)

Library of Congress Cataloguing-in-Publication Data

DeLaune, Valerie.
  Pain relief with trigger point self-help / Valerie DeLaune.
    p. cm.
  Includes bibliographical references and index.
  ISBN 978-1-58394-400-4 (pbk.)
  1. Massage therapy--Popular works. 2. Chronic pain--Alternative
treatment--Popular works. 3. Chronic pain--Exercise therapy--Popular works.
4. Pain--Diet therapy--Popular works. 5. Self-care, Health--Popular works.
I. Title.
  RM722.D45 2011
  615.8'22--dc23
                    2011015831

Contents

Acknowledgements

This book would not have been possible without the lifeworks of Dr. Janet Travell and Dr. David G. Simons, who worked endlessly to research trigger points, document referral patterns and other symptoms, and bring all of that information to medical practitioners and the general public. Together, Doctors Travell and Simons produced a comprehensive two-volume text on the causes and treatment of trigger points, written for physicians. *Pain Relief With Trigger Point Self-Help* is a condensation of those volumes, written for the general public and for practitioners, who do not need the in-depth knowledge to perform trigger point injections.

Dr. Travell pioneered and researched new pain treatments, including trigger point injections. In her private practice, she began treating Senator John F. Kennedy, who at the time was using crutches due to crippling back pain and was almost unable to walk down just a few stairs. Because of television, it had become important for presidential candidates to appear physically fit, and being on crutches probably would have cost President Kennedy the election. Dr. Travell became the first female White House physician, and after President Kennedy died, she stayed on to treat President Johnson. She resigned a year and a half later to return to her passions: teaching, lecturing, and writing about chronic myofascial pain. She continued to work into her nineties and died at the age of 95 on August 1, 1997.

Dr. Simons met Dr. Travell when the latter was lecturing at the School of Aerospace Medicine at Brooks Air Force Base in Texas in the 1960s. He soon teamed up with Dr. Travell and began researching the international literature for any references to the treatment of pain. There were a few others out there who were also discovering trigger points but using different terminology. Dr. Simons studied and documented the physiology of trigger points in both laboratory and clinical settings and tried to find scientific explanations for trigger points. He continued to research the physiology of trigger points, update the trigger point volumes he coauthored with Dr. Travell, and review trigger point research articles until his death at the age of 88 on April 5, 2010.

I am also profoundly grateful to my neuromuscular therapy instructor, Jeanne Aland, who taught me basics about trigger points and introduced me to the books written by Doctors Travell and Simons. I was told Jeanne passed on a few years ago.

All three are well missed, and those familiar with trigger points are extremely grateful for the hard work and dedication of these people. Their work lives on through the hundreds of thousands of patients who have gotten relief because of their research and willingness to train others.

Other Thanks
Many additional researchers have contributed to the study of trigger points, and many doctors and other practitioners have taken the time to learn about trigger points and give that information to their patients. I would like to acknowledge all of them for their role in alleviating pain by making this important information available. In particular, I would like to thank Dr. Juhani Partanen, who kindly explained the "Muscle Spindle" hypothesis to me in lay terms, and also took the time to review the chapter "Trigger Points—What Are They and What Causes Them?" to make sure I had translated scientific language correctly into easier-to-understand terms.

Not least, I would like to thank my publisher, Jonathan Hutchings, of Lotus Publishing, who contacted me and asked me to write this book, and made the incredible artwork possible. Without his help and support, you would not be holding this book in your hands right now. Copyeditor Steve D. Brierley did an excellent job providing organizational suggestions, catching my mistakes, and making various changes to improve the text. Amanda Williams did a fantastic job with the anatomical drawings and referral patterns, and went to great lengths to answer my anatomy questions. Sarah Olsen of Sarahgraphics has done her usual bang-up job on the graphic design work for the pain referral patterns, as she has for my previous books. Wendy Craig put all the pieces together to create a very attractive and useful text. This is a book we can all be proud of; I could not have done it without any of you.

Lastly, I would like to thank the friends who I visited while I was writing this book, who extended Alaskan-style hospitality and let me plug my RV into their electrical outlets for the duration of my stays with them: Joan Pardes, Doug Sturm, Eva the child and Scout the dog of Alaska; Art, Cecily, and Nikki 'the dog' Morris also of Alaska; Judy Lungren and Rick Noll of Washington; Scott Edgerton of Montana; Janet Krivacek, Randy Gage, and Bailey the dog also of Montana; Marc Soderquist of Wyoming; and Lisa Horlick of Colorado. And once again, for my own wolf-dog, Sasha, without whose friendship my life would definitely be both less interesting and less blessed.

Introduction

Pain Cannot Be Effectively Treated Without Understanding Trigger Points

Without a knowledge base of trigger points and referred pain, a health care provider cannot effectively treat pain syndromes. I have treated hundreds of fairly simple cases where people had been told their only recourse was to learn to live with their pain, only because their health care provider didn't know about trigger points. In spite of decades of research, Myofascial Pain Syndrome associated with and caused by trigger points continues to be one of the most commonly missed diagnoses. The most important thing to know about treating pain is that trigger points refer pain to other areas in fairly consistent common patterns. Knowledge of referral patterns gives us a starting point of where to look for the trigger points that are actually causing pain.

I'm frequently contacted by people who are fairly sure trigger point treatment is at least part of the solution to their pain problems, but they are completely frustrated because they cannot find a practitioner who knows about trigger points. At this time, massage therapists, physical therapists, and physiotherapists are the professionals who are most likely to have experience in treating trigger points. However, even if they do know about trigger points, they may have not learned much about perpetuating factors—the things that cause and keep trigger points activated and that absolutely need to be resolved for long-term relief.

That is why learning about trigger points yourself and doing the self-help exercises in this book is so important; with the information in this book, you may be better equipped to treat trigger points than your health care provider. If you cannot find someone who already knows about trigger points, bring your book to your appointments with you. Educate your practitioner about trigger points and your referral patterns.

Do Not Wait to Treat Your Pain

It is important to treat trigger points as soon as possible so that they are less likely to cause chronic pain problems. So often I hear patients say, "I kept thinking it would go away." Sometimes symptoms will go away in a few days and never return. But more often, the longer you wait to see if pain will go away, the more muscles become involved in the chain reaction of chronic pain and dysfunction. A muscle hurts and forms trigger points, then the area of referral (where you feel the pain or other symptoms) starts to hurt and tighten up and forms its own satellite trigger points, then those trigger points refer pain somewhere else, and so on. Or the pain may improve for a while, but the trigger points are really just in an inactive phase and can become active and cause pain or other symptoms once again.

Do Not Assume Your Pain Cannot Be Treated

People often assume that if a parent had the same type of condition, it must be genetic, and they will just have to learn to live with it. You learn many things from your parents—eating habits, exercise habits, how you deal with stressful situations, even posture and gestures—and all of these can influence your health.

I never assume that a condition cannot at least be improved, even if it is genetic. If necessary, I will refer a patient to another provider, such as a chiropractor, naturopath, or surgeon, who can help them. In spite of being told that you have to learn to live with your medical condition, assume you can change it, at least until you have exhausted all treatment options. It may be that you have a systemic perpetuating factor that cannot be completely resolved and will require you to treat your pain over the long term, but at least you can improve the quality of your life by learning how to manage your symptoms.

How Long Will Treatment Take?

When people begin treatment, they commonly ask me, "How long will it take?" The longer the condition has been going on and the more medical conditions you have, the greater the number of muscles that will become involved through central sensitization; this is discussed in chapter 1. This means that treatment will be more complex and take longer. If you are perfectly healthy and have only a recent minor injury, you may not need long-term treatment.

In my experience, people who do self-treatments at home in addition to receiving weekly professional treatments improve at least five times faster than those who only receive professional treatments. As Doctors Travell and Simons said, "Treatments that are done to the patient should be minimized and effort should be concentrated in teaching what can be done by the patient…as patients exercise increasing control [over symptom management,] they improve both physically and emotionally." How quickly you get long-term relief will be determined by how accurately you identify and resolve your perpetuating factors; this is discussed in chapters 2–4.

This is not necessarily a quick fix, though you may get a great deal of relief in a short period of time. There is no such thing as resolving all of your pain in 15 minutes or less, or being pain free in ten easy steps. No technique or practitioner can do that for you. You will need to read the chapters, search for trigger points in your muscles, and use the self treatment techniques on a regular basis until your pain is resolved.

Be sure to read through part I before starting on the pressure techniques and stretches found in part II. Use a highlighter pen to mark any perpetuating factors in chapters 2–4 that you might need to address. You will not get lasting relief until you resolve the things that are causing and aggravating your trigger points. As you address perpetuating factors, pace yourself so that the process is not too overwhelming. Work on your perpetuating factors over time—you likely will not be able to make all the needed changes at once. Then, see chapter 5 for general guidelines for self-treatments, and chapter 6 for the pain guides that will help you determine which muscles might contain trigger points.

> *If we treat myofascial pain syndromes without…correcting the multiple perpetuating factors, the patient is doomed to endless cycles of treatment and relapse…Usually, one stress activates the [trigger point], then other factors perpetuate it. In some patients, these perpetuating factors are so important that their elimination results in complete relief of the pain without any local treatment.*
> —Doctors Janet Travell and David G. Simons

I recommend that, if possible, you have your trigger points identified by a practitioner who has been trained in treating trigger points, such as a neuromuscular massage therapist or a physical therapist, and use the book to supplement their work. It could take longer for you to locate trigger points without the aid of a professional, but with the guidance in this book, you will most likely be able to locate the trigger points yourself.

There are hundreds of suggestions in this book. Plan to devote some time to accomplishing your goals. Resolving pain is like detective work; what causes your pain and what resolves it will be a combination of factors unique to you.

When Should You See a Health Care Provider?

If you cannot get relief by using the self-help techniques in this book, you will need to see a health care provider. It may be that something other than trigger points is causing or contributing to your pain. X-rays, MRIs, and other diagnostic tests can identify some conditions, such as osteoarthritis, stress fractures, and torn ligaments or tendons, that may cause pain.

Referred symptoms due to trigger points can mimic other, more serious conditions, or can occur concurrently with them. It may take some investigation to determine the ultimate cause of the problem. Most muscle chapters in this book contain a section labeled "Differential Diagnosis." Unless you are a health care provider, it is likely you will not understand most of what it says. Do not be too concerned about this; the section has been included so that you can take it to a health care provider and be evaluated for those conditions, though you still ought to read it.

You should see a medical provider immediately to rule out serious conditions if you have pain with any of the following symptoms:

■ Your pain had a sudden onset, is severe, or starts with a traumatic injury, particularly if you heard a noise at the time.
■ Your pain lasts for more than two weeks, unless you have already ruled out more serious conditions.
■ The intensity of pain increases over time, or the symptoms are different; changes can be an indication of a different, more serious cause.
■ Your pain is accompanied by redness, heat, severe swelling, or odd sensations.
■ You develop rashes or ulcers that do not heal.
■ You develop poor circulation, painful varicose veins, and very cold legs, feet, arms, or hands.

Hopefully your health care provider will rule out any serious conditions. If you are diagnosed with pain from structural damage or chronic conditions, chances are you can relieve much or all of your pain with a combination of self-treatment of trigger points and addressing and eliminating the perpetuating factors. Regardless of the diagnosis you receive from a health care provider, my general treatment principle is the same: identify and eliminate all the underlying perpetuating causes to the extent possible, and treat the trigger points.

My Background

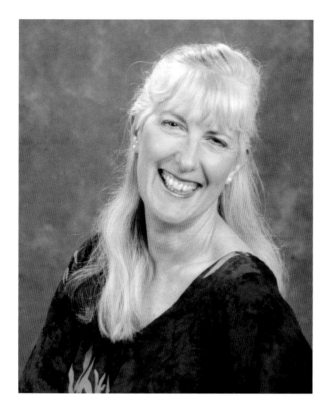

I attended massage school in 1989 and learned Swedish massage. I learned to give a very good general massage, but I did not feel equipped to treat chronic pain. I was very intrigued by a description of a continuing education certificate course called Neuromuscular Therapy, which combines myofascial release (a type of deep tissue massage) with treating trigger points. I attended the class in 1991, taught by Jeanne Aland at Heartwood Institute, and it completely changed my approach to treating patients. Once I had learned about referral patterns, I was able to consistently resolve chronic pain problems.

Over my years of treating thousands of patients, I have added my own observations to those of Doctors Travell and Simons, and developed a variety of self-help techniques. In 1999, I received my master's degree in acupuncture. Since then I have been specializing in dry-needling trigger points, treating pain syndromes with Traditional Chinese Medicine, and writing trigger point books.

www.triggerpointrelief.com

Part I

Trigger Points—What Are They and What Causes Them?

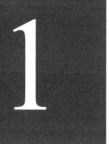

Trigger Points and Chronic Pain

Muscle Anatomy and Physiology

Muscles consist of many muscle cells, or *fibers*, bundled together by connective tissue. Each fiber contains numerous *myofibrils*, and most skeletal muscles contain approximately one thousand to two thousand myofibrils. Each myofibril consists of a chain of sarcomeres connected end to end—it is in the *sarcomere* that muscular contractions take place.

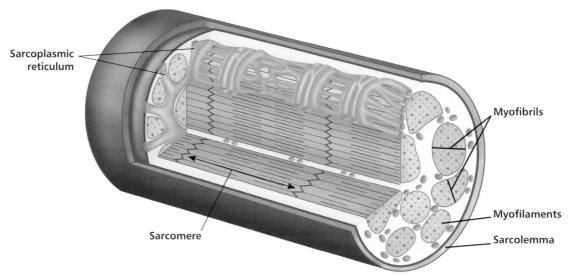

Each skeletal muscle fiber is a single cylindrical muscle cell.

A *muscle spindle* is a sensory receptor found within the belly of a muscle. Muscle spindles are concentrated where a nerve enters a muscle and also around nerves inside the muscles. Each spindle contains three to twelve *intrafusal muscle fibers*, which detect changes in the length of a muscle. As the body's position changes, information is conveyed to the central nervous system via sensory neurons and is processed in the brain. As needed, the *motor end plate* (a type of nerve ending) releases *acetylcholine*, a neurotransmitter that tells the *sarcoplasmic reticulum* (a part of each cell) to release ionized calcium. The *extrafusal muscle fibers* then contract. When contraction of the muscle fibers is no longer needed, the nerve ending stops releasing acetylcholine, and calcium is pumped back into the sarcoplasmic reticulum.

Trigger Point Physiology: Contractions and Inflammation

One of the current theories about the mechanism responsible for the formation of trigger points is the "Integrated Trigger Point Hypothesis." If a trauma occurs, or there is a large increase in the motor end plate's release of acetylcholine, an excessive amount of calcium can be released by the sarcoplasmic reticulum. This causes a maximal contracture of a segment of muscle, leading to a maximal demand for energy and impairment of local circulation. If circulation is impaired, the calcium pump does not get the fuel and oxygen it needs to pump calcium back into the sarcoplasmic reticulum, so the muscle fiber stays contracted. Sensitizing substances are released, causing pain and stimulation of the autonomic nervous system, resulting in a positive feedback system with the motor nerve terminal releasing excessive acetylcholine…and so the sarcomere stays contracted.

Another current theory is the "Muscle Spindle" hypothesis, which proposes that the main cause of a trigger point is an inflamed muscle spindle (Partanen, Ojala, and Arokoski, 2010). Pain receptors activate skeletofusimotor units during sustained overload of muscles via a spinal reflex pathway, which connects to the muscle spindles. As pain continues, sustained contraction and fatigue drive the skeletofusimotor units to exhaustion, and cause rigor (silent spasm) of the extrafusal muscle fibers, forming the "taut band" we feel as trigger points. Because the muscle spindle itself has a poor blood supply, the inflammatory metabolites released will be concentrated inside the spindle and lead to sustained inflammation.

In a ground-breaking study, Shah et al. (2008) were able to measure eleven elevated biochemicals in and surrounding active trigger points, including inflammatory mediators, neuropeptides, catecholamines, and cytokincs (primarily sensitizing substances and immune system biochemicals). In addition, the pH of the samples was strongly acidic compared to other areas of the body. In a study conducted by Issbener, Reeh, and Steen (1996), it was discovered that a localized acidic pH lowered the pain threshold sensitivity level of sensory receptors (part of the nervous system), even without acute damage to the muscle. This means that the more acidic your pH level in a given area, the more pain you will experience compared to someone else. Further investigation is needed to determine whether body-wide elevations in pH acidity and the substances mentioned above predispose people to the development of trigger points.

More studies, therefore, are needed to determine the exact mechanisms of trigger point formation and physiology.

Central Sensitization, Trigger Points, and Chronic Pain

The *autonomic nervous system* controls the release of acetylcholine, along with involuntary functions of blood vessels and glands. Anxiety and nervous tension increase autonomic nervous system activity, which commonly aggravates trigger points and their associated symptoms.

The *central nervous system* includes the brain and spinal cord, and its function is to integrate and coordinate all activities and responses of the body. The purpose of the acute stress responses of our bodies is to protect us by telling us to pull away from a hot stove burner, flee from a dangerous situation, or rest an injured body part due to pain. But when emotional or physical stress is prolonged, even just for a few days, there is a maladaptive response: damage to the central nervous system, particularly to the sympathetic nervous system and the hypothalamus-pituitary-adrenal (HPA) systems. This is called *central nervous system sensitization*.

Pain causes certain types of nerve receptors in muscles to relay information to *neurons* located within part of the gray matter of the spinal cord and the brain stem. Pain is amplified there and is then relayed to other muscles, thereby expanding the region of pain beyond the initially affected area. Persistent pain leads to long-term or possibly permanent changes in these neurons, which affect adjacent neurons through *neurotransmitters*.

Various substances are released: *histamine* (a compound that causes dilation and permeability of blood vessels), *serotonin* (a neurotransmitter that constricts blood vessels), *bradykinin* (a hormone that dilates peripheral blood vessels and increases small blood vessel permeability), and *substance P* (a compound involved in the regulation of the pain threshold). These substances stimulate the nervous system to release even more acetylcholine locally, adding to the perpetuation of trigger points.

Central sensitization may cause the part of the nervous system that would normally counteract pain to malfunction and fail to do its job. As a result, pain can be more easily triggered by lower levels of physical and emotional stressors, and also be more intense and last longer. Prolonged pain caused by central nervous system sensitization can lead to emotional and physical stress. Conversely, prolonged exposure to both emotional and physical stressors can lead to central nervous system sensitization and subsequently cause pain. Just the central nervous system maladaptive changes alone can be self-perpetuating and cause pain, even without the presence of either the original or any additional stressors, creating a vicious cycle of pain and trigger point formation.

Once the central nervous system is involved, because of central sensitization, even if the original perpetuating factor(s) causing trigger points are resolved, trigger points can continue to form and be reactivated. So the longer that pain goes untreated, the greater the number of neurons that get involved and the more muscles they affect, causing pain in new areas, in turn causing more neurons to get involved…and the bigger the problem becomes, leading to the likelihood that pain will become chronic. The problem gets more complex, more painful, more debilitating, more frustrating, and more time-consuming and expensive to treat. The longer you wait, the less likely you are to get complete relief, and the more likely it is that your trigger points will be reactivated chronically and periodically. The sooner pain is treated, including addressing the initiating stressors and perpetuating factors, the less likely it will become a permanent problem with widespread muscle involvement and central nervous system changes.

How Will You Know if You Have Trigger Points?

The two most important characteristics of trigger points that you will notice are tender "knots" or tight bands in the muscles, and referred pain. You may also notice weakness, lack of range of motion, or other symptoms you would not normally associate with muscular problems.

Tenderness, Knots, and Tight Bands in the Muscle

When pressed, trigger points are usually very tender. This is because the sustained contraction of the myofibril leads to the release of sensitizing neurotransmitters via a cascade effect: the sustained contraction elevates metabolites such as potassium ions and lactic acid, which leads to elevated levels of inflammatory agents such as bradykinin and histamine, which activates pain nerve fibers, which then leads to the excretion of pain transmitters, such as substance P.

Pain intensity levels can vary depending on the amount of stress placed on the muscles. The intensity of pain can also vary in response to flare-ups of any of the perpetuating factors discussed in chapters 2–4, and in the presence of central nervous system sensitization (see above). The areas at the ends of the muscle fibers also become tender, either at the bone or where the muscle attaches to a tendon.

Healthy muscles usually do not contain knots or tight bands and are not tender to applied pressure. When not in use, they feel soft and pliable to the touch, not like the hard and dense muscles found in people with chronic pain. People often tell me their muscles feel hard and dense because they work out and do strengthening exercises, but healthy muscles feel soft and pliable when not being used, even if you work out. Muscles with trigger points may also be relaxed, so do not assume you do not have trigger points just because the muscle is not hard and dense.

Referred Pain

Trigger points may refer pain both in the area in which the trigger point is located, and/or to other areas of the body. These are called *referral patterns*. Over 55% of commonly found trigger points are not located within their area of referred pain. The most common referral patterns have been well documented and diagramed, and drawings are provided in the muscle chapters in part II of this book.

Unless you know where to search for trigger points, and you only work on the areas where you feel pain, you probably will not get relief. For example, trigger points in the iliopsoas muscle (deep in your abdomen) can cause pain in your lumbar area. If you do not check the iliopsoas muscle for trigger points and only work on the quadratus lumborum muscle in the lumbar area, you will not get relief. Part II teaches you where to look for trigger points, and how to treat each muscle.

Weakness and Muscle Fatigue

Trigger points can cause weakness and loss of coordination, along with an inability to use the muscle. Many people take this as a sign that they need to strengthen the weak muscles, but you cannot condition (strengthen) a muscle that contains trigger points—these muscle fibers are not available for use because they are already contracted. If trigger points are not inactivated first, conditioning exercises will likely encourage the surrounding muscles to do the work instead of the muscle containing the trigger point, further weakening and deconditioning the muscle containing trigger points.

Muscles containing trigger points are fatigued more easily and do not return to a relaxed state as quickly when you stop using the muscle. Trigger points may cause other muscles to tighten up and become weak and fatigued in the areas where you experience the referred pain, and they also cause a generalized tightening of an area as a response to pain.

Other Symptoms

Trigger points can cause symptoms that most people would not normally associate with muscular problems. For example, trigger points in the abdominal muscles can cause urinary frequency and bladder spasms, bed-wetting, chronic diarrhea, frequent belching and gas, nausea, loss of appetite, heartburn, food intolerance, painful menses, projectile vomiting, testicular pain, and pain that feels like it is in an organ, in addition to causing referred pain in the abdominal, mid back, and lumbar areas.

Trigger points may also cause stiff joints, generalized weakness or fatigue, twitching, trembling, and areas of numbness or other odd sensations. It probably would not occur to you (or your health care provider) that these symptoms could be caused by a trigger point in a muscle.

Sensitization of the Opposite Side of the Body

For any long-term pain, it is not unusual for it to affect both sides of the body eventually; for example, if the right lumbar area is painful, there may be tender points in the left lumbar area. Often the opposite side is actually *more* tender with pressure. This is because whatever is affecting one side is likely affecting the other: poor body mechanics, poor footwear, overuse injuries, chronic degenerative or inflammatory conditions, chronic disease, or central sensitization. For this reason, I almost always treat both sides on patients, and I recommend that you do self-treatments on both sides. You may find that you have trigger points only on one side for any given muscle, but always check both sides before making that assumption.

Active Trigger Points vs. Latent Trigger Points

If a trigger point is active, it will refer pain or other sensations and limit range of motion. If a trigger point is *latent*, it may cause a decreased range of motion and weakness, but not pain. The more frequent and intense your pain, the greater the number of active trigger points you are likely to have.

Trigger points that start with some impact to the muscle, such as an injury, are usually active initially. Poor posture or poor body mechanics, repetitive use, a nerve root irritation, or any of the other perpetuating factors addressed in chapters 2–4 can also form active trigger points. Latent trigger points can develop gradually without being active first, and you do not even know they are there. Most people have at least some latent trigger points, which can easily be converted to active trigger points.

Active trigger points may at some point stop referring pain and become latent. However, these latent trigger points can easily become active again, which may lead you to believe you are experiencing a new problem when in fact an old problem—perhaps even something you have forgotten about—is being reaggravated. Any of the perpetuating factors discussed in chapters 2–4 can activate previously latent trigger points and make you more prone to developing new trigger points initiated by impacts to muscles.

What Causes and Perpetuates Trigger Points?

Trigger points may form after a sudden trauma or injury, or they may develop gradually. Common initiating and perpetuating factors are mechanical stresses, injuries, nutritional problems, emotional factors, sleep problems, acute or chronic infections, organ dysfunction and disease, and other medical conditions; these conditions are discussed in next three chapters.

You will have more control over some perpetuating factors than others. Addressing any pertinent perpetuating factors is so important that you may obtain either substantial or complete relief from pain without any additional treatment. If you do not eliminate perpetuating factors to the extent possible, you may not get more than temporary relief from self-help pressure techniques or practitioners' treatments. Hopefully, you will learn enough about perpetuating factors that at least if you choose not to resolve them, you are making an informed choice about whether the relief of pain is more important to you than continuing to do things that make you feel worse.

You cannot realistically make all of the changes discussed in chapters 2–4 at once, but make a list of the perpetuating factors that might apply to you. Prioritize and work on resolving those you think might be the most important.

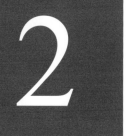

2 Perpetuating Factors: Ergonomics, Body Mechanics, and Clothing

Poorly designed or misfitting furniture, improperly using your body, and ill-fitting clothing causes and perpetuates trigger points, and are nearly always correctable. Investing in well-designed furniture, modifying certain activities, and wearing properly-fitting clothing will greatly speed your healing and provide long-term relief.

Ergonomics

Poorly designed or misfitting furniture causes chronic mechanical stress that leads to the development of trigger points and a self-perpetuating cycle of pain. Modifying your furniture can be one of the most important things to do in order to resolve your pain.

Office Furniture

Misfitting furniture is a major cause of muscular pain, particularly at the office or other workplace. There are many things you can do to minimize the amount of stress placed on your muscles. Even if you do not have a desk job, you may be coming home and spending a fair amount of time on a computer and/or at a desk.

There are companies that specialize in correcting your office arrangement and supplying you with furniture that fits your body. Your employer may balk at the cost, but if they do not change your misfitting furniture, they will end up paying for lost work time and workers' compensation claims. If your employer will not pay for it, you should consider paying for it yourself. What is it worth to you to be pain free?

Solutions

Computer station
Your computer screen should be about 1.5 to 2 feet away, located directly in front of you with the middle of the screen slightly below eye level. The copy should be attached to the side of the screen with a copy-holder so that your head is not tipped up or down, or turned to the side too far. Evaluate your workstation to make sure that you do not have glare on your screen, that your lighting is adequate, and that you have a computer screen that is not bothering your eyes.

If you have a keyboard tray, it should be height-adjustable. Your forearms should be parallel to the floor and your wrists should be straight. You may want to use a wrist rest. Be sure you are close enough to the desk so that you are leaning against the back of your chair, and that your elbows and forearms are supported on armrests or the desk. I see a lot of what I call "mouse injuries"—arm and shoulder pain due to using a computer mouse for extended periods of time without proper arm support. Move and relax your arms when you are not typing. Take frequent breaks and intersperse your computer work with non-computer tasks.

Chair

Your elbows and forearms should rest evenly on armrests of the proper height; the armrests must be high enough to provide support for your elbows without having to lean to the side, but not so high as to cause your shoulders to hike up. Adjustable armrests are ideal, but you can also tape towels or sponges to the armrests if they are too low. Your knees should fit under your desk, and your chair needs to be close enough for you to lean against the backrest. A good chair supports both your lumbar area and your mid back. The chair upholstery needs to be firm, and casters should be avoided. The seat should be low enough for you to keep your feet resting flat on the floor without compression of your thigh by the front edge of the seat, high enough to avoid all the pressure being placed on your gluteal area, and slightly hollowed out to accommodate your buttocks.

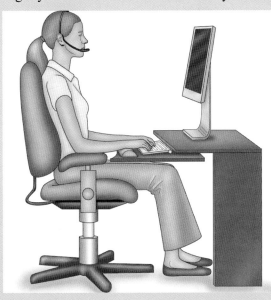

Other office furniture

If you must bend over reading materials or plans, a tilted work surface will alleviate the stress on your back and neck muscles up to a point, but be sure to take frequent breaks.

Headsets

Headsets for phones can be very important in obtaining relief from back, neck, and head pain. Shoulder rests are not adequate, and if you try to hold the phone with one hand, you will end up cradling the phone between your head and shoulder at some point, which is very hard on your neck and trapezius muscles. Get headsets for all of your work, home, and cellular phones.

Lumbar supports

A lumbar support helps correct round shouldered posture. Most chiropractic offices stock lumbar supports of varying thickness. I recommend that you get one for the car and one for your favorite seat or couch at home. You may wish to even take a lumbar support to the movie theatre, or when traveling for use on airplanes and in rental cars.

Try to avoid sitting on anything without back support, which causes you to sit with your shoulders and upper back slumped forward. When going to sporting events, picnics, or other places where you will not have a back support, bring a Crazy Creek Chair® or something similar to provide at least some support. You can get one through most of the major sporting goods suppliers and are not very expensive. They are very lightweight for carrying and a good investment in your back. Or, consider a lightweight collapsible chair, also available at sporting goods stores.

Bedtime Furniture

You probably spend about one third of every day in bed, so it is extremely important to make sure your pillow and bed are right for you. Sleeping on the couch should definitely be avoided.

Solutions

Pillows

If you have a pillow made of stuffed foam rubber or other springy material that will jiggle your neck, get rid of it! Vibrations from these pillows will aggravate trigger points. Memory foam pillows are fine, especially the kind with a hollow in the middle so your neck is supported. Your pillow should support your head at a level that keeps your spine in alignment, and that is comfortable when you are lying on your side—it should not be too high or too low. Chiropractic offices usually stock well-designed pillows. Take your pillow with you when you travel. Try experimenting with pillows until you find one that is right for you.

Beds

Beds that are too soft can cause a lot of muscular problems, and you may not know that it is too soft. People usually insist that their mattress is firm enough, but when queried further, they admit that sleeping on a mat on the floor gives them relief when the pain is particularly bad. Try putting some camp mats on the floor and sleeping on them for a week. If you feel better, your mattress is not firm enough, no matter how much money you spent on it or how well it worked for someone else. Different people have needs for different kinds of mattresses. An all cotton futon is very firm, and may be best for some people. You can put plywood between the box springs and mattress to make a bed firmer. Mattresses really only last about five to seven years, and should then be replaced.

If your partner is heavier, consider that, without realizing it, you may be bracing yourself slightly in order not to roll into them. Some types of mattresses can accommodate couples whose mattress needs differ.

Body Mechanics

If you slouch at your desk or on your couch at home, or if you read in bed, for example, your muscles will suffer. Poor body mechanics (e.g. lifting improperly), long periods of immobility (e.g. sitting at a desk without a break), repetitive movements (e.g. computer use), holding your body in an awkward position for long periods (e.g. dentists and mechanics), and excessively quick and jerky movements (e.g. sports) will all cause and perpetuate trigger points.

Solutions

- **Be aware of your body position.**
- Be sure to sit while putting clothing on your lower body. When having a conversation, turn and face the person, rather than rotating your head in their direction. Use back supports everywhere you sit, and do not read in bed. Do not keep a wallet in your back pocket, since it will tilt your spine and back when sitting. If you are gardening, straighten up frequently, and stand and stretch periodically. Be sure to slide into the center of your car seat. Some bucket seats curve up on each side, and if you are not in the center, your pelvis will be tilted.

Take frequent breaks

Take frequent breaks anytime you must sit or bend over for long periods. Setting a timer placed on the other side of the room can force you to get up periodically to turn it off.

Lift properly
Lift properly by bending your knees rather than your back, and hold objects close to your body.

Be aware of when you are tensing...and relax!
Notice whether you hold your shoulders up or are tightening muscles, such as your butt, arms, or abdomen, when you are under stress. Take a minute to mentally assess your body, noticing where you are holding tension. As you come to each area you are holding tightly, take a deep breath and consciously relax the tense area on your exhalation. Do this several times each day. You will need to retrain yourself to break the habit of holding tension in certain areas.

Gently increase range of motion
If you have a habit of immobilizing your muscles to protect against pain, you will need to start gently increasing your range of motion as you inactivate trigger points. Do not keep stressing the muscle to see if it still hurts or to demonstrate to your treating practitioners where you have to move it to in order to get it to hurt; if you keep repeating this motion, you will just keep the trigger points activated.

Sports
If you ride a bike, sit as upright as possible by adjusting the handlebars or replacing them with ones with a taller stem. If you are using a stationary bike, try to sit upright. If you lift weights, avoid excessive amounts of weight and keep your head straight and pulled back over your shoulders. Avoid head-rolling exercises, sit-ups, and squats. Swimming provides good aerobic exercise, but you need to vary your strokes so that you do not unduly stress the trapezius muscle. More suggestions for trigger points and sports modifications are included in each of the individual muscle chapters in part II.

Do not read in bed
Reading in bed is not a good idea, but if you are not willing to give this up, then keep your head facing in the same direction as your torso, rather than turned to the side. A comfortable chair next to the bed is even better. Make sure that your reading light is positioned so that you are not turning or tilting your head.

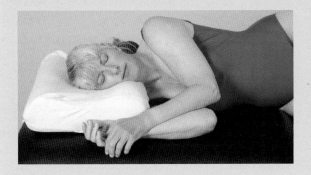

Sleeping position and getting up
When sleeping, try to keep your head facing in the same direction as your torso, rather than turned to the side. When turning over in bed at night, roll your head on the pillow, rather than lifting your head. When getting up from a lying position, do not get up by leading with your head. First roll onto your side or front, then use your arms to start pushing yourself up.

Clothing

What you wear and how you wear it is easily correctable and may provide a substantial amount of relief without any other intervention.

Solutions

Is it too tight?
Constricting clothing can lead to muscular problems. My rule of thumb is—if the clothing item leaves an elastic mark or indentation in the skin, it is too tight and cutting off proper circulation. Check your bras, socks, ties, and belts to see if they are too tight. Jogging bras work great for medium or small-breasted women. Have the salesperson help you find a bra that fits properly; many of them really know their products.

Purses and daypacks/backpacks
If you carry a purse, get one with a long strap and put the strap over your head, so that you are wearing it diagonally across your torso, rather than over one shoulder. Keep its contents light. If you use a daypack, put the straps over both shoulders. Without realizing it, you are hiking up one shoulder at least a little to keep the straps from slipping off no matter how light your purse or pack may be. If you backpack, try to put most of the weight on your hip strap.

Footwear
Do not wear high heels or cowboy boots. Do not wear clogs, because, without realizing it, you need to grip with your toes to keep them on. Only wear shoes that lace up or have a strap across your instep. Avoid shoes with pointed toes and inadequate room across the top of the toes. Your feet get wider as you get older, and shoes that may once have fit properly may now be too narrow. Any shoes that do not fit or are worn unevenly on the bottoms should be discarded. Buy shoes that have wide soles, such as athletic shoes.

If your foot *supinates* (more weight shifted to the outside of your foot), you will likely see excessive wear on the outside edge of the sole of your shoe. If your foot *pronates* (more weight shifted to the inside of your foot), you will likely see excessive wear on the inside edge of the sole of your shoe. While for some people correcting foot supination and pronation is essential, I think it is beneficial for almost everyone to use some kind of foot support, since it affects your muscles all the way up the body, and shoes rarely have adequate arch support. Properly designed custom orthotics will shift your weight slightly to the balls of your feet. This will shift your head back over your shoulders and restore normal cervical and lumbar curves, bring your shoulders back, and open up your chest. My favorite non corrective orthotics are the Superfeet® brand. They have a deep heel cup which helps prevent pronation and supination, and they also have excellent arch support. Superfeet® has a variety of models, including cheaper non custom "Trim to Fit" footbeds, and moderately priced custom molded footbeds to provide support in a variety of footwear. See www.Superfeet.com to learn more about their products. If you find you need corrective orthotics, you will need to see a podiatrist.

Muscular imbalances in the foot, along with misaligned joints, may lead to problems in the knee, hip, pelvis, and spine; therefore, treating trigger points in the feet and resolving the associated perpetuating factors may be crucial to resolving problems in other areas of the body. See chapters 71 and 72 for more information.

Glasses

Visual stress plays a significant role in the development of trigger points during computer work, and that role is even greater when combined with postural stresses. If you wear glasses, make sure your eyeglass prescription is current and you can see far enough with your reading glasses. Do not tilt your head down to look through bifocals. If you are getting a reflection on your eye glasses that causes you to tilt or tip your head, try changing the location of your light.

Hearing aids

If you need a hearing aid, get one and wear it. If you cannot hear properly, you will constantly turn your head to one side and stress your trapezius and neck muscles.

Case Study in Resolving a Mechanical Perpetuating Factor

I had a patient who came in with a backache, knee, and left foot pain. Her symptoms were worse in summer because she waited tables four nights per week in addition to her regular work. During the first appointment, I recommended that she stop wearing clogs and get orthotics plus a different pair of shoes that either laced up or had straps.

When she came in for her third appointment, she told me she had found a pair of shoes that cost her $278 called "The Anti-Shoe"; even *my* jaw dropped at that price! She said she was a little sore in her calves for the first couple of days when wearing the shoes while her muscles adjusted to them, but by the time she came in for her appointment she could not believe how much better she felt. She was no longer hurting even after being on her feet all night. Even though the shoes were expensive, it cost her much less than repeated treatments. I treated her for a couple of other unrelated conditions a few times over the next month, but her initial concerns were resolved.

She kept thanking me for resolving her pain, but I kept reminding her that she needed to take a lot of the credit herself by actually following my advice. She said, "Why would I pay you all this money and then not take your advice?" Good question! But sadly, so many patients expect me to "fix" them at my office, but do not want to follow up on at least trying my recommendations for resolving perpetuating factors, and are then upset when their relief does not last. You *must* resolve perpetuating factors to gain lasting relief!

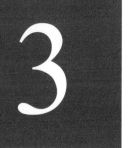

3 Perpetuating Factors: Nutrition, Food, and Beverages

What you eat and drink, or *do not* eat and drink, may cause and perpetuate trigger points. If diet is a factor, improving your nutrition, drinking enough water, and avoiding certain foods and drinks may greatly decrease both the intensity and frequency of your symptoms from trigger points.

Changing your diet will likely take some time, but you can easily start with little effort by taking a multivitamin supplement as well as a multimineral supplement, and drinking enough water. As you identify which foods you need to avoid, start replacing them with foods high in the needed vitamins and minerals. Be sure you are getting enough protein.

Inadequate Nutrition

It is easy and relatively inexpensive to improve your nutrient intake to see if it will decrease your symptoms. Doctors Travell and Simons found that almost **half** of their patients required treatment for vitamin deficiencies or insufficiencies* to obtain lasting relief from the pain and dysfunction of trigger points, and thought it was one of the most important perpetuating factors to address. The more deficient in nutrients you are, the more symptoms of all kinds you will have, and your trigger points and nervous system will be more hyperirritable. Even if a blood test for vitamin and mineral levels determines that you are at the low end of the normal range, you may still need a greater quantity of some nutrients, since your body will pull nutrients from the tissues before it will allow a decrease in the blood levels. Building up sufficient levels of vitamin B_{12}, vitamin D, and iron may take several months; do not get discouraged if you do not see immediate results, though you may start gradually feeling better within a few weeks from taking multivitamin and multimineral supplements.

Several factors may lead to nutrient deficiency or insufficiency, including an inadequate intake of a nutrient, impaired nutrient absorption, inadequate nutrient utilization, an increased need by the body, a nutrient leaving the body too quickly, and a nutrient being destroyed within the body too quickly.

What Should I Take and When?

Even if you have a fairly healthy diet, you may need to take supplements. The soils in many agricultural fields have been depleted of nutrients by repeatedly planting the same crop in the same location, rather than rotating them. Use of chemical fertilizers and pesticides can also adversely affect both crops and the soil. Shipping food over long distances or storing it for long periods also depletes the nutritive value; too much time passes between when the crop is picked and when it is consumed. Most people need to take some kind of multivitamin and multimineral supplement to ensure proper nutrition, especially if you fall into one of the high-risk groups mentioned below.

* *A nutrient insufficiency means that levels are within the lower 25% of the normal range, which may cause subtle clinical signs and symptoms. Most health care providers will dismiss lower levels of a vitamin or mineral as being irrelevant, since results are within a "normal" range. However, insufficiencies can cause and perpetuate chronic pain.*

Do not mega-dose on supplements unless a doctor or other qualified health care provider has determined your condition warrants it, since taking too many vitamins A, D, and E, and folic acid can cause symptoms similar to deficiencies. Some people are not able to absorb certain nutrients, and need to have them injected or mega-dosed. For example, some people cannot absorb vitamin B_{12} and need to get intramuscular injections to provide that necessary vitamin. See the section "Helpful Laboratory Tests" on page 39 for more information.

Take your vitamins with food, since some need to bind with substances found in food in order to be absorbed. Herbs do not need to be taken with food.

Self-Help Technique

Take supplements. Because some vitamins require the presence of other vitamins, a good multi-supplement helps ensure that the needed combination is present. Be sure to check the label to make certain there are adequate minerals in a multi, because you may need to also take a multimineral. You may need to take some additional quantities of some specific vitamins and minerals listed below. Doctors Travell and Simons found the most important supplements for treating trigger points were the water-soluble vitamins B1, B_6, B_{12}, folic acid, and vitamin C, and the minerals calcium, magnesium, iron and potassium. Other researchers have now added vitamin D to that list.

Impaired Digestive Function and Nutrient Malabsorption

If your digestive system is not functioning well, you do not have enough enzymes or possibly hydrochloric acid to break down food properly. Taking digestive enzymes or hydrochloric acid for long periods is not a good solution, because they will take over the natural function of your body. You need to repair the body's natural function so it can perform its own job properly. Digestive problems can be addressed with the help of an acupuncturist, herbalist, or naturopath. They can give you dietary recommendations based on your unique set of health problems and constitution, and prescribe herbs to rebalance your systems.

Fasting is hard on the digestive system. If you want to do a cleanse, use herbs and psyllium, but do not stop eating. It is also a common misconception that raw foods and whole grains are the healthiest way to eat. It is actually better to cook your food somewhat (but not overcook!), such as steaming your vegetables, in order to start the chemical breakdown process, so your digestive system does not have to work as hard.

If you have chronic diarrhea, you will not retain food long enough in the intestines to absorb nutrients. You will need to identify and eliminate the source of diarrhea. Acupuncture, herbs, and dietary changes can often successfully address this problem.

I have seen many people who have injured their digestive systems by taking too many herbs, or herbs that are improper for their conditions and constitution. Most kinds of herbs should be taken with the advice of a *qualified* practitioner. What may be the correct herb for a friend or a family member may not be the correct herb for you.

High-Risk Groups

You may be in a high-risk group for nutrient deficiency if you are elderly, pregnant or nursing, an alcoholic or other drug user, poor, depressed, or seriously ill. If you tend to diet by leaving out important food groups, or have an eating disorder, you will also deplete yourself of necessary nutrients. Many of us do not have a well-balanced diet high in nutrition. Processed foods do not contain as much nutrition as foods that are freshly prepared.

Vegetarianism and Nutrition

Most people should not be strict vegetarians. The argument I usually hear is "I have been a vegetarian for 20 years and the _____ problem just started 10 years ago!" (fill in the blank). I believe that a lack of high-quality protein causes a progressive problem, and it may take years for some symptoms to show up.

Plant sources contain mainly the pyridoxal form of vitamin B_6, but animal sources contain both the pyridoxal and the pyridoxamine forms and are less susceptible to the loss of the vitamin due to cooking or preserving. Vitamin B_{12} is only found in animal proteins, including dairy products. Brewer's yeast does not contain B_{12} unless the yeast is grown on a special B_{12}-containing substrate.

Self-Help Technique
Improve your protein intake. At the very least you should eat eggs for a high-quality protein source. Most vegetarians are not very good about combining foods, and even if they were, most still seem to feel better within a few months after adding high-quality animal protein back into their diet, whether it comes from just a few eggs or a piece of fish once per week.

Vitamins

Adequate intake of vitamin C and the B-vitamins is important for resolving trigger points. The B-vitamins and folic acid need to be taken together as a complex, since they need each other for proper absorption and use by your body. Recent research on vitamin D has indicated that it is also important for treating myofascial pain. These are the only vitamins that will be addressed for the purposes of this book, but *Prescription for Nutritional Healing* (2000), by James F. Balch, M.D. and Phyllis A. Balch, C.N.C., has a comprehensive list of vitamins, minerals, amino acids, antioxidants, and enzymes, as well as food sources for each. There are sections on common disorders, listing supplements needed to treat each condition, and helpful hints.

Vitamin C

Vitamin C (ascorbic acid) reduces post-exercise soreness and corrects the capillary fragility which leads to easy bruising. (Hint: *if you do not remember how you got a bruise, you are likely bruising too easily.*) This vitamin is essential for collagen formation (connective tissue) and forming bones. It is required for synthesis of the neurotransmitters norepinephrine and serotonin, is needed for your body's response to stress, is important for immune system function, and decreases the irritability of trigger points caused by infection. Vitamin C helps stop diarrhea caused by food allergies, but taking too much of it can lead to watery diarrhea or non-specific urethritis. It is currently known that vitamin C daily doses above 400 mg are not used by the body, and that 1000 mg/day increases the risk of kidney stone formation, so mega-dosing with vitamin C is not necessary, nor recommended. Women taking estrogen or oral contraceptives may need 500 mg/day.

Initial symptoms of vitamin C deficiency include weakness, lethargy, irritability, vague aching pains in the joints and muscles, bruising easily, and possibly weight loss. Severe cases of vitamin C deficiency (*scurvy*) are rare in developed countries, but symptoms include red, swollen, bleeding gums, and teeth may fall out.

Vitamin C is likely to be deficient in smokers, alcoholics, older people (the presence of vitamin C in the tissues decreases with age), infants fed primarily on cows' milk (usually between the ages of 6 and 12 months), people with chronic diarrhea, psychiatric patients, and fad dieters.

Self-Help Technique
Food sources of vitamin C include citrus fruits and fresh juices, raw broccoli, raw Brussels sprouts, collard, kale, turnip greens, guava, raw sweet peppers, cabbage, and potatoes. Do not take vitamin C with antacids. Since vitamin C is ascorbic acid, and the purpose of an antacid is to neutralize acid, antacids will neutralize vitamin C and make it ineffective.

B-Vitamins

Vitamin B_1 (*thiamine*) is essential for normal nerve function and energy production within muscle cells. Diminished pain and temperature sensitivity and an inability to detect vibrations indicate that you are low in thiamine. You may also possibly experience calf cramping at night, slight sweating, constipation, and fatigue. Vitamin B_1 is needed for proper thyroid hormone levels: see the section "Organ Dysfunction and Disease" on page 37. Abuse of alcohol reduces thiamine absorption, and absorption is further reduced if liver disease is also present. The tannin in black tea, antacid use, and a magnesium deficiency can also prevent the absorption of thiamine. Thiamine can be destroyed by processing foods and by heating them to temperatures above 212°F (100°C). Thiamine is excreted too rapidly when taking diuretics or drinking too much water.

Self-Help Technique
Food sources of vitamin B_1 are lean pork, kidney, liver, beef, eggs, fish, beans, and nuts, and also some whole grain cereals if the hull and germ are present.

Vitamin B_6 (*pyridoxine*) is important for nerve function, energy metabolism, amino acid metabolism, and synthesis of neurotransmitters including norepinephrine and serotonin, which strongly influence pain perception. Deficiency of B_6 results in anemia, reduced absorption and storage of B_{12}, increased excretion of vitamin C, and blocked synthesis of B_3 (*niacin*), and can lead to a hormonal imbalance. A vitamin B_6 deficiency will manifest as symptoms of deficiency of one of the other B vitamins, since B_6 is needed in order for all the others to perform their functions. The need for B_6 increases with age and with increased protein consumption. Tropical sprue and alcohol use interfere with its absorption. Use of oral contraceptives increases your requirement for B_6 and impairs glucose tolerance. This can lead to depression if you do not supplement with B_6, particularly if you already have a history of depression. Corticosteroid use, excessive alcohol use, pregnancy and lactation, antitubercular drugs, uremia, and hyperthyroidism also increase the need for B_6.

Self-Help Technique
Food sources of vitamin B_6 include liver, kidney, chicken (white meat), halibut, tuna, English walnuts, soybean flour, navy beans, bananas, and avocados. There is also some B_6 present in yeast, lean beef, egg yolk, and whole wheat.

Vitamin B_{12} (*cobalamin*) and folic acid need to be taken together to form *erythrocytes* (red blood cells) and rapidly dividing cells such as those found in the gastrointestinal tract, and for fatty acid synthesis used in the formation of parts of certain nerve fibers. B_{12} is needed for both fat and carbohydrate metabolism. A deficiency can result in pernicious (megaloblastic) anemia, which would reduce oxygen coming to the site of the trigger point, adding to the dysfunctional cycle and increasing pain. A deficiency of B_{12} may also cause symptoms such as non-specific depression, fatigue, an exaggerated startle reaction to noise or touch, and an increased susceptibility to trigger points. B_{12} deficiencies are common in the elderly and people with chronic trigger points. Several drugs may impair the absorption of B_{12}, as can mega-doses of vitamin C for long periods of time.

Self-Help Technique
Food sources of vitamin B_{12} are only found in animal products or vitamin supplements.

Folate

Folate, also known as *folic acid* when in the synthetic form, is another member of the B-complex. A folate deficiency can cause you to fatigue easily, sleep poorly, and feel discouraged and depressed. It can cause "restless legs," diffuse muscular pain, diarrhea, or a loss of sensation in the extremities. You may feel cold frequently and have a slightly lower basal body temperature than the normal 98.6°F (37°C). A deficiency of folate and/or vitamin B_{12} can also lead to megaloblastic anemia, a condition where the red blood cells are larger than normal.

Worldwide, many people get less than the dietary recommendation of folate: deficiency ranges from 15% to 30% or more of the population, depending on race, culture, and country. Part of the problem is that 50% to 95% of the folate content of foods may be destroyed in food processing and preparation, so even if you eat folate sources, you may not be receiving the benefit. Folate is converted into its active form in the digestive system, but this conversion is inhibited by peas, beans, and acidic foods, so eat these separately from your folate sources. Do not take your folic acid supplement at the same time as an antacid.

You are at the greatest risk of folate deficiency if you are elderly, have a bowel disorder, are pregnant or lactating, or use drugs and alcohol regularly. Certain other drugs will also deplete folic acid, such as anti-inflammatories (including aspirin), diuretics, estrogens (such as birth control pills), and anti-convulsants. You must also have adequate B_{12} intake in order to absorb folic acid, plus taking only B_{12} or folic acid on its own can mask a severe deficiency in the other.

Self-Help Technique
Best food sources of folate are leafy vegetables, brewer's yeast, organ meat, fruit, and lightly cooked vegetables such as broccoli and asparagus.

Vitamin D

Vitamin D is required for both the absorption and the utilization of calcium and phosphorus. It is necessary for growth and thyroid function, it protects against muscle weakness, and helps regulate the heartbeat. It is important for the prevention of cancer, osteoarthritis, osteoporosis, and calcium deficiency. A mild deficiency of vitamin D may manifest as a loss of appetite, a burning sensation in the mouth and throat, diarrhea, insomnia, visual problems, and weight loss. It has been estimated that close to 90% of patients with chronic musculoskeletal pain may have a vitamin D deficiency.

Self-Help Technique
Sources of vitamin D include salmon, halibut, sardines, tuna, and eggs. Other sources include dairy products, dandelion greens, liver, oatmeal, and sweet potatoes. If you take supplements, look for the D_3 form, or fish oil capsules.

Vitamin D_3 is synthesized by the skin when exposed to the sun's UV rays. Unfortunately, many people do not get enough sun exposure, especially if they live at latitudes or in climates with little sun available during the winter months. Exposing your face and arms to the sun for 15 minutes three times per week will ensure that your body synthesizes an adequate amount of vitamin D. Because the amount of exposure needed varies from person to person, and also depends on geographical location, you will need to do some personal research and perhaps consult with a dermatologist to determine the proper amount for you.

Minerals

Calcium, magnesium, potassium, and iron are needed for proper muscle function. Calcium is essential for releasing acetylcholine at the nerve terminal, and both calcium and magnesium are needed for the contracting mechanism of the muscle fiber. Potassium is needed to get the muscle fiber ready quickly for its next contraction, and a deficiency may cause muscle soreness during exercise or other physical activity. Iron is required for oxygen transport to the muscle fibers. Deficiency of any of these minerals increases the irritability of trigger points. Calcium, magnesium, and potassium should be taken together, because an increase in one can deplete the others. Also needed for good health, but not as important for muscle function, are zinc, iodine, copper, manganese, chromium, selenium, and molybdenum.

Calcium

Do not take *Tums* or other antacids as a source of calcium. Stomach acid is needed for the uptake of calcium, but an antacid neutralizes stomach acid. So even if there is calcium present, it cannot be used. If you must take an antacid, take it several hours apart from your calcium/magnesium supplement so you will maximize your mineral uptake. It is especially important to take calcium for at least a few years prior to menopause to help prevent osteoporosis. Vitamin D_3 is needed for calcium uptake (see above).

Calcium channel blockers prescribed for high blood pressure inhibit the uptake of calcium into the sarcoplasmic reticulum of vascular smooth muscles and cardiac muscles. Since this is likely also true for skeletal muscles, calcium channel blockers would also make trigger points worse and more difficult to treat. See your health care provider to find out if you can switch to a different medication. Consider treating the underlying causes of hypertension with acupuncture, diet changes, exercise, or whatever is appropriate to your particular set of circumstances.

Self-Help Technique
Food sources of calcium include salmon, sardines, other seafood, green leafy vegetables, almonds, asparagus, blackstrap molasses, brewer's yeast, broccoli, cabbage, carob, collard greens, dandelion greens, figs, filberts, kale, kelp, mustard greens, oats, parsley, prunes, sesame seeds, tofu, and turnip greens. Dairy products and whey are also good sources, but they are contraindicated if you have fibromyalgia or a "damp-type condition" as diagnosed by Traditional Chinese Medicine.

Magnesium

Magnesium deficiency is less likely to result from an inadequate dietary intake in a healthy diet than from malabsorption, malnutrition, kidney disease, or fluid and electrolyte loss. Magnesium is depleted after strenuous physical exercise, but a proper amount of exercise coupled with an adequate intake of magnesium improves the efficiency of cellular metabolism and improves cardio-respiratory performance. Consumption of alcohol, the use of diuretics, chronic diarrhea, the consumption of fluoride, and high intakes of zinc and vitamin D increase the body's need for magnesium.

Self-Help Technique
Food sources of magnesium include most foods, especially meat, fish and other seafood, apples, apricots, avocados, bananas, blackstrap molasses, brewer's yeast, brown rice, figs, garlic, kelp, lima beans, millet, nuts, peaches, black-eyed peas, sesame seeds, tofu, green leafy vegetables, wheat, and whole grains. Dairy products are also good sources, but they are contraindicated if you have fibromyalgia or a "damp-type condition" as diagnosed by Traditional Chinese Medicine. If you are an athlete, you will probably want to take additional calcium and magnesium supplements.

Potassium

A diet high in fats, refined sugars, and salt causes potassium deficiency, as does the use of laxatives and some diuretics. Diarrhea will also deplete potassium. If you suffer from urinary frequency, particularly if your urine is clear rather than light yellow, try increasing your potassium intake. Frequent urination causes potassium deficiency, and potassium deficiency may cause frequent urination, and so a vicious cycle ensues.

Self-Help Technique

Food sources of potassium include fruit (especially bananas and citrus fruits), potatoes, green leafy vegetables, wheat germ, beans, lentils, nuts, dates, and prunes.

Iron

Iron deficiency can lead to anemia and is usually caused by excessive blood loss from a heavy menses, hemorrhoids, intestinal bleeding, donating blood too often, or ulcers. Iron deficiency can also be caused by a long-term illness, prolonged use of antacids, poor digestion, excessive coffee or black tea consumption, or the chronic use of NSAIDs (non-steroidal anti-inflammatory drugs, such as *ibuprofen*). Calcium in milk and cheese, or as a supplement, can impair absorption of iron—therefore you should take your calcium supplement separately. Do not take an iron supplement if you have an infection or cancer. The body stores iron in order to withhold it from bacteria, and in the case of cancer this may suppress the cancer-killing function of certain cells.

Early symptoms of iron deficiency include fatigue, reduced endurance, and an inability to stay warm when exposed to a moderately cold environment. Worldwide, about 15% of menstruating females are iron deficient, though figures are slightly lower for developed countries.

Self-Help Technique

Food sources of iron include eggs, fish, liver, meat, poultry, green leafy vegetables, whole grains, almonds, avocados, beets, blackstrap molasses, brewer's yeast, dates, egg yolks, kelp, kidney and lima beans, lentils, millet, parsley, peaches, pears, dried prunes, pumpkin, raisins, rice and wheat bran, sesame seeds, and soybeans. Generally food sources are adequate for improving iron levels for most people, unless a health care provider has recommended additional supplementation. Iron is best absorbed with vitamin C.

Salt

Do not entirely eliminate salt from your diet, especially if you sweat. You do need some salt in your diet (unless you have been instructed otherwise by your health care provider for certain medical conditions), though you do not want to overdo it either. Inadequate salt, calcium/magnesium, or potassium can lead to muscle cramping.

Water

It is important to drink enough water, because water is the lubricating fluid of your body. Dehydration can cause a variety of symptoms, including pain, and is very common in people who take diuretic medications or drink a lot of coffee or other diuretic-type beverages.

Room-temperature water is better than cold drinks; if you drink something cold, your stomach has to work harder to warm it up, and it taxes the digestive system. Do not drink distilled water, because you need the minerals found in non-distilled water. If you drink bottled water, make sure that you know its source and that it is not distilled. This industry is not currently regulated, so you may need to do some research on the bottling company.

Self-Help Technique
Drink enough water—about two quarts per day, and more if you have a larger body mass or sweat a lot. A general rule of thumb for people weighing more than 100 pounds is one half of your body weight multiplied by the number of ounces; for example, 140 pounds body weight means 70 ounces of water. Drink at least one extra quart per day if it is very hot outside, and extra water during and immediately after a work-out. Be aware, however, that drinking too much water can deplete vitamin B_1 (thiamine).

Improper Diet

Ingesting foods that aggravate your trigger points is a common and significant perpetuating factor. Changing the foods you eat, including avoiding allergens, can help enormously in relieving your pain. Identifying food allergies is addressed in chapter 4.

Plan on avoiding the foods in question for at least two months, in conjunction with receiving acupuncture treatments and/or taking prescribed herbs and other supplements, in order to determine whether eliminating the specific food is helpful. Many people will stop consuming a certain food or other substance for just a short while, perhaps only a week, then decide it has not made a difference and start consuming it again. Or the foods, beverages, or other substances may be so important to them that they had put up with pain and other medical conditions rather than give up the substances. Reaching a conclusion after only a short trial period is one way to justify continuing to consume the substance.

Foods and Drinks to Avoid

You may be reluctant to give up a favorite food or beverage. However, I suggest that you read this section and *consider* that the listed item(s) could be at least part of the cause of your pain. Then at least you can make an informed decision about how committed you are to getting rid of your pain.

Caffeine
Caffeine causes a persistent contracture, or *caffeine rigor*, of muscle fibers, and increases muscle tension and trigger point irritability, leading to an increase in pain. It causes an excess release of calcium from the sarcoplasmic reticulum and interferes with the rebinding of calcium ions by the sarcoplasmic reticulum. Doctors Travell and Simons found that caffeine in excess of 150 mg daily, which is more than two eight-ounce cups of regular coffee, would lead to caffeine rigor. I suspect for some people it could be even less. In figuring out your daily intake, be sure to count any caffeine in the drugs you are taking, and remember that espresso and similar drinks will have *far* greater amounts of caffeine.

Alcohol and Tobacco
Alcohol aggravates trigger points by decreasing serum and tissue folate levels. It increases the body's need for vitamin C, while decreasing the body's ability to absorb it. Tobacco also increases the need for vitamin C.

4 Perpetuating Factors: Medical Conditions

There are several other perpetuating factors that may be very important in the role they play in causing body-wide trigger points. Treating new injuries promptly can help prevent the formation of trigger points. Treatment of older injuries and treating spinal misalignments and other problems in the skeletal system can help stop the perpetuation of trigger points.

Sleep problems, emotional factors such as anxiety and depression, acute and chronic infections, allergies, hormonal imbalances, and organ dysfunction and disease can all cause and perpetuate trigger points. Some of these conditions need to be diagnosed by laboratory tests, and you may want to ask your health care provider if some of these tests would be helpful in your case. See "Helpful Laboratory Tests" on page 39 for an outline of some possible diagnostic tests.

Injuries

An injury is one of the most common initiators of trigger points in general. A healthy muscle is pliable to the touch when it is not being used, but will feel firm if called upon for action. If a muscle feels firm at rest, it is tight in an unhealthy way, even if you work out. I like to use an analogy of a rubber band or stick. Imagine that a sudden, unexpected force is applied to the "stick," or tight muscle, such as during a fall. Like a stick, the muscle will be damaged. If a sudden force is applied to a pliable muscle, or "rubber band," it will stretch with the force instead, and will be much less likely to be injured. Since latent trigger points restrict range of motion to some degree, and almost everyone has some latent trigger points, a muscle may be tight and restricted without you being aware of it, and can be easily injured if a sudden force is applied.

Solutions

Treat new injuries
If you have an injury, begin treatment as soon as possible. Apply cold during the first 48 hours, and use some form of arnica homeopathic orally and/or topically as soon as possible. There are Chinese herb formulas for trauma that you can get from an acupuncturist or possibly a health food store. Have these available in your medicine cabinet since it may be hard for you to go to the store after you are injured, and because these work best when you start taking them immediately after the injury. See an acupuncturist or massage therapist who is experienced in working with recent injuries. You may also need to see a chiropractor or osteopathic physician.

Treat scar tissue
Both injuries and surgeries will likely leave some amount of scar tissue, which can perpetuate trigger points. Scar tissue can be broken up to some extent by vigorous cross-friction massage, but most people will not work on their own scars vigorously enough due to the pain it causes. You will probably need to see a practitioner for help. Acupuncture can treat scar tissue and help eliminate the pain from trigger points around the area. I recommend using both cross-friction massage and acupuncture as part of the treatment protocol, rather than just one or the other.

Spinal and Skeletal Factors

If vertebrae are chronically out of alignment, or you have skeletal asymmetries, the stress placed on the muscle from tightness, imbalances, and pain can lead to trigger point formation. The chronic pain from herniated and bulging discs, bone spurs, and spinal stenosis (a narrowing of the central spinal cord canal or the holes on the sides of the vertebrae that the nerves come out of) may also lead to trigger point formation. If you do not get relief from trigger point treatment, or your symptoms are severe, see a health care provider who can evaluate you for an x-ray or MRI.

Spinal and Joint Misalignments

There are many causes of spinal and joint misalignments, commonly referred to as *subluxation* by chiropractic doctors.* Poor posture, improper lifting, accidents, chronically tensed muscles, and even passing through the birth canal can cause misalignments, which then further stress the muscles and cause and perpetuate trigger points…and a self-perpetuating cycle ensues.

Solutions

Treat misalignments and scoliosis
Usually there are tight muscles that caused the misalignment or scoliosis to begin with, so a combined approach of trigger point self-help techniques and skeletal mobilization, and possibly also massage or acupuncture, is probably necessary for lasting relief. Some scoliosis will be corrected with the trigger point pressure self-treatment found in part II. Vertebrae and joints can be adjusted by a chiropractor or osteopathic physician. They will likely take x-rays at the initial visit to evaluate your spine. If you have already had x-rays taken, bring them along to the visit so you can avoid unnecessary duplication.

Corrective *orthotics* (custom footbeds) may also be necessary to correct muscular imbalances on a permanent basis. See page 19, "Footwear."

Disc Problems, Bone Spurs, and Spinal Stenosis

Disc problems, bone spurs, and spinal stenosis can also cause chronic pain and lead to the formation of trigger points, and need to be confirmed by an MRI. But in a random sample of the population you will find many people with bone spurs and narrowed disc spaces that have no pain. You will also find many people *with* pain who have no bone spurs or narrowed disc spaces, so do not assume that these are causing your problems, even if a health care provider has made this assumption.

If you have had surgery for one of these problems but your pain continues, trigger points are the likely culprit, and need to be treated for lasting relief. If you still do not get relief, there is a possibility the pain is due to scar tissue from the surgery compressing a nerve root, so you will need to check with your health care provider.

*In this case I am using the World Health Organization definition of subluxation, which is "A lesion or dysfunction in a joint or motion segment in which alignment, movement integrity and/or physiological function are altered, although contact between joint surfaces remains intact. It is essentially a functional entity, which may influence biomechanical and neural integrity."

Solutions

Treat herniated/bulging discs

Discs can be very successfully treated with acupuncture (especially Plum Blossom technique coupled with cupping), but if you do not get some relief fairly quickly, you may want to consider surgery if you have insurance. Spinal surgery has become so sophisticated that many surgeries are fairly minor procedures that have you back on your feet the next day.

Treat spinal stenosis

If you have spinal stenosis, acupuncture will help with pain, but not the spinal stenosis, so surgery may be the best option. With any surgery there is a certain amount of risk, so be sure to discuss this with your operating physician, and make sure you understand the procedure. If you are still unsure, get a second opinion from another surgeon.

Skeletal Asymmetries

A skeletal asymmetry means that one or more of the bones on one side of your body are smaller than those of the opposite side. If you have an anatomical size difference in one bone, it is likely that other bones on the same side are also smaller. Injuries can also potentially cause skeletal differences. Asymmetries will place a lot of uneven stress on your muscles, causing and perpetuating trigger points.

Solutions

Get compensating pads and lifts

See a specialist to be evaluated and fitted properly for any corrective devices, such as corrective orthotics, and compensating lifts and pads. An anatomically shorter leg* and a small hemipelvis (either the left or the right half of the pelvic bone) can be corrected with a pad that goes in one shoe and a pad that goes on your chair under one buttock. Having a big toe that is shorter than the second toe causes excessive pronation, which can be corrected with shoe orthotics. Short upper arms can be corrected with ergonomically correct furniture. See chapter 2 for more information on furniture and orthotics.

If you have an anatomical leg-length inequality, even as little as $1/_8$", you will probably stand with one foot forward with your weight on the short foot, or with your pelvis shifted to the shorter side, and you will probably have pain with walking and standing. If a leg-length inequality is *not* corrected, it can contribute to osteoarthritis of the hip and lumbar spine. Symptoms caused by a leg-length inequality may not show up until it is brought on by an acute trauma, such as a car accident. If you are getting a leg-length inequality corrected with lifts, start with a thin lift and gradually use thicker ones until the proper lift height is reached. Work on the thoracolumbar paraspinal muscles (18) during this process to help the back muscles adjust. If you use compensating lifts, you must use them *all the time and in all shoes*, and do not go barefoot. Evaluation of various body asymmetries is discussed in detail in *Myofascial Pain and Dysfunction: The Trigger Point Manual, Vol. 2, The Lower Extremities* (Travell and Simons 1992, pp. 41–63).

* In this book, a "shorter leg" refers to an anatomical leg-length inequality where the bones are actually shorter on one side, rather than the term many chiropractors use to indicate an asymmetry caused by a spinal misalignment. When a patient is examined face-up, it can appear that the affected leg is shorter than the other, so it is important for the diagnosing practitioner to release the tensor fasciae latae and determine if the leg bone truly is shorter than that of the other leg before prescribing lifts.

Sleep Problems

Pain can interrupt sleep, and interrupted sleep can perpetuate trigger points. It is useful to know whether sleep was interrupted or was sound and restful *before* the pain started. If your sleep was poor prior to the onset of pain, then there is another underlying factor that needs to be addressed to help solve the problem.

Solutions

Trigger point pressure
If pain disturbs you at night, keep your self help ball collection by your bed so that if you wake up, you can work on your trigger points, and hopefully fall back to sleep once the pain is reduced. Be sure that you do not fall asleep on the ball, since it will cut off the circulation for too long and make the trigger points worse. Consider whether you need a new bed and/or pillow (see page 16).

Room temperature
Be sure you are not sleeping poorly due to being too warm or too cold. Adjust the room temperature and covers as needed.

Nutrition/water
If you have problems falling asleep, try improving your nutrition and your water intake first. Take a calcium/magnesium supplement before bedtime. See chapter 3 for more information.

Light or disturbed sleep
If you are waking easily due to noise, try Mack's® soft silicon earplugs, or try breathing deeply until you fall back to sleep. If your mind is racing, you sleep lightly and wake frequently, you wake early and cannot fall back to sleep, or have hot flashes or vivid and disturbing dreams, try acupuncture and Chinese herbs. If urinary frequency is disturbing your sleep, try acupuncture and herbs, and increasing your potassium intake. Do not use your computer in the evening: it stimulates the brain and makes it hard to fall asleep and sleep restfully.

Caffeine and alcohol will disturb sleep or make you sleep more lightly. Even if you drink caffeine only in the morning, it will still disturb your nighttime sleep pattern. If you choose to give up caffeine, it will take about two weeks before your energy starts to even out and you do not feel like you have to use it to get going in the morning.

Consider whether your adrenal glands could be excreting too much adrenaline. If you are continually stressed, or if you are pushing yourself too hard and push through fatigue instead of resting or taking a nap, you will excrete more adrenaline and have more difficulty sleeping at night. A naturopathic doctor can administer a saliva test for adrenal function.

Make sure you are not being exposed to allergens at night. Get inexpensive, soft plastic covers for your pillows and mattress. Many people are allergic to mites, which live in your bedding. If you have a down comforter or pillow, you may be allergic to the feathers, even if you are not exhibiting classic allergic symptoms such as sneezing and itchy eyes.

Emotional Factors

Emotional factors can cause and perpetuate trigger points, and are very important to consider along with physical perpetuating factors. But unfortunately, all too often people are dismissed by their doctors as "just being under stress." They leave the doctor's office without their physical symptoms being assessed or addressed, particularly when it comes to the symptoms of pain and depression.

If you are in pain long enough, of course you will begin to feel fatigued and depressed. If you are depressed long enough, you will probably develop pain. Anything that has gone on long enough will have *both* components; see the discussion of central sensitization on page 11. Antidepressants may be prescribed, which may possibly help with the acute symptoms, but the side effects of some medications can add to the underlying condition causing the symptoms, and a vicious cycle ensues.

Anxiety

If you are extremely anxious, chances are you are holding at least some of your body parts very tense and developing trigger points. You may be clenching your jaw or pressing your tongue against your teeth or the roof or your mouth. You may be hiking your shoulders up around your neck, tightening your forearms or abdomen, or tensing your gluteal muscles. Women tense their gluteal muscles more often than men.

Depression

If you are experiencing an unusual desire to be alone, a loss of interest in your favorite activities, and/or you are neglecting your appearance and hygiene, you may be suffering from depression. Clinical symptoms of depression are insomnia, loss of appetite, weight loss, impotence or a lowered libido, blurred vision, a sad mood, thoughts of suicide or death, an inability to concentrate, a poor memory, indecision, mumbled speech, and negative reactions to suggestions. Having only one of these symptoms will not confirm a diagnosis of depression, because there are other causes for some of these symptoms. It is the *combination* of symptoms that confirms a diagnosis of depression. Depression lowers the pain threshold, increases pain, and adversely affects your response to trigger point therapy.

Solutions

Get help for emotional factors
Often people suffering from severe depression, anxiety, chronic fatigue, and/or extreme pain lack the energy to participate in their own healing. You may have difficulty feeding yourself properly or even getting out of bed, and cannot manage even mild forms of exercise such as walking—the very things that would make you start to feel better. You may have difficulty making it to your appointments.

If you think you may be suffering from anxiety or depression, you will need to do whatever you can to get to the point where you can start taking better care of yourself. This may mean getting antidepressants, acupuncture treatments, homeopathy, counseling, or pain relievers, and/or doing the self help techniques in this book.

One of the things I like most about Traditional Chinese Medicine and homeopathy is that both physical and emotional symptoms are used to develop a diagnosis and are treated simultaneously. With acupuncture there are no side effects, and the response is usually rapid. Consult with a trained professional to obtain the correct herbs and homeopathics for your situation.

See the thyroid section in "Organ Dysfunction and Disease" on page 37, since thyroid problems can be an undiagnosed cause of depression. If you are suffering from depression, be sure to insist that your thyroid levels are tested before starting on anti-depressant medication. I have had more than one patient (especially male) where hypothyroidism was discovered only after they had been medicated for some time.

Get enough exercise
Walking and deep breathing are great relievers of tension and depression. Even walking for ten minutes per day, especially outside, can be extremely beneficial. Just doing one of these things will help get you started in the right direction to improve your energy and outlook.

Acute or Chronic Viral, Bacterial, or Parasitic Infections

Infections are a very prevalent perpetuator of trigger points and are often overlooked. It is extremely important to eliminate or manage infections in order to get relief from pain.

Acute Infections

It is important to head off illness at the first sign in order to avoid perpetuating trigger points. This is critical if you have fibromyalgia, sinusitis, asthma, or recurrent infections, since your trigger points will be activated by illness, and getting sick can set you back months in your treatment and healing.

Solutions

Head off acute illness at the first sign
When you start to get sick, take the Chinese herbs Gan Mao Ling or Yin Chiao, echinacea, and/or homeopathics such as Osillococcinum or other appropriate homeopathics for colds, flu, or sinusitis. You should have these herbs and homeopathics available at home so you can treat your symptoms as soon as you notice the first signs. Once you are past the initial stage of illness, if symptoms progress, the appropriate Chinese herb will be determined by your particular set of symptoms, so at this point you may need professional help to determine the proper herb.

Chronic Infections

Chronic infections such as sinus infections*, an abscessed or impacted tooth, urinary tract infections, and herpes simplex (cold sores, genital herpes, herpes zoster) will perpetuate trigger points and need to be managed if recurrence is frequent.

Very often a patient will tell me that they have a "sinus headache." If the only symptom you are experiencing is pain over the forehead and/or between the cheek and nose, this is most likely due to referred pain from the sternocleidomastoid muscle (see chapter 10), rather than a sinus infection. Never assume you know the underlying cause of your headache based only on the location and severity of your pain. Health care providers can make this mistake also. Trigger points may be the major cause of the pain, or there may be a more serious underlying problem that needs to be diagnosed or addressed.

Solutions

Resolve sinus infections

Any mechanical reasons for sinus infections need to be dealt with for lasting relief. Naturopathic doctors can use a small inflatable balloon to open up the passages, but you may need surgical intervention if the blockage is severe enough. Many people report success using a Neti Pot to flush the sinuses with a warm saline solution; you can get one at your health food store.†

† With both sinus infections and urinary tract infections, antibiotics often will not kill all of the pathogens and you will get a lingering, recurrent infection. However, antibiotics also work quickly, so I often recommend that patients combine antibiotics, acupuncture, herbs, and homeopathics to drive out the infection as quickly and completely as possible so it does not become a chronic problem.

Treat urinary tract infections (UTIs)

These infections need to be dealt with promptly. You may use over the counter western drugs, Chinese herbs, and unsweetened cranberry juice or cranberry pills, but if you do not respond to treatment *immediately*, you will need to see your health care provider. UTIs can turn into life threatening kidney infections very quickly.‡

‡ See note † above.

Treat recurrent herpes outbreaks

There are many pharmaceutical drugs and natural supplements and herbs for treating recurrent herpes infections—some will work better for you than others. If you are having recurrent outbreaks, you will want to figure out what is stressing your immune system, such as allergies, sugar, alcohol, or emotional stress. Sometimes a herpes outbreak is the first sign you are fighting an acute illness, so that is the time to take the above mentioned supplements.

See your dentist

If you suspect an infected or cracked tooth, you will need to see your dentist for an evaluation.

Parasitic Infections

The fish tapeworm, giardia, and occasionally amoeba are the most likely parasites to perpetuate trigger points. The fish tapeworm and giardia scar the lining of the intestine and impair your ability to absorb nutrients, and they also consume vitamin B_{12}. Amoeba can produce toxins that are passed from the intestine into the body. Fish tapeworms can be acquired by ingesting raw fish, whereas giardia is most often associated with drinking untreated water from streams. Giardia can also be passed on by an infected person not washing their hands after a bowel movement, particularly if they are preparing food or have some other hand to mouth contact.

Solutions

Eliminate parasites

Anytime you have chronic diarrhea it is worth testing for parasites. A cheaper alternative is just to treat with herbs like grapefruit seed extract or pulsatilla (a Chinese herb) and see if your symptoms improve. If you have blood in your stools, you should always see your health care provider *immediately* to rule out serious conditions.

Many people report feeling much better on an anti-candida diet, and in any case it is quite a healthy way to eat. There are many herbal products on the market for eliminating candida, including grapefruit seed extract, oil of oregano, echinacea, pulsatilla, and many formulas. Since most of these will also kill off the beneficial intestinal flora, you will need to follow treatment with a good multi-acidophilus supplement, as you would after any antibiotic.

Allergies

Both inhaled and ingested allergens perpetuate trigger points and make them harder to treat due to the subsequent histamine release. Some people with pain may experience significant relief if they are able to minimize allergic responses. Environmental allergies must be controlled as much as possible, and if you see a specialist for a skin test to identify allergens, they will make specific suggestions based on the findings.

Solutions

HEPA air filters
A good HEPA air filter will help substantially—you will need one for each room. Make sure each unit is large enough to cover the needed square footage. Not all air filters are equal, so be sure to research your options.

Ozonators
An ozonator will kill molds, but I do not suggest leaving one running while you or your pets are in the room, even though some are made for that purpose. Get an ozonator that puts out enough ozone to "bomb" the room while you and your pets are absent. Bomb one room at a time and close the door so that you will get a high concentration. After a few hours, hold your breath and open the windows and let the room air out for a couple of minutes before you occupy the room again. You will smell ozone (like lightening) lingering, but the air is fine to breathe after just a few minutes, so do not be concerned.

Allergy tests
There are a few methods for testing for food allergens. One of the best ways is an elimination diet, where you eliminate all foods, add them back in one at a time, and then rotate foods. You can find instructions for this under "Allergies" in *Prescription for Nutritional Healing* (2000) by Balch and Balch. The problem with a rotation diet is that most people are not willing to do it, as it requires a very strict control of your diet and a careful logging of a food diary for a month.

As an alternative, Balch and Balch offer a "quick test." After sitting and relaxing for a few minutes, take your pulse rate for one minute, and then eat the food you are testing. Keep still for 15 to 20 minutes, and then take your pulse again. If your pulse rate has increased more than ten beats per minute, eliminate this food from your diet for one month, then re-test. Naturopathic doctors offer a blood test for food allergens, which I have personally found to be accurate.

See a health care provider for tests to identify environmental allergens.

Hormonal Imbalances

Women are more likely to develop trigger points than men, and I have noticed this is particularly true in menopausal women. Teenagers of both sexes going through puberty also seem to have a tendency to develop trigger points. These observations lead me to believe there is a connection between life-cycle hormonal changes and one potential cause of trigger points. Although you obviously cannot stop yourself from going through hormonal changes, making sure that you are as healthy as possible and addressing any of the other perpetuating factors can make those life transitions as smooth as possible and minimize the role of trigger points in causing pain.

Organ Dysfunction and Disease

Organ dysfunction and disease—such as hypothyroidism, hypometabolism, hypoglycemia, and gout—can cause and perpetuate trigger points, and are the more challenging perpetuating factors to control or eliminate.

Thyroid

Both thyroid inadequacy (also known as *hypometabolism* or *subclinical hypothyroidism*) and hypothyroidism will cause and perpetuate trigger points. Even if a patient is on a thyroid supplement, I have noticed that they are still somewhat prone to trigger points, since it is hard to fine tune the medication to the exact amount your body would produce if you still had a healthy thyroid organ.

Some studies report the prevalence of subclinical hypothyroidism to be as high as 17% in women and 7% in men. People who have a low-functioning hypothyroid gland may experience early morning stiffness, and pain and weakness of the shoulder girdle. Both thyroid inadequacy and hypothyroidism can cause cold (and sometimes heat) intolerance, cold hands and feet, muscle aches and pains (especially during cold, rainy weather), constipation, menstrual problems, weight gain, dry skin, fatigue, and lethargy. Muscles feel rather hard to the touch. Occasionally, people with hypometabolism may be thin, nervous, and hyperactive, and the practitioner may fail to consider subclinical hypothyroidism.

Smoking impairs the action of the thyroid hormone and will make any related symptoms worse. Several pharmaceutical drugs, such as lithium, anti convulsants, glucocorticoid steroids, and those that contain iodine, can also affect thyroid hormone levels, so check with your pharmacist if you have been diagnosed with hypothyroidism and are taking another medication.

Solutions

Test your thyroid function
A simple home test to check your thyroid function is to place a thermometer in your armpit for ten minutes upon waking, but before getting out of bed. Normal underarm temperature for men and post menopausal women is 98°F (36.7°C); for premenopausal women it is 97.5°F (36.4°C) prior to ovulation and 98.5°F (36.9°C) following ovulation. If your temperature is lower than this, you will want to check with your health care provider. Often health care providers will only initially test the TSH (thyroid-stimulating hormone) level, which may be normal if you have hypometabolism rather than hypothyroidism. A radioimmunoassay measures T_3 and T_4 levels, and gives a more complete picture of the thyroid function.

Try vitamin B$_1$

People with low thyroid function may be low in vitamin B$_1$ (thiamine). Before starting on thyroid medication, try supplementing with B$_1$ to see if that corrects your thyroid hormone levels. If you are already on thyroid medication and begin to take B$_1$, you may start exhibiting symptoms of hyperthyroidism, and your medication dosage may need to be adjusted. If you are low in B$_1$ at the time you start taking thyroid medication, you may develop symptoms of acute thiamine deficiency, which may be misinterpreted as an intolerance to the medication. After the B$_1$ deficiency is corrected, you will likely tolerate the medication. You will need to supplement with B$_1$ prior to and during thyroid hormone therapy to avoid a deficiency.

Adjust your potassium intake

Total body potassium is low with hypothyroidism and high with hyperthyroidism, so you may also need to adjust your potassium intake.

Hypoglycemia

Hypoglycemia is an abnormally low level of glucose in the blood, often related to diabetes, but there are several causes. A hypoglycemic reaction to a delayed meal, called fasting hypoglycemia, usually indicates a problem with the liver, adrenal glands, or pituitary gland. Missing or delaying a meal does not cause hypoglycemia in a healthy individual. Postprandial hypoglycemia (also called reactive hypoglycemia) usually occurs two to three hours after eating a meal rich in carbohydrates, and is most likely to occur when you are under a lot of stress. Causes will need to be identified and addressed, if possible.

If you have been diagnosed with hypoglycemia, you probably already know the cause and whether it is reactive or fasting hypoglycemia. The important thing to know for the purposes of this book is that both types cause and perpetuate trigger points, and make trigger points more difficult to treat. Symptoms of both are sweating, trembling and shakiness, increased heart rate, and anxiety. Activation of trigger points in the sternocleidomastoid muscle by a hypoglycemic reaction may lead to dizziness and headaches. If allowed to progress, symptoms can include visual disturbances, restlessness, and impaired speech and thinking.

Solutions

Eat small, frequent meals

Symptoms of hypoglycemia will be relieved by eating smaller, more frequent meals with fewer carbohydrates, more protein, and some fat. Even if you do not have hypoglycemia, if you are waking with headaches or pain or having trouble sleeping, then eating a small snack or drinking a little juice before bedtime usually helps. Low blood sugar is a common trigger for headaches—the lower the blood sugar, the more severe the headache, so eating small, frequent meals may help.

Things to avoid

Avoid all caffeine, alcohol, and tobacco, even second hand smoke.

Try acupuncture

Acupuncture is quite successful in stabilizing blood sugar.

Gout

Gout is a disease characterized by high uric acid levels in the blood. It is caused by dietary factors, genetics, or the underexcretion of urate (the salts of uric acid). Monosodium urate (MSU) crystals form and are deposited in joints, tendons, and the surrounding tissues, which then usually cause swelling and intense pain due to an inflammatory reaction. The joint at the base of the big toe is most commonly affected. Gout often occurs in combination with obesity, diabetes, hypertension, insulin resistance, and/or abnormal lipid levels.

Gout will aggravate trigger points and make them difficult to treat. While Doctors Travell and Simons did not speculate in their books as to why gout is a perpetuating factor for trigger points, it is likely that trigger points are caused and perpetuated by the high acid content, in addition to causing a self-perpetuating cycle of pain from central sensitization. See page 10 for a discussion of tissue acidity, biochemicals, and pain.

Solutions

Treat gout
Keep gout under control by following the instructions from your health care provider. Take vitamin C. Avoid alcohol, sugar, fructose, meat, and seafood. Subsequent treatment of trigger points will be more effective if you follow these suggestions.

Helpful Laboratory Tests

Laboratory tests may be necessary to help diagnose some of the systemic and nutritional perpetuating factors. This information is included so that you can discuss them with your health care provider.

With blood chemistry profiles, an elevated erythrocyte sedimentation rate (SED rate) may indicate a chronic bacterial infection, polymyositis, polymyalgia rheumatica, rheumatoid arthritis, or cancer. A decreased erythrocyte count and/or low hemoglobin point to anemia. A mean corpuscular volume (MCV) of over 92fl indicates the likelihood of a folate or B_{12} deficiency. Eosinophilia may indicate an allergy or intestinal parasitic infection. An increase in monocytes can indicate low thyroid function, infectious mononucleosis, or an acute viral infection. Increased serum cholesterol can be caused by a problem with low thyroid function, and a low serum cholesterol can indicate folate deficiency. High uric acid levels indicate hyperuricemia and possibly gout. See the above section on organ dysfunction and disease for a discussion of thyroid function tests.

Iron deficiency is detected by checking the serum ferritin level. A low serum total calcium suggests a calcium deficiency, but for an accurate assessment of the available calcium, a serum ionized calcium test needs to be performed. Potassium levels can be checked with a serum potassium test. A hair analysis can detect high levels of toxic metals exposure and deficiencies in minerals.

Blood tests can determine serum levels of vitamins B_1, B_6, B_{12}, folic acid, and vitamin C. Any values in the lower 25% of the normal range or below would indicate that supplementation would be helpful in the treatment of trigger points. Remember that even if serum levels of vitamins and minerals are normal, you may still wish to use supplements and/or increase your dietary intake since tissue supplies will drop before the body allows serum levels in the blood to drop.

A fasting blood test is used to diagnose hypoglycemia, and an additional glucose tolerance test or a two hour postprandial blood glucose test may be used to rule out diabetes. Measurement of sensory nerve conduction velocities can help diagnose diabetic neuropathy.

A naturopathic doctor can perform blood tests for food allergies. Stool samples will reveal if parasites are a problem.

Part II

Trigger Point Pressure and Stretch Techniques

Part II is divided into color-coded general sections of muscles in which most of the primary area of pain referral lies, but please note that in many cases referred pain crosses several areas of the body. You will still need to refer to the pain guides found in chapter 6 to ensure that you have considered all of the possibilities of trigger point locations. These sections are:

- Head and Neck Pain (page 57)
- Torso Pain (page 101)
- Shoulder, Upper Arm, and Elbow Pain (page 171)
- Forearm, Wrist, and Hand Pain (page 219)
- Leg, Knee and Foot Pain (page 247)

Each section begins with a chapter on common pain conditions primarily affecting that area of the body, for example migraine headache or tennis elbow (except for the section on gluteal and pelvic area pain). You may want to at least briefly peruse the entire section if you feel pain mostly within that area, but do not forget to consult the pain guides for each area found in chapter 6.

Note that a number in parentheses after a particular muscle or muscle group indicates the relevant chapter to consult for more information.

5 Locating and Treating Trigger Points: General Guidelines

In addition to resolving the perpetuating factors that cause and keep trigger points activated (see part I), self-treatment of trigger points includes applying pressure, stretching, and generally taking care of your muscles. This chapter addresses the general guidelines used to apply the specific treatments contained in each muscle chapter in part II.

As you work on each muscle, return to this chapter to review the general guidelines to ensure that you are performing the self-help techniques correctly. If you are seeing a practitioner, have them check to make sure you are performing the techniques properly—doing them incorrectly could increase your pain. If your symptoms are getting worse, stop doing the self-help techniques, re-read this chapter, and consult with your practitioner.

Where to Start?

Chapter 6 contains the trigger point location guides: these will help you figure out which muscles located in part II may contain trigger points that might be causing your symptoms. First locate your pain or other symptoms for each area, and then refer to the chapters listed.

In each muscle chapter there are drawings demonstrating the most common pain referral areas for each trigger point. The more solid red area indicates the primary area of referral, which is almost always present, and the lighter red area shows the most likely secondary areas of referral, which may or may not be present. Keep in mind that the referral patterns only show the most *common* referral patterns; your referral pattern may be somewhat different, or even completely different. You may also have overlapping referral patterns caused by trigger points in multiple muscles. These areas may be more extensive than the patterns common for individual muscles, and pain may be more intense. For this reason, over time, be sure to search for trigger points in all the muscles that refer pain to that area.

Each muscle chapter contains an anatomical drawing of the muscle or muscles covered in that chapter, with blue dots showing some of the most common locations of trigger points. *There may be additional trigger points or they may be in different places, so search the entire muscle.* Keep in mind that for some muscles, the black dot may just be an *example* of a trigger point location and its associated referral pattern, but they may occur at any level: for example, trigger points in the thoracolumbar paraspinal muscles.

The common symptoms and factors that may cause or perpetuate trigger points are listed in each muscle chapter. Again, these are only the most common; you may experience different symptoms, and your causes and perpetuating factors may be different. If you think you might have trigger points in a certain muscle but do not see any perpetuating factors that apply to you, try to imagine whether anything in your life is similar to something on the list that could be causing the same type of stress on the muscle.

Once you have determined which two muscles most closely fit your pain referral pattern and symptoms, start doing the self-help pressure and stretching, and eliminate the applicable perpetuating factors. Over the next few weeks, search for trigger points in additional muscles and add those into your treatment regime as needed. As you start to feel better, you will develop a clearer picture of which trigger points are causing your pain and which perpetuating factors are reactivating your trigger points.

Other Things to Consider…

When you apply pressure to the trigger point, you can often reproduce the referred pain or other symptoms; however, being unable to reproduce the referred pain or other symptoms by applying pressure does *not* rule out involvement of that specific trigger point. Try treating the trigger points that could be causing the problem anyway, and if you improve, even temporarily, assume that one of the trigger points you worked on is indeed at least part of the problem. For this reason, do not work on all the possible trigger points in one session, since you will not know which of the trigger points treated actually gave you relief.

It is important to note that a *primary*, or *key*, trigger point can cause a *satellite*, or *secondary*, trigger point to develop in a different muscle. The satellite trigger point may have formed for one of three reasons: it lies within the referral zone of the primary trigger point; or it is in a muscle that is either substituting for or countering tension for the muscle that contains the primary trigger point. When doing self-treatments, be aware that if some of your trigger points are satellite trigger points, you will not get lasting relief until the primary trigger points have been treated. This is why it is important to work in the direction of referral (see "DOs" below).

You also need to be aware that central sensitization (see page 11) can cause the referral pattern to deviate from the most common pattern found in each muscle chapter. It may also cause trigger points in several muscles within a region to refer pain to the same area, making it more difficult to determine trigger point locations. This means you cannot absolutely rule out the role of a potential trigger point based *only* on consideration of common referral patterns, since other factors may cause you to have an *uncommon* referral pattern. The more intense the earlier pain, the more intense the emotions associated with it, and the longer pain has lasted, the more likely central sensitization will cause deviation from the most common referral patterns.

A small percentage of people will get worse before they get better, mostly in complex cases. Or the pain may move around, or you may have the perception that the pain moved around only because the most painful areas have improved and now you are noticing the next most painful area more. I have only had a few cases where I was not able to help patients: they were so frustrated after receiving little or no help from one professional after another that they only allowed me to treat them a few times before giving up, *even if they had improved*. If you get a little worse before you get better, you may be inclined to give up in the initial stages of treatment. So with any therapy you try, I encourage you to go to at least five appointments before you decide it is not working, even if your condition initially gets worse. Just give your practitioner some time to learn your body and observe how you use it. However, if your practitioner does not seem to care or have time for you, then by all means look for someone who does care about you getting better.

General Guidelines for Applying Self-Pressure

DON'Ts

- **Do not apply pressure over varicose veins, open wounds, infections, herniated/bulging discs, areas of phlebitis/thrombophlebitis, or where clots are present or could be present. If you are pregnant, do not apply pressure on your legs.**
- **Most importantly**—*do not overdo the self-help techniques!* Many people think that if some feels great, then more will be even better, but you can actually make yourself worse by not following the guidelines. Expect gradual improvement, though you may improve by a greater amount during the first few weeks.

DOs

- **Use a tennis ball, racquetball, golf ball, dog play ball, or baseball, or use your elbow or hand if instructed for particular muscles.** For balls, use the weight of your body to give you the pressure; do not press your back or limb onto the balls. The muscle you are working on should be as passive as possible. Use one ball at a time on your back, not one on each side.
- **Apply pressure for a minimum of eight seconds and a maximum of one minute.** Applying less than eight seconds of pressure may activate trigger points, and more than a minute will cut off the circulation for too long and make it worse. Time yourself first to be sure you are actually counting seconds at the correct speed.
- **It should be somewhat uncomfortable, or "hurt good," but it should not be so painful that you are either tensing up or holding your breath. If it is too painful, use a smaller or softer ball, or move to a softer surface (such as a bed, or a surface padded with a pillow or blanket).** If it does *not* hurt at all, keep looking for tender spots, or try moving to a harder surface. If it is too tender to lie on, try putting a ball in a long sock and leaning against the wall. I only recommend using the wall if you cannot lie on the ball, since you are then using the very muscles you are trying to work on. You may need to use a combination of surfaces, depending on the tenderness of different areas. Over time, as sensitivity decreases, you may need to change ball dimensions and/ or hardness, or move to a harder surface.
- **Search the *entire* muscle for tender points, particularly the points of maximum tenderness.** Use the pictures to make sure you are working on the entire muscle and not just the worst spot. Many times a tendon attachment will hurt because the tight muscle is pulling on it, but if you do not treat the bulk of the muscle, it will keep pulling on the attachment.
- **Be sure to work on both sides of the body to treat and relax the muscles symmetrically, but spend more time on the areas that need it more.** Except for very new one-sided injuries, the same muscle on the opposite side will almost always be tender to applied pressure, even if it has not yet started causing symptoms. If you loosen one side but not the other, this can lead to additional problems. Sometimes problems with the muscles on the opposite side are actually causing the symptoms, so it is always worth working on both sides.
- **Work in the direction of referral.** For example, if your gluteal muscles hurt and the pain is being referred from trigger points in the quadratus lumborum muscle in the lumbar area, work on the lumbar area first, then on the gluteal area.
- **If you have limited time, do one area thoroughly rather than rushing through many areas.** You are more likely to aggravate trigger points than inactivate them if you rush.
- **Do stretches *after* the trigger point work.** If you only have time to do one thing, do the ball/ pressure work and skip the stretches.

■ **Most people should work on their muscles once per day initially.** If you have an appointment with your therapist, do not do your self-help the same day. If you are sore from your therapy appointment or your self-help, skip a day. If you are sore for more than one day or your symptoms get worse, it is likely that either the pressure was too hard or you held points for too long. Review these guidelines if that is the case. Tell your therapist if you are sore from their work. This is not a case of where "if some is great, more is better." Pick a time when you will remember to do your self-help, e.g. when you wake up, when you watch television, or when you go to bed, and keep your balls by the bed (*but do not fall asleep on a ball!*). After a few weeks, you may wish to increase your self-help to twice per day, as long as you are not getting sore. If a particular activity bothers you, you may wish to do the self-help before and after the activity. If you start getting sore or your symptoms worsen, decrease your self-help frequency. Treat your trigger points for as long as they are sensitive, even if active symptoms have disappeared. If trigger points are still tender, they are *latent*, and could easily be reactivated. Most likely you will start forgetting as symptoms disappear; however, the most important thing you will have learned is what to do if your symptoms return.

■ **If you have questions or your symptoms get worse, or you are sore for more than one day, stop the self-help until you have had a chance to consult with your therapist.** They should be able to help you figure out any problems.

■ **Take your balls on trips with you, since travel frequently aggravates trigger points.** You may even wish to keep some balls at your workplace.

General Guidelines for Stretches and Conditioning

It is very important to understand the difference between *stretching* and *conditioning* exercises. *Stretching* means you gently lengthen the muscle fibers; *conditioning* means you are trying to strengthen the muscle. Doctors Travell and Simons found that *active* trigger points benefited from stretching, but were usually aggravated by conditioning exercises. Once trigger points have been *inactivated*, conditioning is beneficial. Make sure your physical therapist or physiotherapist is familiar with trigger points and begins your therapy with stretching exercises.

Usually two weeks of trigger point self-help treatment will be sufficient before adding in conditioning exercises, but if your trigger points are still very irritable, you will need to wait until your symptoms improve. Meanwhile, learn the stretches in this book. If you are not sure whether an assigned activity is a stretch or a conditioning exercise, ask your practitioner. I will not cover guidelines for conditioning exercises in depth here, since your physical therapist or physiotherapist will prescribe them.

DON'Ts

- **Do not bounce on stretches, and avoid stretching when your muscles are tired or cold.**
- **Do not perform a conditioning exercise just because it worked for someone else.** Doctors Travell and Simons said, "Exercise should be regarded as a prescription, much as one prescribes medication. Like a drug, there is a right kind, dose, and timing of exercise." Often a friend will recommend an exercise that worked for them, but you are a different person with a different set of symptoms, and you should no more do their assigned exercises than you would take their prescribed medications. Be sure to tell your therapist about all of the activities and exercises/stretches you are doing, because one of these can be contributing to your trigger point activation.
- **Do not persist with an exercise or stretch that is aggravating your symptoms.** Check with your therapist to determine why it is bothering you and to find out how to proceed.

DOs

- **Stretch slowly and only to the point of just getting a gentle stretch**—*do not force it*. If you stretch the muscles too hard or too fast, you can aggravate trigger points.
- **Hold each stretch for 30 to 60 seconds.** There will be little benefit after 30 seconds, but it will not hurt you to stretch for longer either. You may repeat the stretch after releasing and breathing.
- **For any type of repetitive exercise, breathe and rest between each cycle of the exercise.**
- **If you are sore for more than one day from exercises or stretches, reduce the number of repetitions and try again after the soreness has disappeared.** If you are still sore for two days after the exercise or stretch, it needs to be changed.

General Guidelines for Muscle Care

These are some general suggestions for taking care of your muscles; each muscle chapter will have specific suggestions.

DON'Ts

- **Never put the maximum load on a muscle**—*it is too easy to strain it.*
- **Do not lift anything too heavy**—*ask for help.*
- **Do not keep muscles in positions of sustained contractions, where you are holding them tense or in sustained use.** In order to increase blood flow and bring oxygen and nutrients to the muscles, they need to alternately contract and relax.
- **Do not sit for too long in one position**.
- **Do not expose your muscles** to cold drafts.

DOs

- After treatments, **gently use the muscle normally**, using its full range of motion. Initially, avoid strenuous activities immediately afterward until the trigger points are not so easily reaggravated.
- **Vary your activities** so you are not doing any one thing for too long. Rest and take breaks frequently from any given activity.
- **Lift with your knees bent and your back straight, with the object close to your chest**.
- **Notice where you hold tension** and practice relaxing those areas.
- **Swimming is generally a good exercise**, and bicycling is easier on the body than running, but in both cases, take care to avoid straining the trapezius and neck muscles. A recumbent, stationary, or other bike that allows you to sit more upright is preferable.
- When starting an exercise program, **underestimate what you will be able to do**. Gradually add increments in duration, rate, and effort that will not cause you to be sore or activate trigger points.
- **Warm up adequately for sports activities**.

If you are working with a practitioner, they should be able to help you decide what needs to be done in order of priority. If your practitioner is giving you too many things to do at once, be sure to tell them that you are overwhelmed and need to set priorities. Giving a patient too many assignments is all too easy for a practitioner to do, especially when they are first out of school and brimming with many useful ideas and suggestions.

Be sure to return to this chapter often to review the guidelines to ensure that you are treating the muscles properly, particularly if something is not working for you, or trigger points are being aggravated instead of inactivated. Chances are you have forgotten to follow these guidelines.

Breaking the Pain Cycle: Other Therapies

Something starts to hurt, so you tense up. Then it hurts more, so the muscle tightens up more, perpetuating and escalating the cycle of pain. Any intervention that helps treat trigger points and eliminate perpetuating factors can help break the cycle: trigger point self-treatments, stretching, heat and/or ice, herbs, chiropractic or osteopathic treatments, massage, ultrasound, homeopathy, biofeedback, trigger point injections, counseling, and even analgesics.

People are often surprised that I support the use of analgesics, such as aspirin and ibuprofen, but anything that breaks the pain cycle as soon as possible will help prevent symptoms from getting worse or trigger points developing. Analgesics can also help you tolerate the initial stages of treatment if you are in extreme pain. But be aware that just because your pain level has decreased after taking analgesics, this does not mean the trigger points are gone. You still need to treat trigger points yourself and/or seek treatment, preferably as soon as possible. Analgesics will most likely take the edge off the pain, but unless you plan to take them as a long-term solution, you also need to treat the source of the problem.

Muscle relaxants are of limited value for people with pain caused by trigger points, because muscle spasms are not the cause of the pain. Also, these drugs first release tension in the muscles that contract to compensate for or protect the weakened muscles containing the trigger points. Removing this protective splinting increases the load on the muscles containing trigger points and leads to additional pain.

Ready, Set,…Go!

The techniques taught in this book are one way to treat trigger points and are geared toward easily accessible self-help strategies. You may find one technique or a combination of techniques works best for *you*. No matter which treatment you settle on, you will still need to address the perpetuating factors found in chapters 2 through 4 in order to gain lasting relief.

Be sure to set realistic goals. Focus on a few muscles at a time unless there is a reason that you need to work on several together. Setting unrealistic goals can discourage you and cause you to give up. It is better to pick just a few things and do them well, rather than rush through too many self-help techniques or suggestions and do them poorly. You probably will not be able to apply pressure on five different muscles and stretch them, get orthotics and replace bad shoes, change your diet, and start walking every day all in the first week. Pace yourself so that this is an enjoyable process, and work on the perpetuating factors over time.

6 Trigger Point Location Guides

Any muscle can develop trigger points, potentially causing referred pain and other symptoms. Remember, there are approximately four hundred muscles in the human body, but a few of them may or may not be present in some people. There are also individual variations in fiber or tendon arrangement, so trigger points may be located in different places for different people.

To figure out which muscles to work on first, look at the trigger point location guides and refer to the chapters listed for each. Examine the photos of referral patterns in each chapter and try to find those that most closely match your pain pattern, and read the list of symptoms for each muscle. Refer to chapter 5 for additional instructions on where to start and general guidelines for applying pressure, stretching, and general muscle care.

Blank Body Chart

You may wish to make copies of the blank body chart on page 50 and draw your symptom pattern on one of them with a colored marker. Then you can compare your pattern with the pain referral pictures in chapters 8 through 72. Out to the side of each painful area, note your pain intensity on a scale of 1 to 10 and the percent of time you feel pain in that area—for example, 6.5/80%.

I recommend that you fill out a body chart at least a couple of times per week. Date them so you will be able to keep them in order. This chronological record will come in handy in several ways. It will:

- make it easier for you to discern which patterns fit your pain referral most closely;
- help you recognize the factors that cause and perpetuate your symptoms by matching fluctuations in the level and frequency of your symptoms;
- allow you to track your progress (or lack thereof) and provide a historical record of any injuries.

As your condition improves, you may forget how intense your symptoms were originally, and you may think you are not getting any better. You will be able to see that you are improving, even if you have an occasional setback. One thing to note, however, is that not everyone can accurately draw their pain location, due in part to lack of familiarity with anatomy, so take that possibility into consideration and check muscles with adjacent referral patterns just in case your drawing is inaccurate.

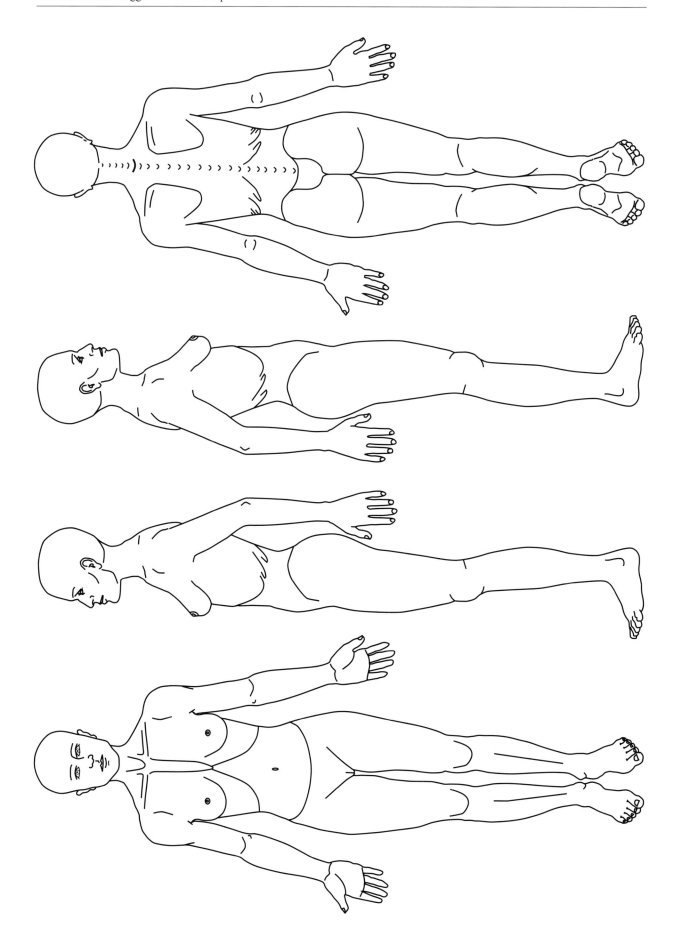

Head and Neck Pain

The muscle names are followed by the chapter number

1. Sternocleidomastoid (10)
Splenius capitis (9)

2. Trapezius (8)
Sternocleidomastoid (10)
Posterior neck (9)
Occipitalis (12)
Digastric (16)
Temporalis (11)

3. Trapezius (8)
Sternocleidomastoid (10)
Temporalis (11)
Posterior neck (9)

4. Sternocleidomastoid (10)
Semispinalis capitis (9)
Facial / Scalp (12)

5. Sternocleidomastoid (10)
Temporalis (11)
Posterior neck (9)
Masseter (13)
Facial / Scalp (12)
Trapezius (8)

6. Lateral pterygoid (15)
Masseter (13)
Sternocleidomastoid (10)
Medial pterygoid (14)

7. Sternocleidomastoid (10)
Masseter (13)
Lateral pterygoid (15)
Trapezius (8)
Digastric (16)
Medial pterygoid (14)
Facial / Scalp (12)

8. Temporalis (11)
Masseter (13)
Digastric (16)

9. Trapezius (8)
Cervical multifidi (9)
Splenius cervicis (9)
Levator scapula (19)
Infraspinatus (35)

10. Sternocleidomastoid (10)
Digastric (16)
Medial pterygoid (14)

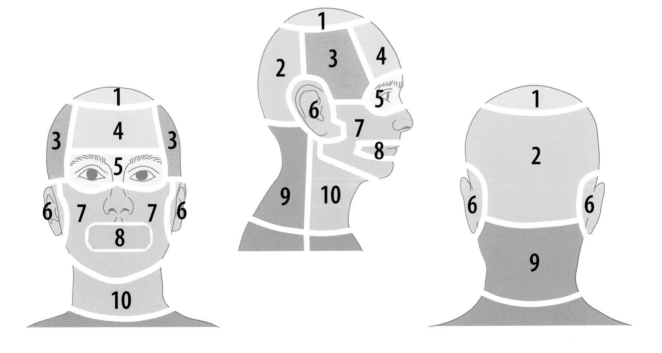

Upper Torso and Upper Arm Pain

The muscle names are followed by the chapter number

11. Scalene (42)
Levator scapula (19)
Supraspinatus (34)
Trapezius (8)
Multifidi (18)
Rhomboid (20)
Splenius cervicis (9)
Triceps brachii (41)
Biceps brachii (46)

12. Scalene (42)
Latissimus dorsi (38)
Levator scapula (19)
Paraspinals (18)
Rhomboid (20)
Serratus posterior
superior (36)
Infraspinatus (35)
Trapezius (8)
Serratus anterior (26)
Pectoralis major (23)

13. Paraspinals (18)
Serratus posterior inferior (21)
Rectus abdominis (25)
Intercostals / Diaphragm (27)
Latissimus dorsi (38)
Iliopsoas (22)

14. Serratus anterior (26)
Intercostals / Diaphragm (27)
Latissimus dorsi (38)

15. Deltoid (44)
Levator scapula (19)
Scalene (42)
Supraspinatus (34)
Teres major (40)
Teres minor (39)
Subscapularis (37)
Serratus posterior
superior (36)
Latissimus dorsi (38)
Triceps brachii (41)
Trapezius (8)
Iliocostalis thoracis (18)

16. Scalene (42)
Triceps brachii (41)
Deltoid (44)
Subscapularis (37)
Supraspinatus (34)
Teres major (40)
Teres minor (39)
Latissimus dorsi (38)
Serratus posterior
superior (36)
Coracobrachialis (45)

17. Infraspinatus (35)
Deltoid (44)
Scalene (42)
Supraspinatus (34)
Pectoralis major /
Subclavius (23)
Pectoralis minor (43)
Biceps brachii (46)
Coracobrachialis (45)
Sternalis (24)
Latissimus dorsi (38)

18. Scalene (42)
Infraspinatus (35)
Biceps brachii (46)
Brachialis (52)
Triceps brachii (41)
Supraspinatus (34)
Deltoid (44)
Sternalis (24)
Subclavius (23)

19. Pectoralis major /
Subclavius (23)
Pectoralis minor (43)
Scalene (42)
Sternocleidomastoid (10)
Sternalis (24)
Intercostals / Diaphragm (27)
Iliocostalis cervicis (18)
External abdominal
oblique (25)

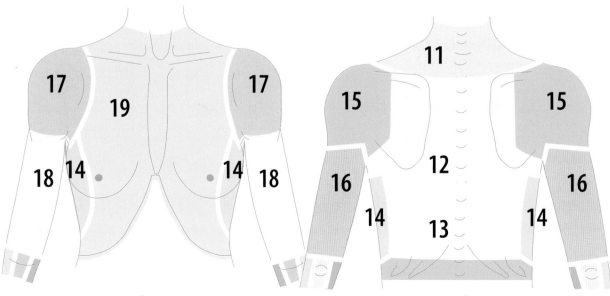

Front   Back

Lower Torso and Thigh Pain

The muscle names are followed by the chapter number

20. Paraspinals (18)
Iliopsoas (22)
Rectus abdominis (25)
Gluteus medius (31)
Iliolumbar ligament (28)

21. Pelvic floor (32)
Gluteus medius (31)
Quadratus lumborum (28)
Gluteus maximus (30)
Multifidi (18)
Rectus abdominis (25)
Soleus (59)

22. Gluteus medius (31)
Quadratus lumborum (28)
Gluteus maximus (30)
Paraspinals (18)
Semitendinosus /
Semimembranosus (56)
Iliolumbar ligament (28)
Piriformis (29)
Gluteus minimus (62)
Rectus abdominis (25)
Soleus (59)
Pelvic floor (32)

23. Gluteus minimus (62)
Hamstrings (56)
Piriformis (29)
Obturator internus (29)

24. Gluteus minimus (62)
Quadriceps femoris (65)
Piriformis (29)
Quadratus lumborum (28)
Tensor fasciae latae (63)
Gluteus maximus (30)

25. Pectineus (68)
Vastus medialis (65)
Adductor muscles
of the hip (67)
Sartorius (66)

26. Abdominals (25)
Paraspinals (18)
Quadratus lumborum (28)

27. Abdominals (25)
Paraspinals (18)
Quadratus lumborum (28)

28. Pelvic floor (32)
Adductor magnus (67)
Piriformis (29)
Abdominals (25)

29. Adductor muscles
of the hip (67)
Iliopsoas (22)
Quadriceps femoris (65)
Pectineus (68)
Sartorius (66)
Quadratus lumborum (28)
Tensor fasciae latae (63)

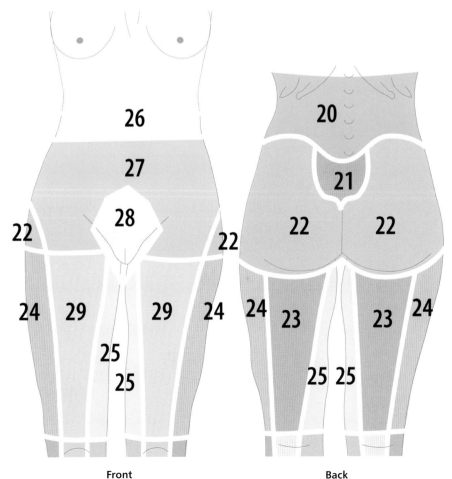

Front   Back

Elbow, Lower Arm and Hand Pain

The muscle names are followed by the chapter number

30. Triceps brachii (41)
Serratus posterior
superior (36)

31. Supinator (49)
Hand / Finger extensors (48)
Triceps brachii / Anconeus (41)
Supraspinatus (34)

32. Triceps brachii (41)
Pectoralis major (23)
Pectoralis minor (43)
Serratus anterior (26)
Serratus posterior
superior (36)

33. Triceps brachii (41)
Teres major (40)
Hand / Finger extensors (48)
Coracobrachialis (45)
Scalene (42)
Trapezius (8)

34. Infraspinatus (35)
Scalene (42)
Brachioradialis (48)
Supraspinatus (34)
Subclavius (23)

35. Latissimus dorsi (38)
Pectoralis major (23)
Pectoralis minor (43)
Serratus posterior
superior (36)

36. Hand / Finger extensors (48)
Subscapularis (37)
Coracobrachialis (45)
Scalene (42)
Latissimus dorsi (38)
Serratus posterior
superior (36)
First dorsal interosseous (54)
Trapezius (8)

37. Supinator (49)
Scalene (42)
Brachialis (52)
Infraspinatus (35)
Hand / Finger extensors (48)
Adductor / Opponens
pollicis (53)
Subclavius (23)
First dorsal interosseous (54)
Flexor pollicis longus (51)

38. Finger extensor digitorum (48)
Hand interosseous (54)
Scalene (42)
Pectoralis major (23)
Pectoralis minor (43)
Latissimus dorsi (38)
Subclavius (23)

39. Brachialis (52)
Biceps brachii (46)

40. Palmaris longus (50)
Pronator teres (51)
Serratus anterior (26)
Triceps brachii (41)

41. Hand / Finger flexors (51)
Opponens pollicis (53)
Pectoralis major (23)
Pectoralis minor (43)
Latissimus dorsi (38)
Palmaris longus (50)
Serratus anterior (26)

42. Flexores digitorum superficialis
and profundus (51)
Hand interosseous (54)
Latissimus dorsi (38)
Serratus anterior (26)
Subclavius (23)

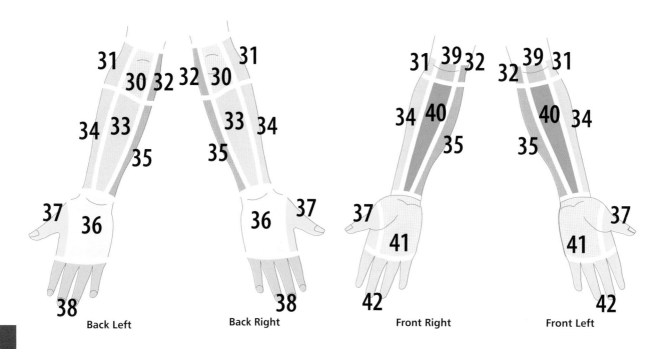

Back Left   Back Right   Front Right   Front Left

Knee, Lower Leg, Ankle and Foot Pain

The muscle names are followed by the chapter number

43. Quadriceps femoris
muscles (65)
Adductors longus &
brevis (67)

44. Vastus lateralis (65)

45. Gastrocnemius (58)
Hamstring muscles (56)
Popliteus (57)
Soleus (59)

46. Quadriceps femoris
muscles (65)
Adductor muscles of
the hip (67)
Sartorius (66)

47. Tibialis anterior (69)
Adductors longus &
brevis (67)

48. Gastrocnemius (58)
Gluteus minimus (62)
Peroneus longus & brevis (64)
Vastus lateralis (65)

49. Soleus (59)
Gastrocnemius (58)
Gluteus minimus (62)
Semimembranosus &
Semitendinosus (56)
Flexor digitorum longus (61)
Tibialis posterior (60)

50. Tibialis anterior (69)
Peroneus tertius (64)
Long extensor muscles
of the toes (70)

51. Peroneal muscles (64)

52. Soleus (59)
Tibialis posterior (60)

53. Abductor hallucis (71)
Flexor digitorum longus (61)

54. Extensors digitorum brevis
and hallucis brevis (71)
Long extensor muscles of
the toes (70)
Deep intrinsic foot
muscles (72)
Tibialis anterior (69)

55. Tibialis anterior (69)
Extensor hallucis longus (70)
Flexor hallucis brevis (72)

56. Foot interossei (72)
Extensor digitorum
longus (70)

57. Soleus (59)
Quadratus plantae (72)
Abductor hallucis (71)
Tibialis posterior (60)

58. Gastrocnemius (58)
Flexor digitorum longus (61)
Deep intrinsic
foot muscles (72)
Soleus (59)
Abductor hallucis (71)
Tibialis posterior (60)

59. Deep intrinsic foot
muscles (72)
Superficial intrinsic foot
muscles (71)
Long flexor muscles
of the toes (61)
Tibialis posterior (60)

60. Flexor hallucis longus (61)
Flexor hallucis brevis (72)
Tibialis posterior (60)

61. Flexor digitorum longus (61)
Tibialis posterior (60)

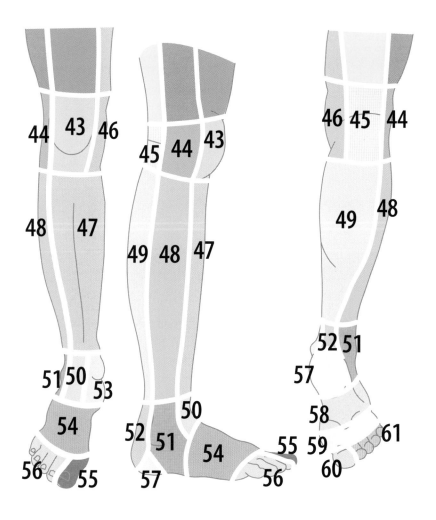

7

Head and Neck Pain

There are several general self-help techniques that will assist you in treating trigger points in your head and neck. Retraining yourself to hold your head properly and breathe correctly will help treat several muscles in the neck and torso. There are also a few techniques that will help resolve temporomandibular joint dysfunction and headaches and migraines, including checking all of the muscles in the head and neck section for trigger points.

Improper Breathing and Trigger Points

Learning to breathe properly is important for resolving trigger points in several muscles, including the posterior neck muscles (9), sternocleidomastoid (10), thoracolumbar paraspinal muscles (18), serratus posterior inferior (21), abdominal muscles (25), serratus anterior (26), intercostals and diaphragm (27), and pectoralis minor (43).

Solutions
Place one hand on your chest and the other on your belly. When you inhale, both hands should rise. As you exhale, both hands should fall. You need to train yourself to notice when you are breathing only into your chest and make sure you start breathing into your belly.

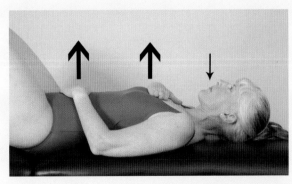 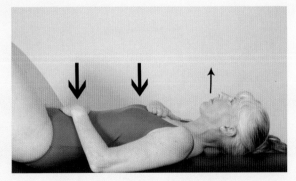

Head-Forward Posture and Trigger Points

Head-forward posture leads to the development and perpetuation of trigger points. Have someone look at your side profile to see if your head is further forward than your trunk. The further you hold your head forward of your shoulders, the greater the likelihood that you will develop a larger number of trigger points. Head-forward posture can be aggravated while sitting in a car, at a desk, or in front of a computer, or while eating dinner or watching TV.

Solutions

Get lumbar supports and orthotics

Head-forward posture can be caused and aggravated by common daily activities such as sitting in a car or watching TV. Using a good lumbar support everywhere you sit will help correct poor sitting posture, while orthotic inserts in your shoes may improve your standing posture. See chapter 2, "Ergonomics" and "Body Mechanics."

Retrain yourself

Postural exercises can help eliminate head-forward posture. To learn proper posture and correct a head-forward position, stand with your feet about four inches apart, with your arms at your sides and thumbs pointing forward. Tighten your buttocks to stabilize your lower back, then, while inhaling, rotate your arms and shoulders *out* and *back* by rotating your thumbs backward, and squeeze your shoulder blades together in the back. Keep holding this position while dropping your shoulders down and exhaling. Move your head back to bring the ears in line with the shoulders and hold this position for about six seconds while breathing normally.

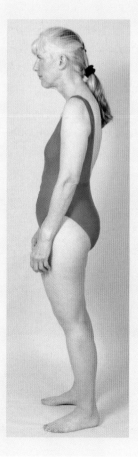
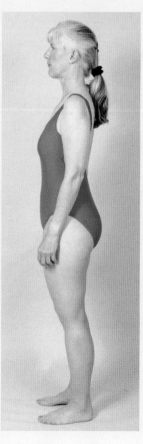

When moving your head, do not move your nose up or down, or open your mouth. Relax, but then try to maintain good posture once you release the pose. If holding this position feels uncomfortable or "stiff," try shifting your body weight from your heels to the balls of your feet, which causes your head to move backward over your shoulders. This exercise should be repeated frequently during the day in order to retrain yourself in good postural techniques, at least every one to two hours. It is better to do one repetition six or more times per day than to do six repetitions in a row.

Temporomandibular Joint Dysfunction and Trigger Points

Temporomandibular joint (TMJ) dysfunction can be caused by problems in the joint itself due to alignment problems and inflammation and/or untreated trigger points in the muscles in and around your mouth. Trigger points can eventually lead to changes in the joint or to *malocclusion*, which means that the teeth in the upper and lower jaws do not fit together properly.

People without jaw restrictions can get at least two knuckles vertically between their top and bottom front teeth. If you cannot do this, you do not have a normal range of motion. If your jaw deviates to one side when you open your mouth, the side it deviates toward is the one more likely to contain trigger points. If you experience a great deal of pain when you press right over the joint and inside your ear, the joint itself is probably inflamed. A displaced jaw disc may cause a feeling of pressure, leading you to bite down in an attempt to relieve the pressure, and subsequently adding to the problem.

Trigger points can be caused by clenching or grinding your teeth, pressing your tongue against your teeth or the roof of your mouth, abnormal head and neck postures, or direct trauma to your face. If your jaw makes grating or popping sounds, you may have disc erosion, bone on bone, or arthritis. This can be caused by long-term trigger points that have not been relieved, so it is important to inactivate trigger points before permanent damage results. Latent trigger points may cause symptoms other than pain, so it is wise to treat the likely trigger points even if you are not experiencing the pain of active trigger points.

Solutions
Tongue rolls

Tongue rolls help relax the muscles of the mouth. First, take three deep breaths, and continue breathing deeply through your nose during the entire exercise. Keeping your lips sealed, begin rolling your tongue in big circles on the outside of your teeth, but inside your lips. Roll your tongue ten times in each direction, or if you cannot do this many initially, do as many as are comfortable.

Supplements

Take calcium, magnesium, and folic acid, as a deficiency can play a role in grinding your teeth, called *bruxism*. See chapter 3 for more information.

Try adjustments and acupuncture

Your jaw may need an adjustment from a chiropractor or osteopath. Acupuncture very successfully treats both emotional tension and TMJ problems. Even if there is degeneration or arthritis of the jaw joint, acupuncture is still helpful for pain control, but will not restore the joint to its original condition.

See a dentist for evaluation

Always ask to use a bite block during dental procedures, such as when getting a filling.

Since changes in your bite can be either the cause of *or* the result of trigger points, it is wise to first identify and relieve your trigger points before making *any* kind of permanent dental corrections. Since working on your muscles can change your bite, perform the self-help techniques for at least four weeks before being fitted for any dental appliances. Work on *all* trigger points in the neck and head, including the sternocleidomastoid muscle pressure (chapters 8 through 16). You do not want to have to pay for a second night guard or occlusal splint because your bite has changed, or have your bite adjusted irreversibly.

You may need to be fitted with a night guard or occlusal splint with a flat occlusal plane which can change your bite. While bite guards and splints will not prevent you from clenching, they will help protect your teeth and relieve some of the muscular fatigue. The soft plastic bite splints available over the counter in pharmacies are too soft and will not help TMJ dysfunction. You need to be fitted by your dentist for a hard, acrylic bite guard. If your teeth contact prematurely (your bite is off), your dentist may recommend an occlusal splint. Your dentist may have other solutions for your particular situation. If the above suggestions do not work, then you may need to have a dentist adjust your bite, but this should be a last resort since it is irreversible. Be sure to choose a dentist who has experience with trigger points and TMJ dysfunction, and will take the time to make sure corrective devices fit properly. Improperly fitted devices can make trigger points worse and can cause additional jaw joint problems. You may need to see a specialist in TMJ evaluation.

For more information on trigger points and TMJ dysfunction, see *Trigger Point Therapy for Headaches & Migraines: Your Self-Treatment Workbook for Pain Relief* (DeLaune, 2008).

Headaches, Migraines and Trigger Points

A headache is defined as aching or pain in one or more areas of the head or neck. Both the frequency and the pain level can vary greatly. About 90% of all headaches fall into three categories: tension headaches, migraines, and cluster headaches.

People who have headaches are almost twice as likely to have postural abnormalities, such as head-forward posture, and to have trigger points in the back of the neck, particularly in the suboccipital muscles (9). The greater the number of active trigger points, the more frequent and severe the headaches.

People with migraine headaches have the same prevalence of postural abnormalities and number and location of trigger points as people with tension headaches, even when they tend to have one-sided migraines. With one-sided headaches, a greater number of active trigger points are located on the same side as the headache. People who suffer from both migraine and tension-type headaches are far more likely to have a greater number of active trigger points than those who only have one kind of headache. This means that the probability of trigger points being part or the entire problem in the majority of headaches is likely to be high.

Solutions
Trigger point self-work
If you have headaches, they can be a composite of trigger point pain referrals from neck and chewing muscles. Be sure to check all the muscles found in this section of the book ("head and neck pain") to eliminate all sources of referred pain. Trigger points will be more tender during a headache and will probably be more tender just prior to and immediately after the headache.

For more information on trigger points and headaches and migraines, see *Trigger Point Therapy for Headaches & Migraines: Your Self-Treatment Workbook for Pain Relief* (DeLaune, 2008); for headache symptoms and perpetuating factors tables, and a headache diary worksheet form, see www. triggerpointrelief.com.

Each muscle chapter in this section will contain additional solutions for these conditions and others affecting this part of the body.

8 Trapezius

As you can see from the muscle drawing, the *trapezius* is a large diamond-shaped muscle. It is the most superficial muscle and covers much of the mid and upper back, and the back of the neck, attaching near the base of the skull, to the collarbone (*clavicle*), shoulder blade (*scapula*), and the C6 to T12 vertebrae. There are three main parts to the muscle—the upper, middle, and lower trapezius—and each part has its own attachments, actions, and common symptoms.

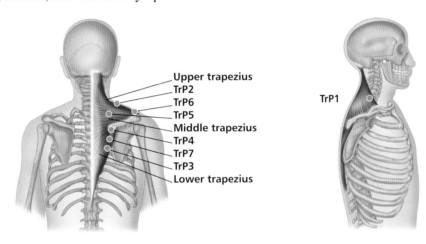

The main function of the trapezius is to move the shoulder girdle and the shoulder blade in various directions, depending on which fibers are being used. This muscle commonly contains trigger points, and referred pain from these trigger points compels people to seek help more often than pain caused by any other trigger points.

Common Symptoms

Upper Trapezius
- Headaches on the temples (TrP1).
- Facial, temple, or jaw pain (TrP1).
- Pain behind the eye (TrP1).
- Severe neck pain (TrP1 and TrP2).
- Dizziness or vertigo (in conjunction with the sternocleidomastoid muscle) (TrP1), a stiff neck (TrP1 and TrP2), limited range of motion (TrP1 and TrP2), and intolerance to weight on the shoulders (TrP1 and TrP2).

Middle Trapezius
- Mid back pain.
- Headaches at the base of the skull.
- TrP5 refers superficial burning pain close to the spine.

- TrP6 refers aching pain to the top of the shoulder near the joint.

Lower Trapezius
- TrP3 can cause mid back, neck, and/or upper shoulder region pain.
- TrP7 can possibly cause referral on the back of the shoulder blade, down the inside of the arm, and into the ring and little fingers, very similar to a serratus posterior superior referral pattern.
- TrP3 can cause headaches at the base of the skull.
- TrP3 can refer a deep ache and diffuse tenderness over the top of the shoulder.

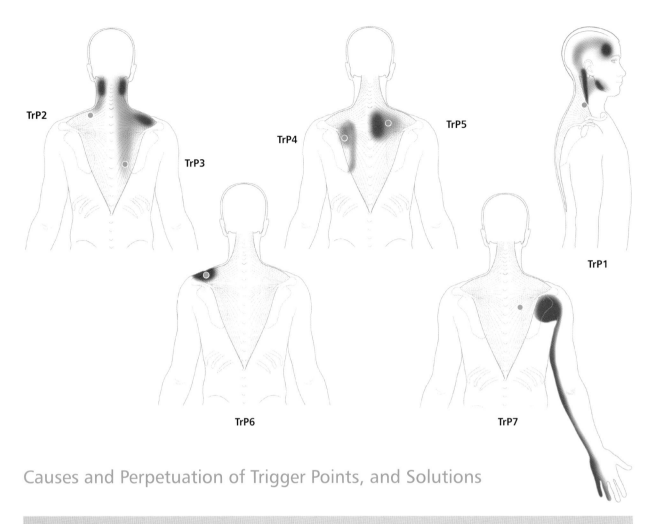

Causes and Perpetuation of Trigger Points, and Solutions

■ Poor posture and ergonomics at your desk workstation, such as sitting in a chair without armrests or with armrests that are too high, typing with a keyboard that is too high, cradling a phone between your ear and shoulder, or sitting slumped without a firm back support. Any profession or activity that requires you to bend over for extended periods, such as a dentist/hygienist, architect/draftsman, and secretary/computer user. Walking with a cane that is too long.

Solutions
■ Modify or replace your misfitting furniture and pillows. See chapter 2, "Ergonomics," for detailed information. If you use a walking cane, be sure it is not so high that it hikes up your shoulder.

■ Other poor postural positions, such as tensing your shoulders, sewing on your lap with your arms unsupported, sleeping on your front or back with your head rotated to the side for a long time, turning your head to one side for long periods to have a conversation, playing a violin, or head-forward posture.

Solutions
■ Retrain yourself to relax your shoulders, repeatedly noticing tension and relaxing. When having a conversation, turn and face the person, rather than rotating your head in their direction. Putting your hands in your pockets takes the weight off the trapezius muscle. See the exercise for postural retraining in chapter 7.

- Anything that puts constricting pressure on the muscles, such as shoulder or torso bra straps that are too tight, a purse or daypack/backpack that is too heavy, or a heavy coat. Carrying a daypack or purse over one shoulder—even if you think you are not hiking up one shoulder, you *are*, no matter how light the item.

Solutions

- Putting shoulder pads in a heavy coat can help take the weight off the upper trapezius. See page 19, "Clothing," for more information on how to resolve other clothing issues.

- Sports such as jogging, bike-riding, kayaking, and weight lifting, turning your head to one side to breathe while swimming, and activities with sudden one-sided movements.

Solutions

- You may need to modify or stop doing these activities until trigger points are inactivated. Swimming provides good aerobic exercise, but you need to vary your strokes so you do not unduly stress the trapezius muscle. See page 17, "Body Mechanics," for more information.

- Structural problems such as one leg anatomically shorter than the other, a hemipelvis that is smaller on one side (either the left or the right half of the pelvic bone), large breasts, or short upper arms (which causes you to lean to one side to use the armrests).

Solutions

- If you have a body asymmetry or short upper arms, see a specialist to get compensating lifts or pads. If your breasts are large enough that they cause backaches, your insurance company may cover breast reduction surgery if your health care provider recommends it. Carefully consider the risks of surgery if you are considering this option.

- Fatigue.

Solutions

- See page 32, "Sleep Problems." If you suffer from chronic fatigue syndrome, see an acupuncturist or naturopathic doctor.

- Injuries such as whiplash caused by a car accident, falling on your head, or any sudden jerk of the head, or tight pectoralis major muscles.

Solutions

- Work on the muscles listed at the end of this chapter for associated trigger points.

Self-Help Techniques

Applying Pressure

Thoracolumbar Paraspinal / Trapezius Pressure
See chapter 18 for how to use a ball to apply pressure to most of the thoracolumbar paraspinal muscles and the mid to lower trapezius muscle.

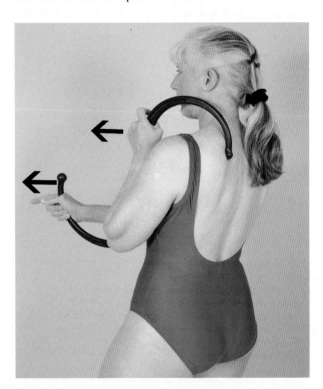

Backnobber®
If you are at work and unable to lie on the floor, I recommend using a Backnobber® from Pressure Positive Company to apply pressure to the trapezius muscle. Note how both hands are pulling the Backnobber® away from the body in the direction the arrows are pointing, rather than pressing it into the front of the trunk to lever pressure onto the back.

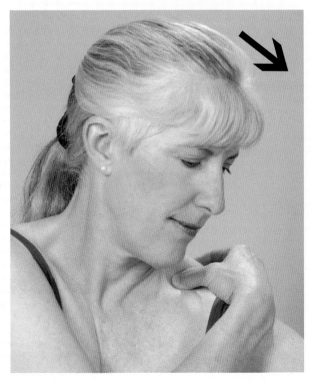

Trapezius Pinch
Place your elbow and forearm on a surface high enough to support the weight of your arm. With the opposite hand, reach across your front and pinch the upper portion of the trapezius muscle. Be sure to stay on the meat of the muscle and *do not dig your thumb into the depression directly above the collarbone.* You may need to tilt your head slightly toward the side you are working on, to keep the muscle relaxed enough to be able to pinch it.

Supraspinatus Pressure
The supraspinatus pressure (34) will also help treat the upper trapezius.

Posterior Neck Pressure
Perform the self-help posterior neck pressure (9) on the back of your neck with a golf ball.

Stretches

Trapezius Stretch

This stretch benefits the middle and lower trapezius. Start with your arms at your sides and then move them through the positions indicated in the photographs. End with your arms at your sides and take two deep breaths. Repeat three to five times.

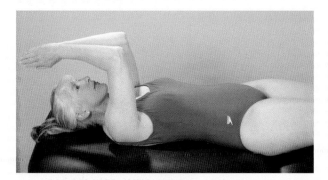
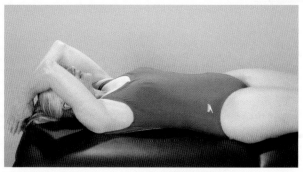

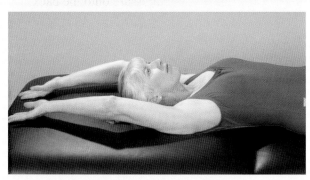
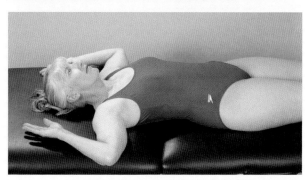

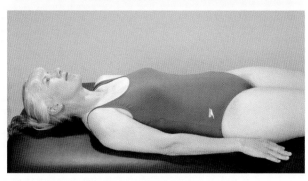

Posterior Neck Stretch

See the posterior neck muscles (9) and perform the self-help stretch for the back of your neck.

Pectoralis Stretch

The pectoralis stretch (17) will benefit the trapezius muscle.

Also Check

Supraspinatus (34). Sternocleidomastoid (10). Levator scapula (19). Infraspinatus (35). Pectoralis major (23). Pectoralis minor (43). Rhomboid (20). Temporalis (11, satellite trigger points). Facial and scalp muscles (12, occipitalis – satellite trigger points). Posterior neck muscles (9, satellite trigger points). Masseter (13, satellite trigger points).

Differential Diagnosis

If you are unable to relieve your symptoms with trigger point self-help techniques, you may need to see a health care provider to rule out occipital neuralgia and cervicogenic headaches. Or, you may need to see a chiropractor or osteopathic physician to be evaluated for vertebrae that are out of alignment.

Posterior Neck Muscles

Cervical Multifidi, Semispinalis Cervicis, Semispinalis Capitis,
Splenius Capitis, Splenius Cervicis, Suboccipital, Longissimus Capitis

The muscles on the back of the neck are complex in their fiber arrangements and attachments, but generally attach at or near the base of the skull and to the cervical and upper thoracic vertebrae. Their main function is to rotate the head and to bring the head back up from a forward position, generally moving and stabilizing the head.

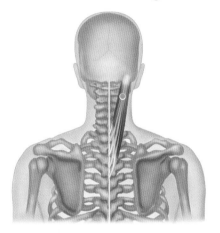

Splenius capitis

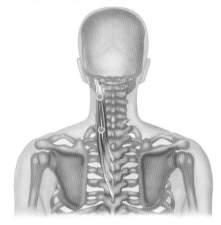

Splenius cervicis

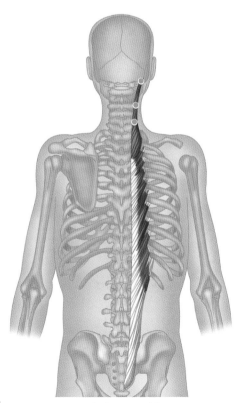

Longissimus capitis

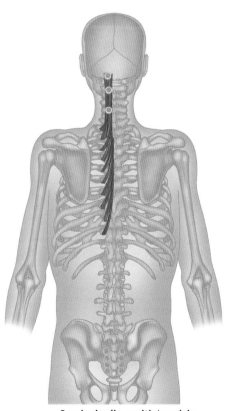

Semispinalis capitis/cervicis

Trigger points in these muscles are extremely common, particularly in people whose jobs require them to hold their heads in awkward positions for long periods of time. Fortunately, some simple ergonomic workstation corrections combined with pressure and stretching techniques can make a great deal of difference.

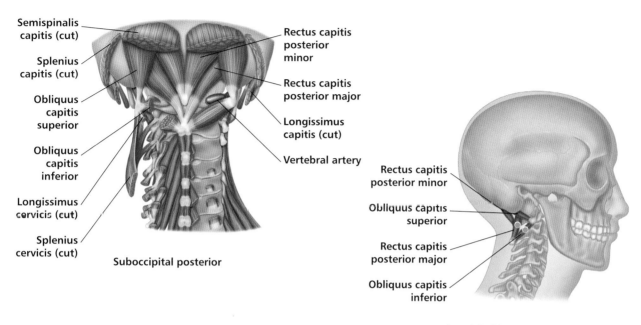

Suboccipital posterior

Suboccipital lateral

Common Symptoms

Splenius Capitis
■ Pain referred to the top of the head, but slightly toward the side of the trigger point.

Splenius Cervicis
■ Diffuse pain referred throughout the inside of the head.
■ Pain may feel like it is focused behind the eye or shooting through the head to the back of the eye.
■ Pain may also refer to the back of the skull.
■ Pain may be referred to the junction of the neck and top of the shoulder, and up the back of the neck.
■ Trigger points may cause a stiff neck, and/or limited range of motion, or blurred vision on the same side of the trigger point, but without dizziness.

Cervical Multifidi, Semispinalis Cervicis, Semispinalis Capitis
■ Pain and tenderness over the back of the head and neck.
■ Painful, restricted range of motion in all directions, with the pain worsening when bending the head forward.
■ The pressure of lying on a pillow is too painful.
■ If the greater occipital nerve becomes entrapped, symptoms may also include numbness, tingling, and burning pain on the back of the head.

Suboccipital
■ Pain referred inside the head, but it is difficult to define a specific area.
■ Pain is vaguely more localized from the back of the skull, over the ear, and to the temples, forehead, and eye.
■ Soreness just below the base of the skull, and the pressure of lying on a pillow is too painful.

Longissimus Capitis
■ Pain around, just behind, and/or below the ear. Pain may also extend down the neck, or behind the eye.

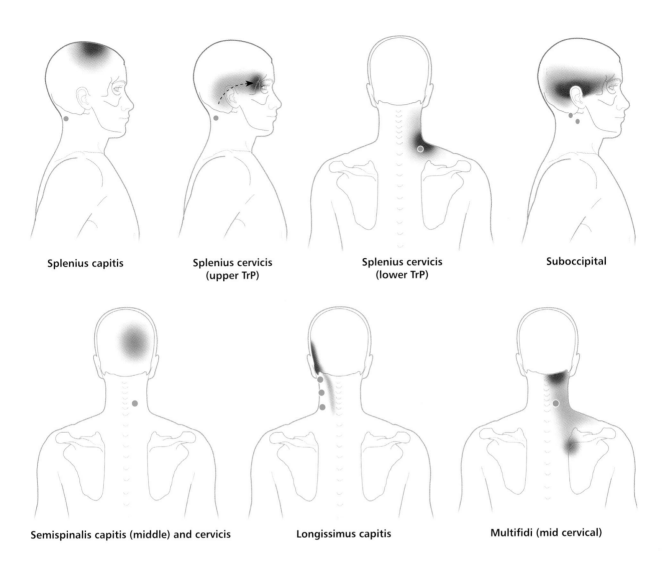

Splenius capitis

Splenius cervicis (upper TrP)

Splenius cervicis (lower TrP)

Suboccipital

Semispinalis capitis (middle) and cervicis

Longissimus capitis

Multifidi (mid cervical)

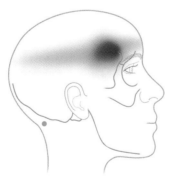

Semispinalis capitis (upper)

Causes and Perpetuation of Trigger Points, and Solutions

■ Poor posture, such as holding your neck in awkward positions, as when bird-watching, playing some musical instruments, looking up for long periods of time, falling asleep on the couch with your head propped up on the arm of the couch, or lying face-down on the floor while propped up on your elbows to watch TV. Poor posture and ergonomics at your work desk, including lack of lumbar support, having your copy where you have to tilt or rotate your head, or glasses that have too short a focal length.

Solutions

■ Sit upright, with your head held directly over your trunk and your back well supported by a lumbar support. Get a copy-holder for the side of your computer screen, so your head is not tipped down or turned to the side too far. Make sure your computer monitor is at eye-height. If there is a reflection on your eye glasses that causes you to tilt or tip your head, try changing the location of your light. Make sure your eyeglass prescription is current and you can see far enough with your reading glasses. Read chapter 2 for a full list of suggestions for proper body mechanics and ergonomically designed furniture.

■ Get a pillow that keeps your spine in alignment and is not made with a springy material that will jiggle your neck. Chiropractic offices usually sell well-designed pillows.

■ Head-forward posture.

Solutions

■ See the exercise for postural retraining in chapter 7.

■ Structural problems, such as compensation for an excessive outward spinal curve in the mid back (known as *kyphosis*, which can be aggravated by tension in the pectoralis major muscles), or having a long neck, a laminectomy surgery, or cervical facet joint osteoarthritis, which particularly affects the semispinalis capitis.

Solutions

■ Any body asymmetries need to be corrected, such as an anatomical short leg or a small hemipelvis (either the left or the right half of the pelvic bone). See a specialist to get compensating lifts and pads. If you use a walking cane, be sure it is not so high that it hikes up your shoulder.

■ Check the pectoralis major muscles (23) to make sure tightness is not putting too much strain on the mid and upper back.

■ Exposure to a cold draft or air conditioner when the muscle is fatigued.

Solutions

■ Avoid cold drafts and keep your neck warm by wearing a scarf, turtle neck, or neck gaiter, even in bed at night.

■ Injuries such as whiplash (especially if your head was rotated at the time of the accident), falling on your head, and vertebrae that are out of alignment with nerve entrapment.

Solutions

■ See a chiropractor or osteopathic doctor, and check and treat all of the muscles in this section for trigger points.

■ Sports activities such as diving into a pool, pulling on a rope, or lifting heavy exercise or other weights, particularly with your head rotated or held forward.

Solutions

■ Avoid head-rolling exercises. If you ride a bike, sit as upright as possible by adjusting the handlebars. If you are using a stationary bike, try to sit upright. If you lift weights, avoid excessive amounts of weight and keep your head straight and pulled back over your shoulders.

■ Restrictive clothing items such as a bathing cap, coat, shirt, or necktie that is too tight.

Solutions

■ If any clothing item is leaving a mark on your skin, it is too tight. Replace the item with something more loosely fitting. See page 19, "Clothing."

■ Depression.

Solutions

■ If you are depressed, you may be rounding your shoulders with your head held forward. Treat the underlying cause of depression with counseling, acupuncture, homeopathics, and/or herbs. See page 33, "Emotional Factors," for more information.

Self-Help Techniques

Applying Pressure

I find it is best to treat the trapezius muscles first and the posterior neck muscles second. Be sure you have looked at the trapezius muscle (8) and have performed at least the thoracolumbar paraspinal / trapezius pressure technique (18) prior to working on the back of the neck.

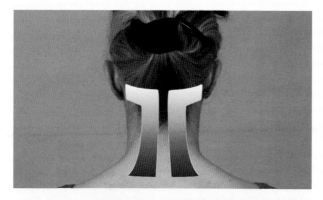

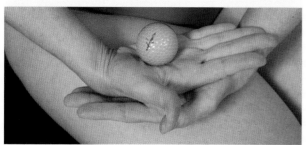

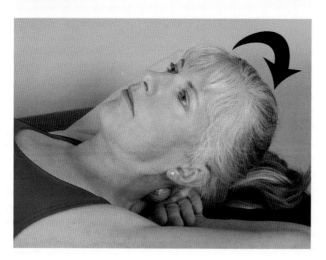

If you have headaches, they can be a composite of trigger point pain referrals from neck and chewing muscles. Make sure that you check all the muscles found in this section of the book to eliminate all sources of referred pain.

Posterior Neck Pressure

The shading in the picture marks the area to work on. You may work along the base of the skull and down the back of the neck. Try to get all the way to the base of the neck where it intersects the top of the shoulder, in order to work on the entire splenius cervicis muscle.

To treat the back of your neck, use a golf ball and lie face-up with your hands behind your neck. One palm should be squarely over the other palm, with the golf ball in the center of your top palm, and *not* where the fingers join the palm.

Keep your head relaxed throughout the self-treatment. To apply pressure, rotate your head toward the ball. Be sure to work on the muscles to the *side* of the spine—do not put the ball directly *on* the spine. To move the ball, roll your head away from the side you are working on, move the ball a small amount, and then rotate your head back toward the side you are working on. If you want more pressure, rotate your head toward the side you are working on even more; rotate your head less if you want less pressure. *Do not raise your head to move the ball.* This will cause additional stress on the muscles, so be sure to move the ball by *rotating* your head away from it.

Stretches

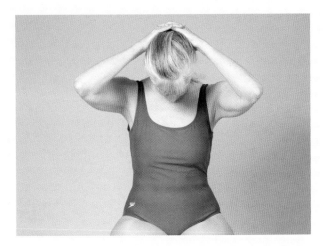

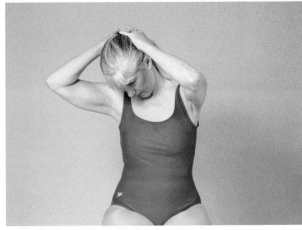

Posterior Neck Stretch
You may do this stretch under a hot shower and, if possible, seated on a stool. Lock your fingers behind your head and pull your head gently forward. Turn your head to one side at a 45-degree angle and gently pull your head in that direction. Place one hand on the top of your head and gently pull your head down to that side. Repeat on the opposite side.

Side-Bending Neck Stretch
See the scalene muscles (42) and perform this stretch.

Also Check

Levator scapula (19). Pectoralis major (23). Thoracolumbar paraspinal muscles (18). Digastric (16, posterior portion). Infraspinatus (35). Sternocleidomastoid (10). Trapezius (8).

Differential Diagnosis
If you are unable to relieve your symptoms with trigger point self-help techniques, you may need to see a health care provider to rule out several types of arthritis, herniated or bulging discs, and spinal stenosis. Or, see a chiropractor or osteopathic physician to evaluate for vertebrae out of alignment.

10 Sternocleidomastoid

The *sternocleidomastoid* has two parts to the muscle—the sternal and clavicular divisions—and both attach at the base of the skull to the mastoid process. The sternal division attaches to the breastbone (*sternum*); the clavicular division attaches to the collarbone (*clavicle*). One side used alone functions to rotate the head and tilt it upward. When both sides are used together, they function to bring the head and neck down in front, and keep the head from rolling backward unchecked. They also assist in taking a breath.

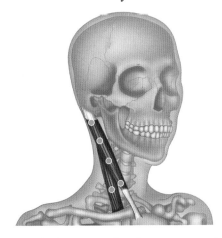

Trigger points in each division have their own referral patterns and common symptoms. Both divisions frequently contain multiple trigger points and can have symptoms other than pain; the sternal division causes symptoms in the eyes and sinuses, while the clavicular division causes symptoms in the forehead and ear.

Common Symptoms

- A tension headache.
- Muscles may be sore to the touch.
- A persistent, dry, tickling cough.
- Entrapment of cranial nerve XI by the sternocleidomastoid may cause partial paralysis of the trapezius on the same side.

Sternal Division

- Pain referred to the top of the head, the back of the head, the cheek, and/or over the top of or behind the eye.

- Sinus congestion on the affected side, or a chronic sore throat due to referred pain to the throat and back of the tongue when swallowing, rather than due to infection.
- Profuse tearing of the eye, reddening of the eye whites and the insides of the lids, visual disturbances including blurred vision and/or dimming of perceived light intensity, and/or a drooping upper eyelid or eyelid twitching.
- One-sided deafness or a crackling sound in the ear.

Clavicular Division

- Headaches on the forehead, possibly across the whole forehead rather than just on one side.
- Earaches with deep pain.
- Pain in the cheek and molar teeth on the affected side.
- Referred symptoms to the eye and sinuses (self-treatment can help clear the sinuses).
- Dizziness and disturbed balance (disorientation) or vertigo (a spinning sensation), especially when changing position.

- Seasickness or car sickness.
- Nausea and loss of appetite.
- Veering into doorjambs or objects on the affected side, or an inability to drive a car without veering to the side.
- Inability to gauge differences in weights held in the hands.
- Sweating, blanching, and a cool sensation on the forehead.

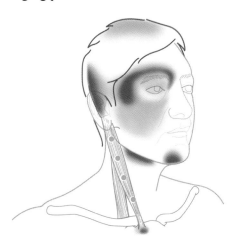

Sternal division

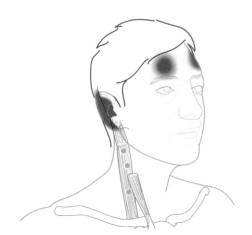

Clavicular division (Sternal division cut away)

Causes and Perpetuation of Trigger Points, and Solutions

- Activities that stress these muscles such as overhead work (e.g. painting a ceiling), looking up for long periods of time, swimming strokes that require you to turn your head to breathe, or horseback riding and horse handling. A necktie or collar that is too tight can put pressure on the muscles and cause trigger points.

Solutions

- Avoid any overhead work that requires you to bend your head backward. *Do not do head-rolling exercises!* In particular, do not bend or roll your head backward. If you are a swimmer, avoid the crawl stroke or any stroke that requires you to turn your head to one side to breathe.

- Make sure your collar or tie is not too tight—your finger should fit comfortably inside your shirt collar, even when your head is turned. See chapter 2 for more information.

- Poor posture or ergonomics such as head-forward posture, reading in bed with a lamp off to the side, sleeping with a pillow that is too high, or constantly tilting your head to avoid light reflection on glasses or contacts, or to improve hearing. This includes any profession or activity that requires you to tilt your head back or turn it to the side for long periods.

Solutions

- See chapter 2, "Ergonomics" and "Body Mechanics," for more information. See chapter 7 for a postural retraining exercise.

- Injuries, such as whiplash caused by a car accident, a fall on your head, or any sudden jerk of the head.

Solutions

- See a chiropractor or osteopathic doctor and check and treat all of the muscles in this section for trigger points.

- Breathing improperly, or a tight pectoralis major muscle (23) pulling down and forward on your collarbone.

Solutions

- See chapter 7 for a proper breathing technique. Be sure to check the pectoralis major muscle (23) to make sure it is not causing the sternocleidomastoid to be pulled tight. If you are doing the pectoralis stretch (17), be sure to bring your head back straight over your shoulders and look straight forward.

- Suffering from a chronic cough or chronic infection, such as sinusitis, a dental abscess, or oral herpes (cold sores). Acute infections, such as the common cold or flu, can activate latent trigger points. "Hangover headaches" may be the result of alcohol stimulating trigger points in the sternocleidomastoid. Leakage of cerebrospinal fluid following a spinal tap may activate sternocleidomastoid points, and subsequently cause a chronic headache that may last from weeks to years.

Solutions

- Chronic infections must be eliminated or controlled as much as possible. You will probably need to work on your sternocleidomastoid muscles after illnesses such as a cold, flu, or facial herpes (cold sores) outbreak. The chronic cough from asthma and emphysema can aggravate trigger points, as can breathing improperly. See chapter 7 for proper breathing techniques, and chapter 4 to address chronic infections.

- Any structural problems, severe deformity, or injury that restricts upper-body movement, forcing the neck to overcompensate to keep balance, such as severe *scoliosis* (a curved and/or rotated spine), an anatomical leg-length inequality, or unequal hemipelvis size (either the left or the right half of the pelvic bone).

Solutions

- If you have a body asymmetry, such as a small hemipelvis or anatomically short leg or upper arm, see a specialist to get compensating lifts or pads. Trigger point self-help techniques, chiropractic adjustments, acupuncture, and massage can help reduce scoliosis.

Self-Help Techniques

Applying Pressure

Sternocleidomastoid Pressure

It is best to do this self-treatment lying down, but you can do it sitting up, which comes in handy at work. Tilt your head just a little toward the side you are working on (bringing the ear closer to the shoulder) and then rotate your head slightly *away* from that side.

To work the lower half of the muscle, grasp *both* parts of the muscle with your hand of the same side (i.e. the right hand grasps the right sternocleidomastoid), but *do not dig your fingers deep into the neck!* Pinch and pull at the same time, holding each tender spot for eight seconds to one minute.

To work the upper half of the muscle, switch hands (i.e. the left hand grasps the right sternocleidomastoid) and pull the muscle outward in the middle. Then use the hand of the same side to work your way up to the attachment behind the ear. For most people, this is the tightest part, but also the most critical to work on. If your sternocleidomastoid is particularly tight, it may be hard to get a hold of it at first, but after you have worked on it a few times, it should become easier to grasp. Remember that you may have to work this muscle again after an illness, because sternocleidomastoid trigger points will likely be reaggravated.

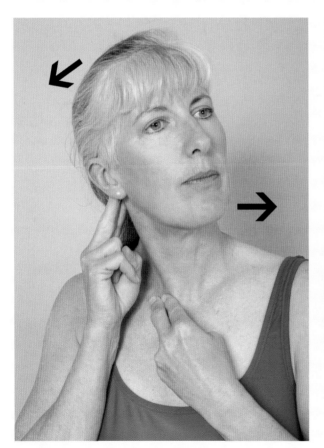
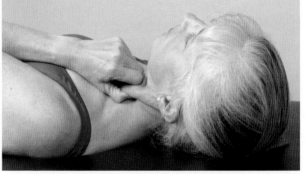
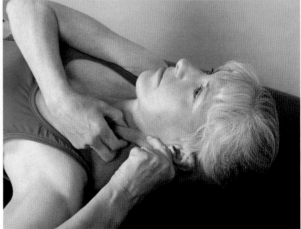

Stretches

Side-Bending Neck Stretch
See chapter 42.

Also Check

Trapezius (8). Masseter (13, satellite trigger points). Facial (12, platysma). Scalene muscles (42). Posterior neck muscles (9). Levator scapula (19). Sternalis (24, satellite trigger points). Temporalis (11, satellite trigger points). Facial and scalp muscles (12, satellite trigger points). Pectoralis major (23).

Differential Diagnosis
If you are unable to relieve your symptoms with trigger point self-help techniques, you may need to see a health care provider to rule out non-trigger point related headaches, atypical facial neuralgia, trigeminal neuralgia, dizziness caused by problems within the ears, Ménière's disease, tic douloureux, arthritis of the sternoclavicular joint, and wryneck (where the neck is twisted to the side due to muscle spasming).

Temporalis

The *temporalis* muscle is located on the side of the head, attaching to the skull above and to a part of the jaw bone (*mandible*) on the other end. The primary function of this muscle is to close the jaw, but some of the fibers also assist in moving the jaw in various directions.

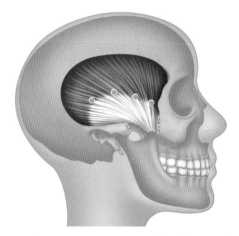

Trigger points in the temporalis muscle are very common. Tenderness in the muscle may indicate trigger points, but there can be an absence of tenderness even though trigger points are present and causing symptoms. Try putting the knuckles of the index and middle fingers of your non-dominant hand in your mouth; if you cannot get both in, you have trigger points in the temporalis and/or masseter (13) muscles.

Common Symptoms

- Pain referred on and above the temple and ear, over the eyebrow, to the upper teeth on the affected side. Occasionally pain is referred to the face and jaw joint, usually experienced as a headache or toothache.

- Your teeth can become sensitive to heat or cold, or achy.
- Improper bite alignment. Your jaw may "zigzag" during opening and closing.
- Teeth clenching (although often this is a cause of trigger points).

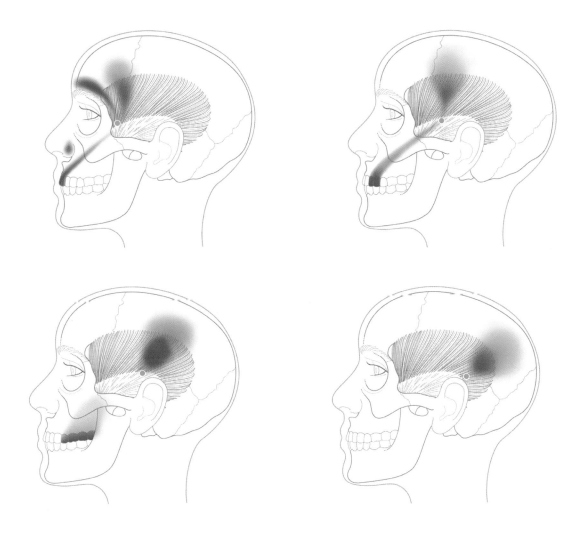

Causes and Perpetuation of Trigger Points, and Solutions

■ Chronic stressors to the muscles operating the jaw, such as clenching and teeth grinding, your teeth hitting other teeth and throwing off the bite (this may start after dental work), or long periods of keeping your mouth open or closed (as in dental work or cervical traction without a bite splint).

Solutions
■ See chapter 7, "Temporomandibular Joint Dysfunction," for more information.

■ Injuries or chronic irritations, such as a direct blow to the side of the head, constantly chewing gum, wearing a surgical mask, or a cold draft on the side of the head from, for example, a car window or air conditioner.

Solutions
■ Apply a hot pack to the temple area and sides of your face. Protect your head from drafts by wearing a scarf or hat that covers the side of your head. Avoid chewing gum or other chewy or hard foods. If you wear a face mask, remove it periodically and stretch your jaw. Get a pillow that supports the jaw, such as the kind with higher edges and a curve in the middle for support of the neck. These can usually be obtained at chiropractic offices.

■ Satellite trigger points that develop secondary to trigger points in the trapezius (8) and/or sternocleidomastoid (10) muscles, and head-forward posture.

Solutions

■ Work on trigger points in the trapezius, posterior neck muscles, and sternocleidomastoid first, and then the temporalis. You may even need to work on trigger points in the lower extremities. See chapter 7 to correct head-forward posture.

■ Body asymmetries need to be corrected by lifts, massage, chiropractic treatment, or good quality orthotic footbeds, since structural inequalities activate posterior neck trigger points which then cause satellite trigger points in muscles used for chewing.

■ Systemic perpetuating factors, such as a folate deficiency, hypothyroidism, and low-normal serum levels of T_3 to T_4 thyroid hormones, or chronic infections or inflammation, even after the infection or inflammation has been resolved.

Solutions

■ Be sure to evaluate and eliminate any systemic perpetuating factors, such as reduced thyroid function and nutritional deficiencies. Folic acid deficiency may be a cause of teeth grinding. See chapters 2 and 3 for more information.

■ Mouth breathing needs to be eliminated by correcting the causes, such as nasal obstruction.

Self-Help Techniques

Applying Pressure

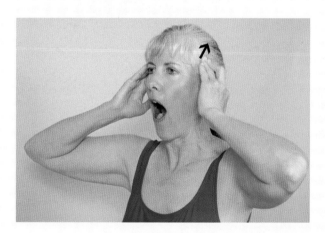

Temporalis Pressure

Using your fingertips, apply pressure to the areas above your temple and ear. While holding tender points, slowly open and close your jaw. Look at the muscle illustration and the referral pattern illustrations to make sure you are working on the whole muscle—it covers most of the side of your head.

Stretches

Yawning
Yawn widely to stretch the temporalis muscle.

Supine Mandible Stretch
After applying hot packs to the sides of your head, lie face-up and insert your index finger behind your lower front teeth, and pull forward and down, giving a gentle stretch. This is a good stretch to do just before bedtime.

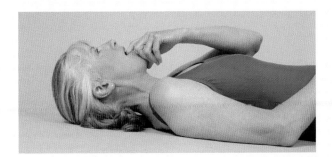 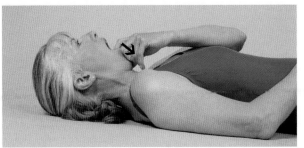

If your jaw deviates to one side, for example to the left, place your right fingers on the right upper cheek over your upper teeth, and place your left fingers on your lower jaw on your left side, and push your lower jaw toward the right. If your jaw deviates toward the right, do the opposite motion.

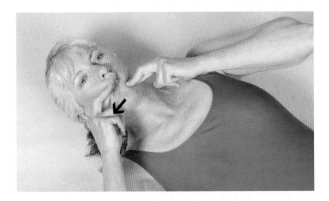 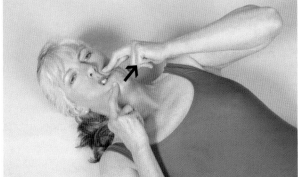

Exercises

Tongue Rolls
Tongue rolls help relax the muscles of your mouth (see chapter 7 for this exercise).

Also Check

Trapezius (8, upper portion). Sternocleidomastoid (10). Masseter (13). Medial pterygoid (14). Lateral pterygoid (15).

> **Differential Diagnosis**
> If you are unable to relieve your symptoms with trigger point self-help techniques, you may need to see a dentist or health care provider to rule out temporomandibular joint internal derangements, diseased teeth, polymyalgia rheumatica, temporal arteritis, or temporal tendinitis.

12 Facial and Scalp Muscles

Orbicularis Oculi, Zygomaticus Major, Platysma, Buccinator, Frontalis, Occipitalis

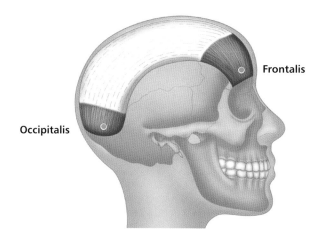

There are several muscles in your face that can cause or contribute to head and facial pain. The *orbicularis oculi* muscle closes the eye tightly. The *zygomaticus major* muscle raises the corner of the mouth for smiling. The *platysma* muscle tenses the skin on the front of the neck and pulls the corner of the mouth downward, as in frowning. The *buccinator* muscle is used for moving food around the mouth while chewing. All of these muscles attach to subcutaneous fascia (connective tissue) rather than bone.

The *occipitofrontalis* consists of a flat, tendinous sheet running from the eyebrow area to the occipital bone at the back. It attaches to the skin and slides over the skull, and has two muscle bellies: the *frontalis*, which underlies the forehead and front of the skull, and the *occipitalis*, which is above the base of the skull at the back. The frontalis muscle belly raises the eyebrow and wrinkles the forehead, such as when you are surprised. When the frontalis and occipitalis are used together, they open the eyes very widely, producing an expression of horror and causing the hair on the front of the skull to stand up. Anxiety causes these muscles to tense.

Common Symptoms

Orbicularis Oculi

- Pain referred from the orbicularis oculi travels over the eyebrow and down the nose, and possibly spills off the nose and into the upper lip.
- There may be an inability to close the eyelid tightly, causing eye dryness, and it may be difficult to look up without tilting the head backward, since the eyelid will not go all the way up. Tears may not drain properly.
- When reading text with strong black and white contrast such as a book, the letters seem to "jump."

Zygomaticus major

- Pain referred from below the cheek, up next to the nose, and into the forehead.
- Difficulty smiling or laughing.
- Restriction of normal jaw opening by 0.4"–0.8" (10–20 mm).

Platysma

- A strange prickling pain over the cheek and lower part of the face like multiple pinpricks. A trigger point close to the collarbone may refer hot prickling pain across the front of the chest.

Buccinator

- Referred pain feels both superficial and deep under the cheekbone, and is worse when chewing.
- Difficulty whistling or playing a wind instrument.
- Perceived difficulty swallowing, even though swallowing is actually normal.

Frontalis

- Referred pain over the forehead on the same side.
- Trigger points in the middle half of the frontalis can entrap the supraorbital nerve, causing a frontal headache.

Occipitalis

- One-sided headaches.
- Referred pain between the top of the ear and top of the head, or deep pain inside the head.
- Intense referred pain deep behind the eye, in the eye, and on the eyelid.
- Referred pain with pressure against the muscles when lying on a pillow.

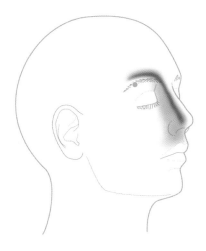

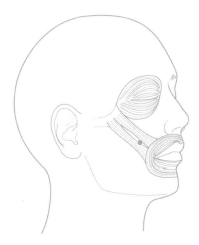

Orbicularis oculi

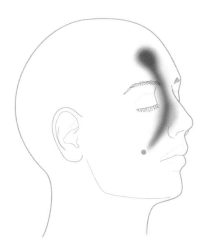

Zygomaticus major

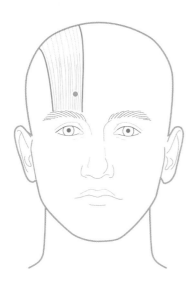 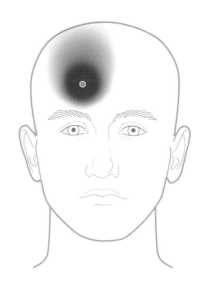

Frontalis

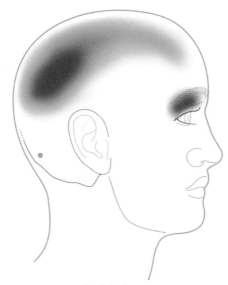

Occipitalis

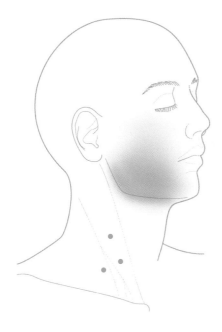 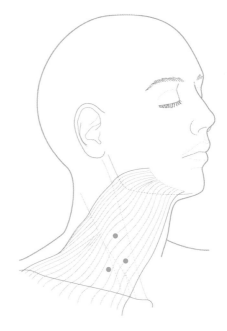

Platysma

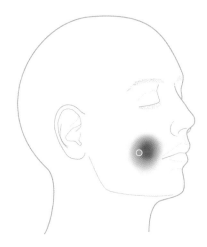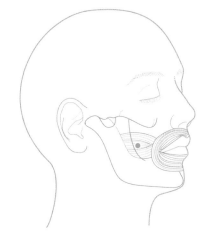

Buccinator

Causes and Perpetuation of Trigger Points, and Solutions

■ Habitual frowning or squinting may cause trigger points in the orbicularis oculi. Chronically raised eyebrows and wrinkling the forehead may cause trigger points in the frontalis. Occipitalis trigger points form as a result of squinting due to glaucoma or deterioration of vision.

Solutions

■ Avoid holding facial expressions for long periods of time, such as wrinkling your forehead, raising your eyebrows, and frowning. You are probably not aware you are doing this, so you will need to train yourself to realize it and relax. Have your vision checked.

■ Trigger points from the sternal division of the sternocleidomastoid (10) may cause satellite trigger points in the orbicularis oculi. Trigger points in the muscles used for chewing may activate trigger points in the zygomaticus major. Trigger points in the sternocleidomastoid or scalene muscles (42) can activate trigger points in the platysma. Trigger points in the frontalis are likely to develop as satellite trigger points as a result of referral from the clavicular division of the sternocleidomastoid, and satellite trigger points can form in the occipitalis due to referral from trigger points in the posterior neck muscles (9).

Solutions

■ Pain from trigger points in the orbicularis oculi, buccinator, and zygomaticus is frequently diagnosed as a tension headache, and may also be misdiagnosed as temporomandibular joint (TMJ) dysfunction. Pain from trigger points in the occipitalis and frontalis is also frequently diagnosed as a tension headache. Check all of the other muscles listed in this chapter for associated trigger points.

Trigger points in the buccinator may be activated by dental appliances (such as night guards), that do not fit well.

Solutions

See a dentist for re-evaluation and a re-fit after working on trigger points for at least four weeks, since that will change your alignment. See chapter 7, "Temporomandibular Joint Dysfunction," for more information.

Self-Help Techniques

Be sure to check the sternocleidomastoid (10), digastric (16, posterior portion), and semispinalis cervicis (9) muscles for trigger points since referred pain can activate trigger points in the forehead or back of the head. Trigger points in the platysma are rarely present without trigger points in the sternocleidomastoid, scalene muscles (42), or muscles used for chewing (masseter, digastric, medial pterygoid, lateral pterygoid, and temporalis), so be sure to check those muscles for trigger points also.

Applying Pressure

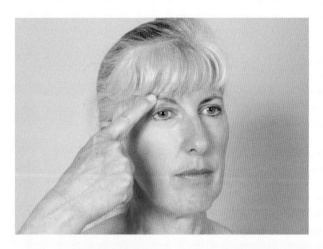

Orbicularis Oculi Pressure

To treat the orbicularis oculi, use the tip of your index finger to press in the area below the eyebrow, on the bone above your eye. You may also pinch and roll the muscle between your thumb and index finger—just pinch as close to the bone as possible, to be sure you are getting a hold of the muscle in addition to the skin.

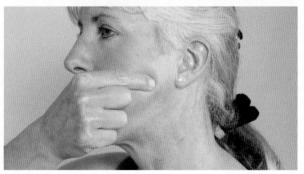

Buccinator and Zygomaticus Major Pressure

To treat the buccinator and the zygomaticus major, put your opposite thumb inside your mouth and your index finger outside your mouth, and pinch from just below the lower rim of your cheekbone, down to close to the bottom of your jaw. You may stretch your cheek outward as you do this, and open your mouth wider as the trigger points release.

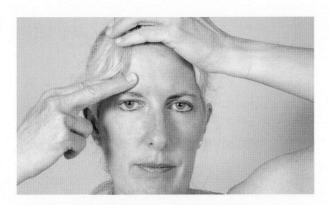

Frontalis Pressure
Use your fingers to press on the frontalis trigger points on your forehead.

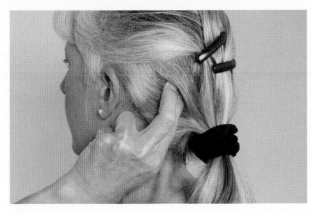

Occipitalis Pressure
Use your fingers to search for trigger points on the back of your head in the occipitalis muscle. You may also rest your head on a tennis ball.

Platysma
It is probably best to have a trained therapist treat the platysma, due to the delicate structures in the front of your neck.

Stretches

Tongue Rolls
Tongue rolls help relax the muscles of your mouth. See chapter 7.

Also Check

Sternocleidomastoid (10). Scalene muscles (42). Masseter (13). Lateral pterygoid (15). Medial pterygoid (14). Digastric (16). Trapezius (8). Temporalis (11). Posterior neck muscles (9, semispinalis cervicis).

Differential Diagnosis
If you are unable to relieve your symptoms with trigger point self-help techniques, you may need to see a dentist to rule out TMJ dysfunction.

13 Masseter

The *masseter* is a very powerful muscle, used primarily for chewing. It attaches to the cheekbone above (*zygomatic arch* and *zygomatic process* of the *maxilla*) and to the jawbone (*mandible*) below.

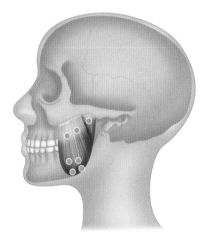

Trigger points are very common in the masseter, due in part to chewing gum and/or teeth grinding (*bruxism*). Dental work can change the bite, even with the most careful dental work. Long procedures that require overstretching cause trauma to the muscles, and the removal of wisdom teeth can be particularly problematic. Difficulty in opening your mouth very far is most likely due to trigger points in the masseter and/or temporalis muscles. Try putting the knuckles of the index and middle fingers of your non-dominant hand in your mouth—if you cannot get both in, you likely have trigger points in one or both muscles.

Common Symptoms

- Pain referred to the eyebrow, ear, jaw joint, mouth, and cheek region.
- The upper or lower molar teeth can be sensitive to pressure or temperature changes.
- Difficulty opening the mouth; you should be able to get the knuckles of your index and middle fingers of your non-dominant hand between your front teeth. The jaw may deviate to one side when opening.
- One-sided ringing or other noise in the ear, often described as a "low roaring." If the ringing is on both sides, fluctuation in its intensity is likely to be one-sided, as opposed to two-sided tinnitus that has a cause other than trigger points (such as drug-induced tinnitus).
- Pressure in the sinus area can be mistaken for a sinus infection.
- Puffiness/bags under the eyes on the affected side, due to restriction of venous flow from the area around the eyes, and the eyelid muscles may spasm.
- Trigger points may play a role in "tension headaches."

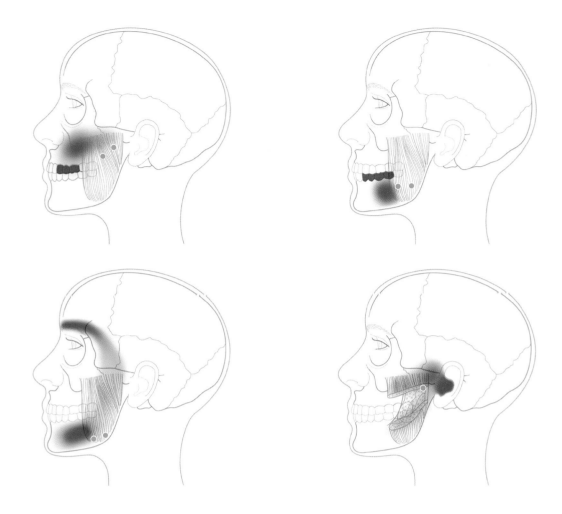

Causes and Perpetuation of Trigger Points, and Solutions

■ Teeth grinding, which may occur at night when you are not aware of it. Constantly chewing gum, clamping a pipe or cigarette holder in your teeth, constantly biting off threads, cracking nuts or ice between your teeth, or thumb sucking late in childhood.

Solutions

■ If you are clenching your jaw or grinding your teeth, see a dentist for help. Try taking calcium/ magnesium, folic acid, and B-complex supplements, and practice stress-reduction techniques. Do not chew gum or hold a pipe or cigarette holder clamped between your teeth. Avoid foods that require a lot of prolonged chewing or cracking of hard objects.

■ Changes in your bite, through either dental work or natural changes, or dentures that are worn out and need to be replaced.

Solutions

■ See chapter 7 for information on temporomandibular joint dysfunction and corrective measures. If you must have a long dental procedure, see if your dentist is willing to give your mouth periodic rest breaks, or use a bite block. Perform your self-help techniques before and after the appointment. If you wear dentures, replace them if they are worn out.

■ Extreme or moderate emotional tension and/or depression, possibly due to high-stress jobs or relationships, where feelings cannot be safely expressed, for example holding back anger or "biting your tongue." This perpetuating factor is perhaps the most common cause of masseter trigger points, and a major contributor to temporomandibular joint dysfunction.

Solutions

■ See a counselor, learn relaxation and coping techniques, and otherwise reduce stress to eliminate emotional causes of teeth grinding. See page 33, "Emotional Factors," for more information.

■ Systemic factors, such as vitamin deficiencies (especially B-vitamins), low thyroid function, anemia, electrolyte imbalances (sodium, potassium, calcium, and magnesium), or chronic infections of the mouth or rest of the body.

Solutions

■ See a health care provider or naturopathic doctor to determine if you have a low-functioning thyroid, anemia, a vitamin deficiency, or an electrolyte imbalance. A deficiency in calcium, magnesium, potassium, and sodium is easily remedied with supplements, and will usually relieve symptoms within one to two weeks. Chronic infections must be eliminated or controlled as best you can. See chapter 4 for more information.

■ Mouth breathing, structural imbalances, or head-forward posture.

Solutions

■ Treat the cause of mouth breathing. Mechanical problems such as nasal polyps or a deviated septum may require surgery. Chronic sinusitis or allergies can be treated with acupuncture, herbs, and homeopathics. Neti pots are helpful and are available at health food stores. Naturopaths use a small inflatable balloon to open up sinus passages. See page 34 for more information on chronic infections and allergies.

■ If one leg is shorter than the other it may help to see a specialist to get compensating lifts. If you have a longer second toe, a footbed orthotic will help stabilize the foot. See chapter 7 for an exercise to correct head-forward posture.
■ Activation of satellite trigger points in the sternocleidomastoid (10) or upper trapezius (8), or trauma, such as prolonged overstretching during dental work, or direct trauma from an accident.

Solutions

■ Difficulty in opening your mouth may be due to trigger points found in other muscles. If you cannot find trigger points in the masseter or other mouth muscles, or you have relieved them and still cannot open the mouth fully, search for trigger points in the legs (especially if you have a second toe longer than the big toe), and the sternocleidomastoid, trapezius, and scalene muscles.

Self-Help Techniques

Applying Pressure

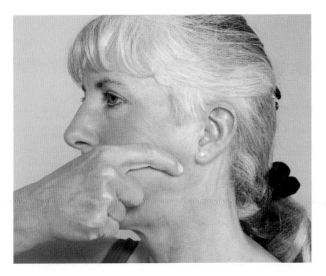

Masseter Pressure
Using the hand opposite the side you are working on, insert your thumb inside your mouth, but outside your gums. You may relax your jaw once your thumb is in place. With your index and middle fingers, press on the outside of your cheek, pinching your masseter in between your fingers and thumb. Be sure to work all the way from the bottom of your jaw up to your cheekbone, and all the way back toward your ear. See the picture of referral patterns so you will know what you are aiming for.

Stretches

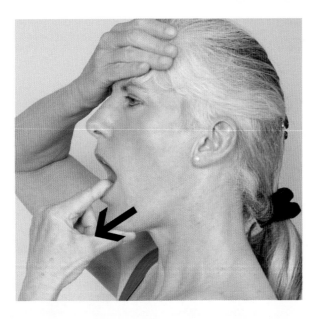

Mandible Stretch
Warm your face with hot moist towels if possible. Place one hand on your forehead, and use two fingers of your other hand to gently pull your jaw down and forward. Count to eight and then relax. Repeat five to six times.

Exercises

Tongue Rolls
Tongue rolls help relax the muscles of the mouth. See chapter 7.

Yawning
Yawning is a good exercise to stretch and condition the masseter muscle.

Also Check

Temporalis (11, satellite trigger points). Medial pterygoid (14, satellite trigger points). Sternocleidomastoid (10). Facial and scalp muscles (12, satellite trigger points). Trapezius (8).

Differential Diagnosis
If you are unable to relieve your symptoms with trigger point self-help techniques, you may need to see a dentist to rule out problems with the teeth or jaw joint discs. If your jaw is spasmed shut (lockjaw), you will need to see a health care provider to eliminate the possibility of an infection or a tumor.

14 Medial Pterygoid

The *medial pterygoid* is a muscle deep inside your mouth; it attaches to the sphenoid bone (forming the very back of the roof of your mouth) and the inside of your jawbone (*mandible*). Use of the muscle on only one side allows you to deviate your jaw toward the opposite side. When both are used at the same time, they allow you to close your mouth and to jut out your jaw.

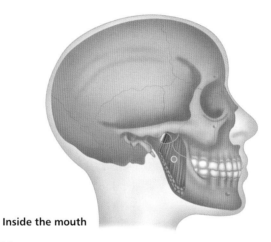

Inside the mouth

Common Symptoms

- Pain referred to the back of the mouth, tongue, and throat, below and around the jaw joint, and deep in the ear.
- Pain or difficulty with swallowing, or a sore throat.
- Pain when chewing or clenching your jaw, and/or pain when opening your jaw, with some restriction; usually you will only be able to barely open your mouth wide enough to fit two knuckles between your teeth (normally your mouth should open wide enough for almost three knuckles).
- The jaw may deviate to the same or opposite side if only one side is involved, and deviation mainly happens at the end of the movement.
- Stuffiness in your ear, because trigger points prevent another muscle from opening the Eustachian tubes.

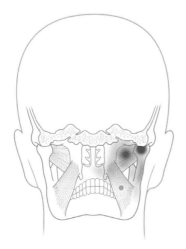

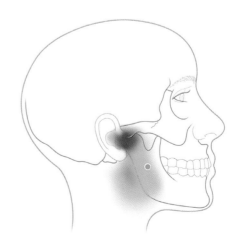

Causes and Perpetuation of Trigger Points, and Solutions

■ Teeth grinding or clenching (most likely due to anxiety and emotional tension), chewing gum, or thumb sucking after infancy.

Solutions

■ See a counselor, learn relaxation and coping techniques, and otherwise reduce stress to eliminate emotional causes of teeth grinding. See chapter 4 for more information.

■ Do not chew gum, and avoid foods that require a lot of prolonged chewing or cracking of hard objects.

■ Trigger points in the lateral pterygoid (15).

■ Improper bite alignment may cause or *be caused by* trigger points.

Solutions

■ See chapter 7, "Temporomandibular Joint Dysfunction," for a discussion of bite alignment. If those suggestions do not work, then you may need to have a dentist adjust your bite, but this should be a last resort since it is irreversible.

■ Buy a pillow that supports the jaw, such as the kind with higher edges and a curve in the middle for support of the neck (see page 16). Try chiropractic or osteopathic treatment, and/or acupuncture. Your jaw may need an adjustment, and acupuncture very successfully treats temporomandibular joint problems and emotional tension.

■ Head-forward posture.

Solutions

■ See chapter 7 for an exercise to correct head-forward posture.

■ Systemic perpetuating factors.

Solutions

■ Evaluate for and treat chronic nutritional deficiencies (see chapter 3). Chronic infections in the neck and shoulder area need to be identified and treated, including oral herpes (cold sores); see page 34 for more information.

Self-Help Techniques

If you continue to have difficulty swallowing, try the sternocleidomastoid (10) and digastric (16) muscles. Also check for trigger points in the neck muscles (9), shoulder girdle muscles (see shoulder, upper arm and elbow pain section), pectoralis major (23), and pectoralis minor (43), and sometimes even in the lower extremities.

Applying Pressure

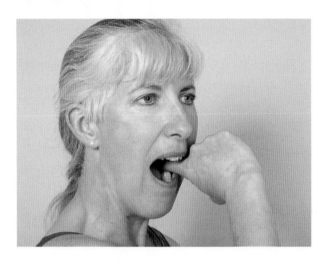

Medial Pterygoid Pressure
Using your opposite index finger, reach inside your mouth, inside your teeth, and all the way behind the top set of molars. Sweep downward along the soft tissue behind your molars to the floor of your mouth. Press and hold anything that is tender. If this causes a gag reflex, take a deep breath and hold it while you are treating trigger points.

Stretches and Exercises

The stretches and exercises are the same as those for the lateral pterygoid muscle in chapter 15.

Also Check

Digastric (16). Sternocleidomastoid (10). Lateral pterygoid (15). Masseter (13). Pectoralis major (23). Pectoralis minor (43).

15 Lateral Pterygoid

The superior (upper) division of the *lateral pterygoid* muscle attaches to the sphenoid bone in the face, and the inferior (lower) division of the muscle attaches to the lateral pterygoid plate. Both divisions attach to the jawbone at the "neck" of the mandible, adjacent to the *temporomandibular joint* (TMJ). The lateral pterygoid allows you to open your mouth, jut your jaw forward, and deviate your jaw to the side.

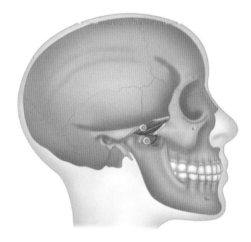

Trigger points in this muscle are frequently the cause of the jaw not tracking properly, resulting in TMJ dysfunction. Often treatment by dentists that has focused on treating the joint or teeth has been unsuccessful, because the actual problem was trigger points in the muscles.

If your jaw zigzags when opening, do this simple test. Place the tip of your tongue as far back in the roof of your mouth as you can. If your jaw opens straight this time, it is mainly the lateral pterygoid that is causing the problem. If your jaw still zigzags, other chewing muscles are involved, or there may be a problem with the TMJ itself, and the lateral pterygoid may or may not be involved.

Common Symptoms

- Pain referred deep into the TMJ and over the cheek.
- Pain when chewing.
- The jaw wobbles back and forth when opening and closing the mouth, usually deviating away from the affected side.
- A small amount of loss of range of motion, probably imperceptible.
- Trigger points may cause the nose to run, and patients describe the referred pain as "sinus pain," and can be misdiagnosed with sinusitis.
- Tinnitus (ringing in the ears) in either one or both ears.
- A possible "weird tingling" or numbness in the cheek, caused by entrapment of the buccal nerve.

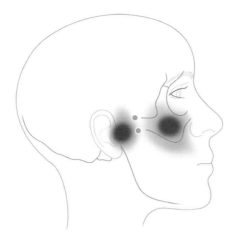

Causes and Perpetuation of Trigger Points, and Solutions

- Teeth grinding or clenching (most likely due to anxiety, stress, and emotional tension), chewing gum, nail biting, playing a wind instrument or violin, or thumb sucking after infancy.

Solutions
- See a counselor, learn relaxation and coping techniques, and otherwise reduce stress to eliminate emotional causes of teeth grinding. See chapter 4 for more information.
- Do not chew gum, and avoid foods that require a lot of prolonged chewing or cracking of hard objects. If you play a wind instrument or violin, do the self-help techniques before and after playing.

- Trigger points in the sternocleidomastoid muscle (10) can cause satellite trigger points in the lateral pterygoid.
- Trigger points can be the cause *or* the result of premature tooth contact, *or* possibly they can be the cause or the result of TMJ degenerative arthritis.

Solutions
- It is wise to first identify and relieve your trigger points before making permanent dental corrections, so work on *all* trigger points in the neck and head first for at least four weeks, including the sternocleidomastoid muscles. See "Temporomandibular Joint Dysfunction" in chapter 7 for more information.

- Inadequate folic acid or B-vitamin intake.

Solutions
- Take a good B-vitamin complex, with folic acid. Evaluate for and treat chronic nutritional deficiencies. See chapter 4 for more information.

- Head-forward posture or an anatomical leg-length inequality or unequal hemipelvis size (either the left or the right half of the pelvic bone).

Solutions
- See chapter 7 for an exercise to correct head-forward posture. Have an evaluation for anatomical leg length and hemipelvis size, and use corrective lifts if necessary.

Self-Help Techniques

Applying Pressure

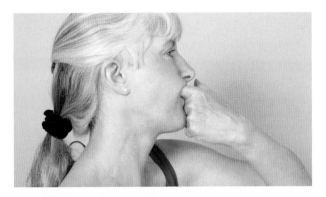

Lateral Pterygoid Pressure

Using the index finger of the same side, place your finger between the cheek and the upper molars, slide it all the way to the back, behind the last molar, and press toward your nose. You will not be able to access the entire muscle, so it may be impossible to entirely eliminate trigger points in this muscle without the assistance of someone trained in trigger point injections specifically in this area, or acupuncture treatments.

Stretches

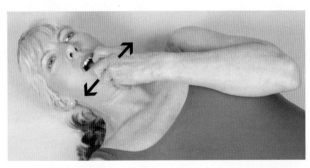

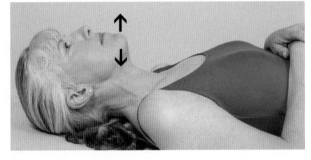

Lateral Pterygoid Stretch

After applying a hot pack to your cheeks, while resting your head against a firm support, relax the jaw and gently push back and rock gently side to side.

Next, increase your range of motion by jutting out the jaw and pulling it back all the way, with no assistance from your fingers.

Then place your index finger on the inside of the lower teeth and the thumb under the jaw, and gently pull down and forward.

Exercises

Tongue Rolls

Tongue rolls help relax the muscles of your mouth (see chapter 7 for this exercise).

Also Check

Medial pterygoid (14). Masseter (13). Sternocleidomastoid (10).

16 Digastric

The posterior belly of the *digastric* muscle attaches to the mastoid process, just behind the earlobe. The anterior belly attaches to the inside of the jawbone (*mandible*) just under the tip of the chin. The two bellies meet at the hyoid bone, or *Adam's apple*, and are attached end to end by a common tendon, and to the hyoid bone via a fibrous loop. The digastric muscles open the mouth when other muscles in the front of the neck stabilize the position of the hyoid bone.

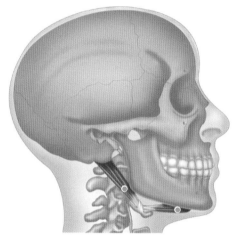

Because trigger points in the posterior digastric can refer to the area around the upper end of the sternocleidomastoid muscle at the mastoid process, it is important to check the digastric muscle if you have inactivated trigger points in the sternocleidomastoid (10) but still have pain in that area.

Common Symptoms

- The part of the muscle closest to the ear, the *posterior digastric*, refers pain and tenderness below the ear and sometimes into the back of the skull.

- The part closer to the front of the jaw, the *anterior digastric*, refers pain to the four front lower teeth and just below those teeth.
- Possibly difficulty swallowing or a sensation of a lump in the throat.

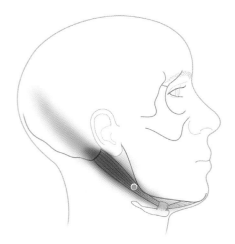
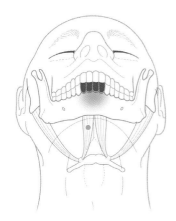

Causes and Perpetuation of Trigger Points, and Solutions

▪ Teeth grinding or jutting out the jaw.

Solutions
▪ See a counselor, learn relaxation and coping techniques, and otherwise reduce stress to eliminate emotional causes of teeth grinding. See chapter 4 for more information.
▪ Do not chew gum or other chewy or hard to chew foods. If you grind or clench your teeth, see chapter 7, "Temporomandibular Joint Dysfunction," for more information.

▪ Trigger points in the masseter (13) or sternocleidomastoid (10) muscles.

Solutions
▪ Because referral from the posterior portion of the digastric is easy to confuse with referral from the sternocleidomastoid muscle, check the sternocleidomastoid first. If trigger points and referred pain are not relieved, check the digastric. Also work on the masseter and temporalis muscles, particularly on the *opposite* side.

▪ Mouth breathing due to mechanical or other problems with the nasal passages.

Solutions
▪ Treat the cause of mouth breathing. Mechanical problems such as nasal polyps or a deviated septum may require surgery. Chronic sinusitis or allergies can be treated with acupuncture, herbs, and homeopathics. Neti pots are helpful and are available at health food stores. Naturopaths use a small inflatable balloon to open up sinus passages. See chapter 4 for information on chronic infections and allergies.

▪ In the space below the earlobe there is a little point of bone that can become calcified and lengthened— this is called *Eagle syndrome*. It can cause problems such as pain, dizziness, and blurred vision on the affected side, especially when the head is turned all the way to the affected side.

Solutions
▪ If you have Eagle syndrome, you will need to get it x-rayed for confirmation and possibly have it surgically removed.

Self-Help Techniques

Applying Pressure

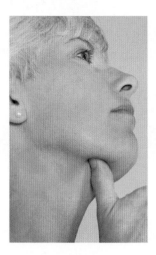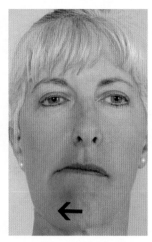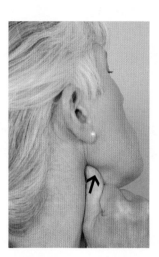

Digastric Pressure
Hook your thumb under the rim of your jaw and push toward the top of your head. Start in the front and work your way back, working around the back angle of your jaw below your earlobe.

Once you get around the angle of your jaw, press toward your nose. It will be easier to treat this portion of the muscle if you deviate your jaw toward the side on which you are working. *Do not push deep into your neck muscles*, particularly in the area below your earlobe, as you can break that little bony point.

Stretches

Mandible Stretch
Perform the mandible stretch found in the masseter muscle chapter (13).

Exercises

Tongue Rolls
Tongue rolls help relax the muscles of your mouth (see chapter 7).

Also Check

Sternocleidomastoid (10). Temporalis (11). Masseter (13).

Differential Diagnosis
Difficulty swallowing, pain when talking, a mysterious sore throat, and head, neck, throat, tongue, and mouth pain may be caused by trigger points in other deep neck muscles such as the stylohyoid, mylohyoid, geniohyoid, omohyoid, thyrohyoid, sternothyroid, longus colli, rectus capitis anterior, rectus capitis lateralis, and longus capitis muscles. You would need to see a practitioner trained in deep anterior neck muscles in order to explore the possibility of trigger points in these muscles.

17 Torso Pain

There are several general self-help stretches that will assist you in treating trigger points in your torso.

Solutions

In-Bathtub Stretch

With your head hanging forward, lean forward and reach your hands down toward your toes, until you are feeling a gentle stretch. Relax and then repeat, moving your hands further down each time, but only as far down as you can feel a gentle stretch. Do this in a hot bath if you can. If you have trigger points in the iliopsoas muscle, even if they are latent, this stretch can cause a reactive cramp, and you will need to work on and stretch the iliopsoas (22) first.

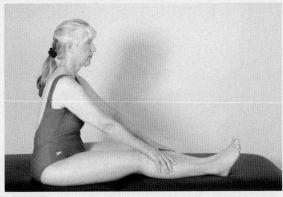
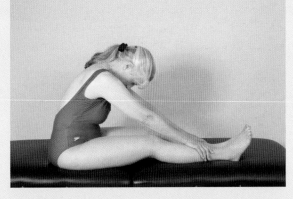
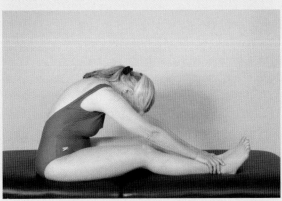
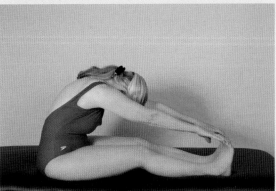

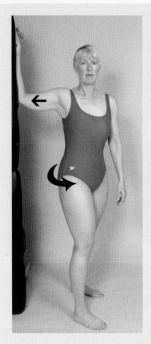 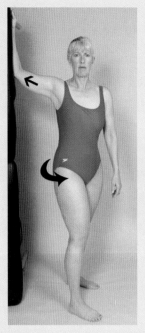 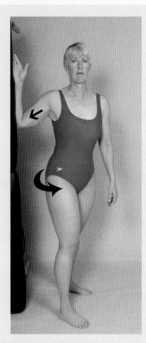

Pectoralis Stretch

The pectoralis stretch will benefit the trapezius muscle. Stand in a doorway and place your forearm along the door frame, including your elbow. With the foot of the same side placed about one step forward, rotate your body gently away from the side you are stretching.

Move your forearm up to about a 45-degree angle and repeat.

Bring the forearm down below the first position and repeat. The different forearm positions will stretch different parts of the muscle.

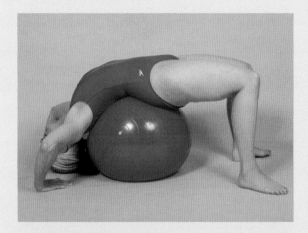

Abdominal Stretch

Use something round such as a large inflatable therapeutic exercise ball (from a chiropractor or physical therapist) or a concrete form tube (from a building supply store). Lie face-up over it with your arms outstretched over your head and touch your palms to the floor. Be careful not to fall over, and do not do this stretch if you are elderly or pregnant. I find the concrete form tube easier to use, since you cannot roll off to the side. You may not be able to perform this stretch if you have back problems.

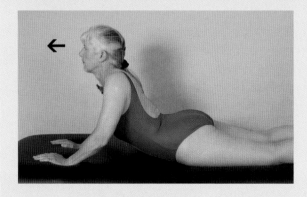

Hip-Extension Stretch

As an alternative to the Abdominal Stretch, lie face-down on a flat surface, such as the floor. Using your arms, push your torso off of the surface with your head looking straight ahead at the wall, but keep your pelvis on the surface. If you can only rest on your elbows, you will still get a stretch. Breathe deeply to expand your abdomen. You may not be able to do this stretch if you have neck or shoulder girdle problems.

Each muscle chapter in this section will contain additional solutions.

18 Thoracolumbar Paraspinal Muscles

Iliocostalis Lumborum, Iliocostalis Thoracis, Longissimus Thoracis, Multifidi

The thoracolumbar paraspinal muscle group includes the *iliocostalis lumborum, iliocostalis thoracis, longissimus thoracis,* and *multifidi*. Part of this muscle group runs the entire length of the spine, and some of the muscles run most of the length of the spine. Yet others (multifidi) are small muscles that attach one vertebra to the next.

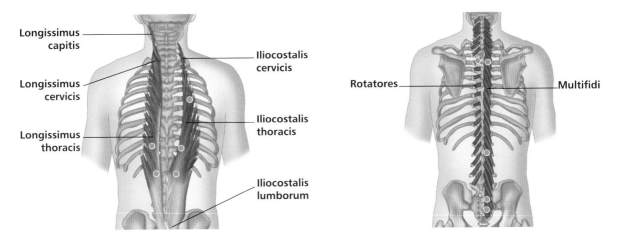

The paraspinal muscles allow you to stand up straight from a bending position, assist in rotating your trunk, and provide stability.

Common Symptoms

- See the pictures for all the pain referral patterns. Please note that these pictures show common trigger points, *but trigger points can develop at any level and cause similar referral patterns at any level.* Also note that in many cases the pain can refer to the front side of the body, causing you or your practitioner to think you are having organ problems, particularly with the heart. Trigger points in these muscles are an often-overlooked cause of gluteal area pain.
- Deep, aching pain that feels like it is in the spine.
- Pain that may increase with coughing, or straining to have a bowel movement.

- Stiffness in the spine, mostly from longissimus thoracis trigger points.
- Restricted range of motion or restricted rotation of the trunk, possibly severe.
- Possibly difficulty climbing stairs or getting out of a chair.
- Possibly nausea, belching, and gastrointestinal pain and cramping.
- Entrapment of spinal nerves can cause increased or decreased sensitivity and/or uncomfortable sensations on the skin of the back.

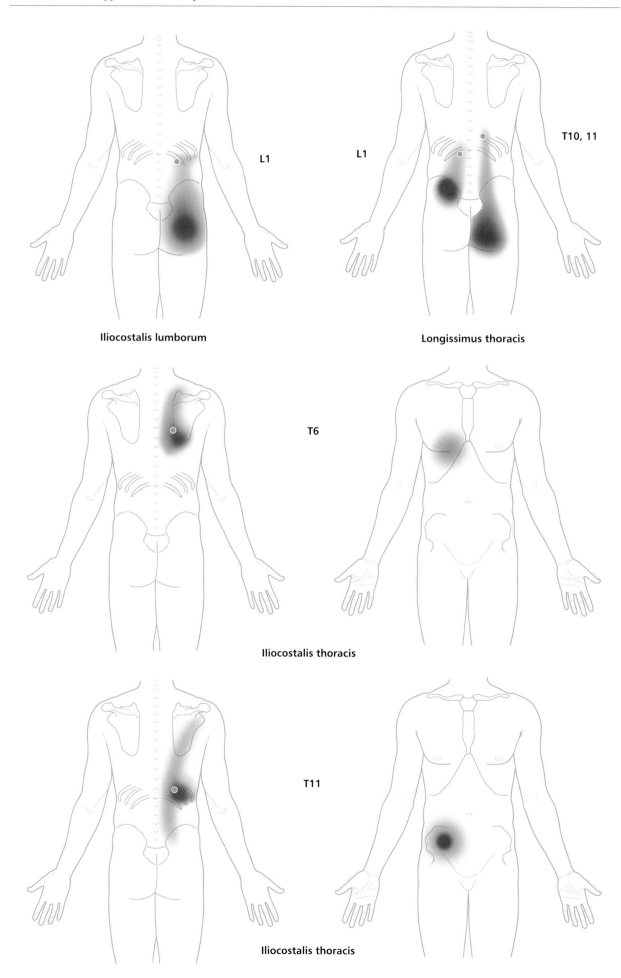

L1

L1

T10, 11

Iliocostalis lumborum

Longissimus thoracis

T6

Iliocostalis thoracis

T11

Iliocostalis thoracis

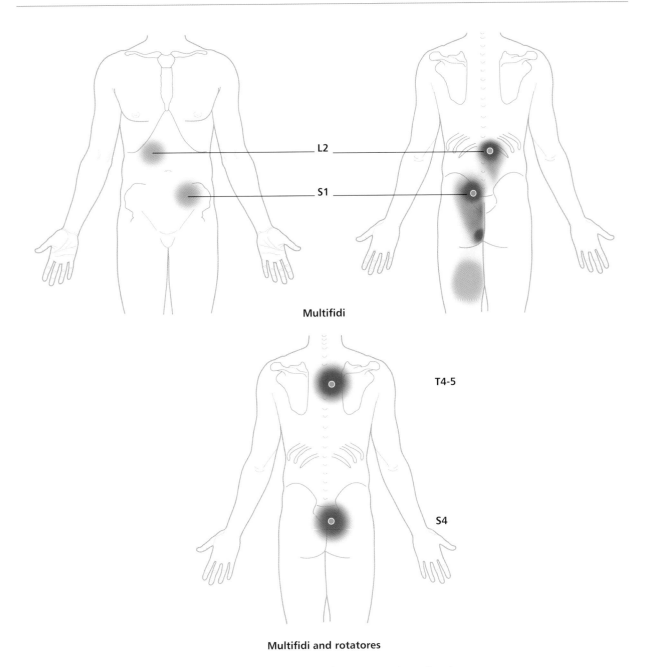

Multifidi

Multifidi and rotatores

Causes and Perpetuation of Trigger Points, and Solutions

■ A sudden overload, often when bending, lifting, and twisting at the same time (people frequently say they were moving boxes), or catching yourself from falling, such as when slipping on ice. Injury is more likely when the muscles are chilled or fatigued.

Solutions

■ Lift properly by bending your knees rather than your back, and hold objects close to your body. When climbing stairs or a ladder, rotate your entire body 45 degrees and keep your back straight. Be sure to keep your trunk warm, especially if you are working in cold weather.

■ If you have difficulty getting up, roll over onto your hands and knees and crawl to where you can grab onto something and pull yourself up. When standing up from a chair, slide your butt to the front of the chair, turn your entire body a little sideways, put one foot under the front edge of the chair, then stand with the torso erect so that your thighs take the load. You can use your hands to assist you if necessary. Sit down in the opposite sequence.

■ Poor posture such as head-forward posture, sitting on a wallet in your back pocket, bending over while gardening, or sitting for long periods without moving can aggravate trigger points in as little as half an hour or less for some people.

Solutions

■ Restoration of proper posture, especially head positioning, is critical to treating trigger points since head-forward posture can both cause *and* perpetuate trigger points (see chapter 7). See "Ergonomics" and "Body Mechanics" in chapter 2 for more information.

■ Mattresses that are too old or too soft, or sleeping next to someone who is heavier and trying to avoid rolling into them.

Solutions

■ See chapter 2, "Bedtime Furniture."

■ A tight belt or bra strap.

Solutions

■ See chapter 2, "Clothing."

■ Car accidents, especially with a whiplash injury.
■ Trigger points in the latissimus dorsi (38).

Solutions

■ If you have had a car accident, be sure to treat the posterior neck (9), sternocleidomastoid (10), and scalene (42) muscles. Check the latissimus dorsi (38).

■ Structural problems, such as one leg anatomically shorter than the other, or an unequal hemipelvis size (either the left or the right half of the pelvic bone).

Solutions

■ If you have a body asymmetry or an anatomically shorter leg, see a specialist to get compensating lifts or pads.

Self-Help Techniques

Also check the latissimus dorsi (38), quadratus lumborum (28), serratus posterior inferior (21), serratus posterior superior (36), and iliopsoas (22), since these muscles often contain related trigger points.

Applying Pressure

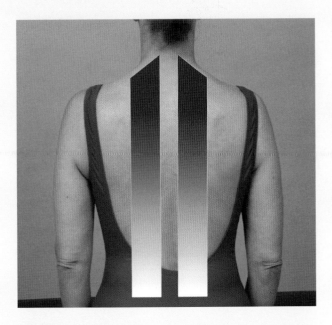

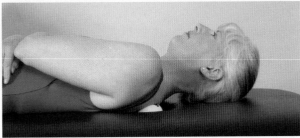

Thoracolumbar Paraspinal / Trapezius Pressure
The shading on the picture marks the area you will want to work on.

Lie face-up on a firm bed or the floor, with your knees bent. Using a tennis ball or racquet ball, start at the shoulder, about one inch out to the side of the spine, and hold pressure for eight seconds to one minute per spot. Shift a small amount to the next spot further down the back by using your legs to move your body over the ball, and continue to hold pressure on each spot. Continue working down all the way to the top of the pelvis in order to treat both the trapezius and the paraspinal muscles (the "back strap" muscles). You may want to repeat this on a second line further out from the spine, especially if you have a wide back or if you have tender points further out. *Do not do this directly on the spine!* I recommend using one ball at a time, rather than using a ball on each side at the same time. By performing this technique lying down, as opposed to standing and leaning into the wall, you keep the muscles as passive as possible, so that you are not using them to hold you upright while you are applying pressure.

If you are at work and unable to lie on the floor, I recommend using a Backnobber® from Pressure Positive Company (see chapter 8).

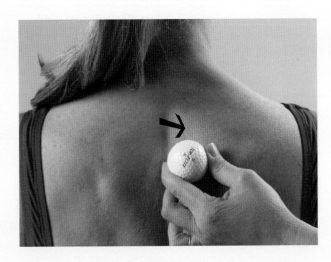

Longissimus Thoracis Pressure
To work on the longissimus thoracis, which is very close to the spine, you will need to lie on a hard floor and use a golf ball. Place the golf ball *in between* your spine and the muscle (not *on* the spine—see photograph), and then move your body just a little *away* from the side you are working on. This presses on the muscles at a 45-degree angle, the only really effective way to get this muscle. Do this from the bottom of the neck, down to the top of the pelvis. As a neuromuscular therapist, I perform this treatment by standing on the opposite side and leaning across, pressing the muscle out at a 45-degree angle.

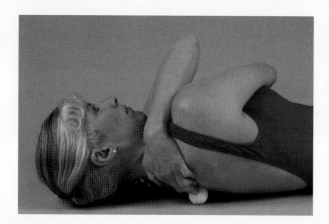
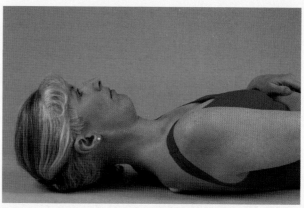

Multifidi Pressure

To treat the multifidi (the little muscles that attach one vertebra to the next), you will need the assistance of another person, as even a golf ball is too large. They will need a tool, such as a rubber-tipped wooden dowel (available at a massage supply store), or an eraser that is rounded off. Working next to the spinous process (the pointy part of the vertebra), massage in the groove next to it. Your assistant may be able to use their thumb, but a gadget works better and is easier on the person administering the treatment.

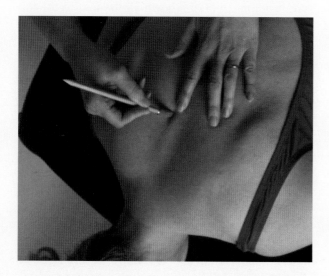

Posterior Neck Pressure
See chapter 9.

Stretches

In-Bathtub Stretch
See chapter 17.

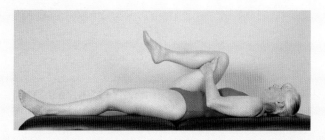

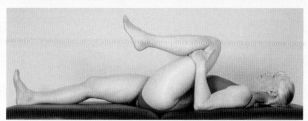

Low Back Stretching Exercise
Lying on your back, with your hands clasped *behind* one knee, gently bring that knee toward your chest until you are just feeling the stretch. Repeat with the opposite knee and then both legs at the same time.

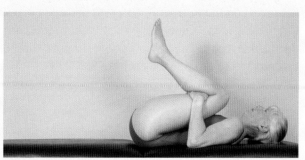

Also Check

Latissimus dorsi (38). Quadratus lumborum (28). Serratus posterior inferior (21). Serratus posterior superior (36). Iliopsoas (22).

Differential Diagnosis
If you are experiencing pain in the spine, you will need to see a health care provider to rule out herniated discs, spinal stenosis (narrowing of the hole the spinal cord goes through, or of one of the holes the nerves go out through), infections, tumors, cancer, or other more serious problems. Other diagnoses that should be considered are fibromyalgia, organ disease, osteoarthritis, fat lobules, strain of spinal ligaments, retrocecal appendicitis, a dissecting aortic aneurysm or saddle thrombus, kidney stones, torsion of the kidney, pelvic inflammatory disease, endometriosis, ankylosing spondylitis, Paget's disease, leukemia, Hodgkin's disease, prostatitis and seminal vesiculitis, or sacroiliitis. A finding of osteoarthritis in itself may not account for the pain felt, since you can have pain without degenerative changes to the spine, and you can have degenerative changes without pain. Lumbar zygapophysial (facet) joints may refer pain in the same pattern as multifidi muscles.

Vertebrae may be out of alignment and need to be adjusted by a chiropractor or osteopathic physician. Combining acupuncture or massage with adjustments is more helpful, since tight muscles will keep pulling vertebra out of alignment.

19

Levator Scapula

The *levator scapula* muscle attaches to vertebrae C1 to C4 on one end, and to the corner of the shoulder blade (*scapula*) on the other end. It moves the scapula up and down over the rib cage, and also assists in rotation of the neck to the same side. When both muscles are used together, they help control the neck when bending the head forward. This muscle very commonly harbors trigger points, and people will often report a stiff neck and an inability to rotate their head.

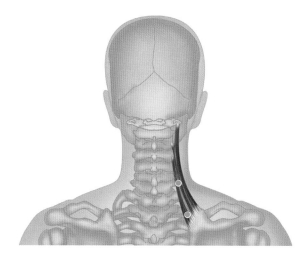

Common Symptoms

- Pain referred to the intersection of the neck and shoulders and down the mid back, and possibly out over the shoulder joint.

- Pain is more common with movement, but it can also be painful without movement.
- Limited rotation of the head, so you have to turn your whole body to look behind you.

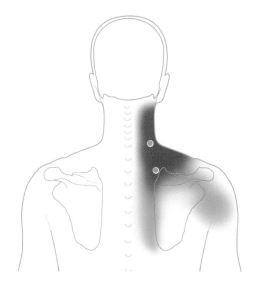

Causes and Perpetuation of Trigger Points, and Solutions

- Poor posture such as sitting for long periods of time with your head rotated to one side, as when using a computer screen at the wrong angle or with the copy to the side, or when talking to a person sitting next to you. Cradling the phone between your shoulder and ear (even with a shoulder cradle), or carrying a purse or pack over one shoulder. Sleeping with your head at an angle when sitting up, tilted with a pillow that is too tall, or tilted on a couch arm, especially when the muscle is fatigued or exposed to a cold draft.
- Raising your shoulders toward your head in response to stress, which you may not even realize you are doing.
- Poor ergonomics such as sitting in a chair with armrests that are too high or walking with a cane that is too long.

Solutions

- Turn your body or furniture to face the person to whom you are speaking. When reading, try to position the music or book at eye level and make sure your vision does not need correction. See chapter 2, "Ergonomics" and "Body Mechanics."
- Do not sleep sitting up or on the couch or on an airplane, unless you have head support that will keep the neck as straight as possible. Your pillow should be of a height that will keep your spine straight. Chiropractor offices often sell well-designed pillows with cervical support.
- Notice if you are raising your shoulders toward you head and relax them. Keep noticing and relaxing, as you will need to retrain yourself to keep your shoulders relaxed. Deal with the source of tension, using acupuncture, herbs, homeopathics, and/or counseling. See chapter 4.
- Apply a heating pad or hot pack to your neck, especially at the end of the day. Keep cold drafts off of your neck by using a scarf or neck gaiter.

- Swimming using the crawl stroke.

Solutions

- When swimming, either vary your stroke or use a snorkel if doing the crawl stroke.

- The initial onset of a cold, flu, or cold sores (oral herpes simplex) can activate levator scapula trigger points, even before other viral symptoms become apparent.

Solutions

- At the onset of a cold or flu, an acupuncturist will perform cupping or Gua Sha, which will relax the shoulder muscles and help get rid of the achiness. See page 34 "Acute Infections" in chapter 4 for suggestions on how to minimize the symptoms of acute infections.

- Injury from car accidents.
- Trigger points in the serratus anterior (26) or upper portion of the trapezius (8).
- Structural imbalances in the lower body such as calf muscle weakness, one leg anatomically shorter than the other, a flattened arch, or a shortened quadratus lumborum muscle (28).

Solutions

- Work on all the muscles in the "Also Check" list below. Check all of the muscles in chapters 8 to 16 if you have been in a car accident or suffered any kind of whiplash injury. Check the quadratus lumborum muscle in chapter 28. If your calves are tight, see chapters 58 and 59. If your calves are weak, you will need to do conditioning exercises, which are not included in this book. See a trainer or physical therapist for assistance in learning how to condition properly. If you have a body asymmetry, see a specialist to get compensating lifts or pads. Consider buying foot bed orthotics if you have a flattened arch.

Self-Help Techniques

Applying Pressure

Posterior Neck Pressure
The posterior neck pressure will also benefit levator scapula trigger points (see chapter 9).

Stretches

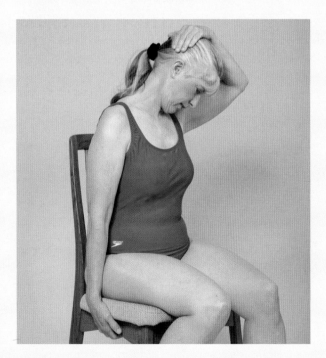

Levator Scapula Stretch
Sit on a chair or stool and hook the fingers of one hand around the edge of the seat bottom. Use your other hand to pull your head down to about a 45-degree angle, or until you feel a gentle stretch; just be sure to feel the stretch on the back of your neck. You may also do this stretch under a hot shower while seated on a stool.

Also Check

Posterior neck muscles (9). Scalene muscles (42). Serratus anterior (26). Trapezius (8, upper portion).

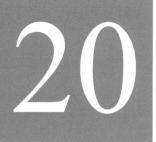

20 Rhomboid

The *rhomboid* muscle attaches to the spine (C7 to T5) and to the middle edge of the shoulder blade (*scapula*). It stabilizes the scapula and moves it toward the spine, with some rotation.

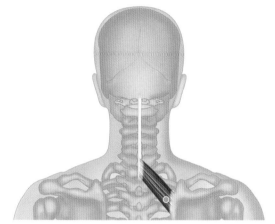

Rhomboid minor

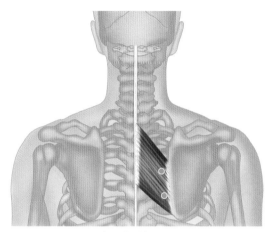

Rhomboid major

Most of the time, trigger points are formed in the rhomboid muscles due to tight pectoralis major and/or pectoralis minor muscles. Even though you may not be experiencing the referral patterns of the "pecs," there may be tightness and/or latent trigger points in those muscles that are pulling on the rhomboids. I often find that physical therapists and chiropractors want to focus on strengthening the rhomboids, rather than eliminating trigger points and tightness in the pectoralis muscles. When working on yourself, it is important to check and work on the pectoralis muscles first, followed by the rhomboids.

Common Symptoms

- Pain is usually fairly localized in the mid back, close to the scapula, and often feels fairly superficial and achy, and pain may also spread over the top edge of the shoulder blade.
- Symptoms may be aggravated by lying on the same side, or by reaching forward or stretching to reach for something.

- Snapping and crunching noises during movement of the shoulder blade may be due to trigger points in the rhomboid muscle.
- Often the shoulder will appear rounded forward, indicative of pectoralis major and/or pectoralis minor involvement.

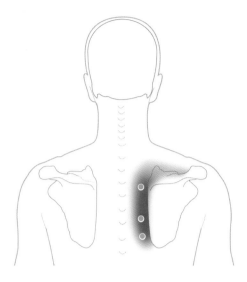

Causes and Perpetuation of Trigger Points, and Solutions

■ Poor posture, such as leaning forward with the shoulders rounded forward for long periods of time (e.g. sewing), or holding your arms out for a long time, such as when painting a ceiling.

Solutions
■ See chapter 2, "Ergonomics" and "Body Mechanics."

■ Tightness or trigger points in the pectoralis major and/or pectoralis minor muscles.

Solutions
■ See chapters 23 and 43 to work on those muscles.

■ Chronic discouragement and/or sadness may cause you to slump your shoulders forward and breathe improperly.

Solutions
■ Learn to breathe properly again (see chapter 7). If you are suffering from depression, discouragement, or sadness, see chapter 4.

■ Structural problems, such as upper thoracic scoliosis (curvature of the spine in the mid to upper back area).

Solutions
■ Some scoliosis will be corrected with the trigger point pressure self-treatment. See page 30, "Spinal and Skeletal Factors," for more information. If you have an anatomically shorter leg or a small hemipelvis (either the left or the right half of the pelvic bone), be sure to see a specialist to get compensating lifts and pads.

Self-Help Techniques

Check the pectoralis major (23) and pectoralis minor (43) muscles for any needed self-treatment, and do that first. Be sure to also check the levator scapula (19), trapezius (8), scalene (42), latissimus dorsi (38), and infraspinatus (35) muscles, since these can also cause symptoms in the same area. Trigger points in the rhomboids will likely only be noticeable when trigger points in these other muscles are inactivated.

Applying Pressure

Rhomboid Pressure
Use a tennis ball or racquet ball. Lie face-up, and hold your arm across your chest to pull the scapula out of the way and access the trigger points along the edge of the scapula. Then, while leaning over onto the ball with however much pressure you want to apply, work from the top edge of the scapula to the bottom. It is just easier to work in this direction, but not critical. It is also easier to move from spot to spot if your legs are bent, and

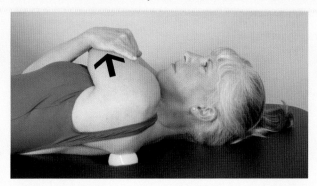

you shift yourself to the next spot by using your legs to slide your body over the ball, rather than moving the ball with your hand. As you lean onto the ball, be sure not to let your arm drop back down, as this closes up the space next to your shoulder blade, and you will miss some of the worst spots. Patients will often sense they "just cannot seem to get to the main spot," so if you think you might be missing the rhomboid muscle, check your arm positioning and make sure the ball is close to the edge of the scapula.

Stretches

Trapezius Stretch
See chapter 8 for a stretch that benefits the middle and lower trapezius, which will also help treat the rhomboid muscles.

Pectoralis Stretch
See chapter 17 for a stretch that relaxes the pectoralis muscles, which will also benefit the rhomboids.

Also Check

Pectoralis major (23). Pectoralis minor (43). Levator scapula (19). Trapezius (8). Infraspinatus (35).

Differential Diagnosis
If you have received a diagnosis of scapulocostal syndrome, be sure to check for trigger points in the rhomboid muscle. You may need to see a chiropractor or osteopathic physician for vertebral misalignments from C7 to T5.

21 Serratus Posterior Inferior

The *serratus posterior inferior* muscle attaches toward the midline of the body to connective tissue coming from T11 to L2, and to the bottom four ribs (nine through twelve) further out toward the side where the rib cage starts to curve toward the front. Though some literature says its function is to assist in breathing, Travell and Simons (1999) report that a study documenting electrical activity during use showed that this is not the case. They surmise that it assists in trunk rotation and bending forward at the waist.

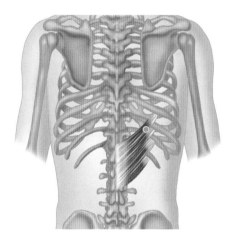

Usually you will not feel symptoms from trigger points in this muscle alone, since activation is usually because of some kind of back strain. If you have pain remaining in this area after treating the other involved muscles (likely the thoracolumbar paraspinals), be sure to check this muscle just in case you missed it with the thoracolumbar paraspinal muscle self-treatment (18).

Common Symptoms

- Nagging, achy pain over and around the muscle which is on the back of the trunk, near the bottom of the rib cage, and occasionally the pain will feel like it is going through the trunk to the front.

- Restricted rotation of the trunk.

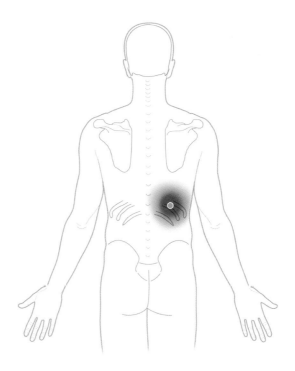

Causes and Perpetuation of Trigger Points, and Solutions

■ Straining the back while lifting, twisting, and reaching, or by working overhead.

Solutions
■ Lift properly by bending your knees rather than your back, and hold objects close to your body. If you must work overhead, take frequent breaks.

■ Use a lumbar support wherever you are sitting. Buy a firm mattress and replace it every five to seven years. Modify or replace your misfitting furniture. See chapter 2, "Ergonomics" and "Body Mechanics."
■ Improper breathing techniques, or coughing from an acute or chronic illness.

Solutions
■ Learn proper breathing techniques (see chapter 7). If you are suffering from a chronic cough, see chapter 4.

■ One leg anatomically shorter than the other.

Solutions
■ See a specialist to correct any body asymmetries, such as an anatomically shorter leg or small hemipelvis (either the left or the right half of the pelvic bone).

Self-Help Techniques

Be sure to check the thoracolumbar paraspinal muscles, particularly the iliocostalis thoracis and longissimus thoracis (18).

Applying Pressure

Serratus Posterior Inferior Pressure
If you have already worked on the thoracolumbar paraspinal muscles you have probably already treated this muscle, but be sure you work out toward the side, almost to where the ribs start to curve around to the front.

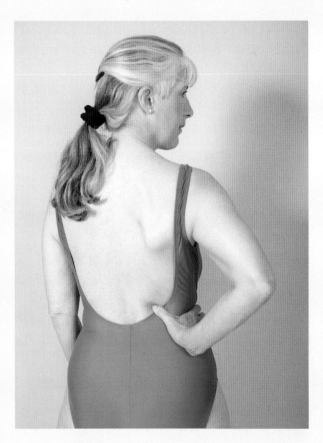 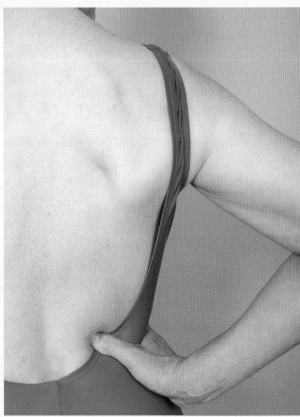

Also Check

Thoracolumbar paraspinal muscles (18).

Differential Diagnosis
If you are unable to relieve your symptoms with trigger point self-help techniques, you may need to see a health care provider to rule out diseases of the kidney, such as caliectasis, pyelonephritis, or ureteral reflux, or a lower thoracic nerve root irritation. You may need to see a chiropractor or osteopathic physician to be evaluated for T10 to L2 vertebral misalignments, or the last four ribs out of alignment.

22 Iliopsoas

The *iliopsoas* consists of two muscles that are joined together: the *iliacus* and the *psoas*. The psoas attaches above to the fronts of the T12 to L5 vertebrae and to all the discs in between the vertebrae; it is positioned adjacent to and forward of the quadratus lumborum muscle (28), which attaches to the back side of the vertebrae. Inside the pelvis, the psoas joins the iliacus muscle, where it mostly becomes a tendon, crosses the hip joint, and attaches to the femur bone in the thigh. The *psoas minor*, present in only about 50% of humans, does not cross the hip joint. The iliacus muscle lines the wall of most of the pelvis, also crosses the hip joint, and attaches to the femur. These muscles primarily allow you to bend at the hip or bring the thigh toward the trunk, and help to maintain an upright posture.

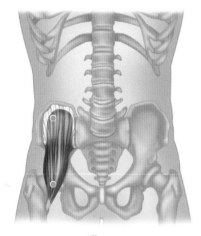

Iliacus

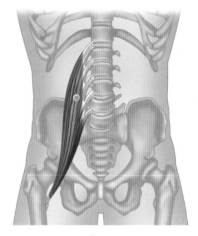

Psoas

Trigger points are very common, but without knowledge of trigger point referrals, a health care provider could easily misdiagnose lumbar pain and attribute it to another cause. Pain unresolved by surgery may be caused by trigger points in the iliopsoas *or* the quadratus lumborum muscles.

Common Symptoms

■ The psoas primarily refers pain to the back of the body, in the lumbar region close to the spine and perhaps a little lower. The iliacus refers pain to the front of the thigh and groin. If both right *and* left iliopsoas muscles are affected, then pain may feel more like it is running *across* the lumbar area, rather than *vertically*, similar to a quadratus lumborum trigger point pain referral distribution.

■ Pain is worse when standing, but may still be felt as a slight nagging backache when sitting or reclining, and may be aggravated by constipation. The most comfortable lying positions are on the side with the knees drawn up, or face-up with the knees bent. You may be unable to straighten up enough to stand erect, unable to do sit-ups, or have difficulty standing up from a seated position.

■ In teenage girls, if the growth of this muscle does not keep pace with the growth of the pelvis, it can cause appendicitis-like symptoms. Pain can occur on either side, but the girl would likely only be evaluated for appendicitis if the pain was right-sided. The iliopsoas may also be susceptible to easy bruising, even with minor injuries.

■ If you are taking anticoagulant drugs, the iliopsoas may be particularly susceptible to hematomas (bruising) and can cause pain, swelling, and difficulty walking. Hematomas can also cause problems with the femoral nerve, which can be diagnosed by ultrasound.

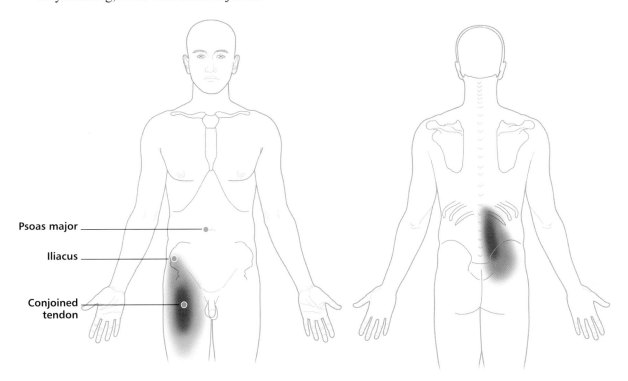

Psoas major

Iliacus

Conjoined tendon

Posterior referred pain distribution

Causes and Perpetuation of Trigger Points, and Solutions

■ Poor posture such as sitting for long periods of time with the knees at an angle of less than 90 degrees (knees higher than the hips), for example in a car or sleeping in the fetal position.

Solutions
■ When sitting, increase the angle between your thighs and trunk by leaning back against a slightly reclined backrest. If you must sit for long periods of time, stand up frequently to stretch. If you are unable to stand, you may be able to crawl on your hands and knees until you are able to treat the muscles.

■ Sleep with a pillow under your knees. Avoid sleeping curled up tightly in the fetal position. Buy a firm mattress and replace it every five to seven years. You can put plywood between the box springs and the mattress to make the surface firmer. See chapter 2.

■ Vertebrae out of alignment in the T10 to L1 area for the psoas portion, or L5 vertebra out of alignment for the iliacus portion.

Solutions

■ Misalignments in the lumbar vertebrae and sacroiliac joint (the joint where the sacrum and big pelvic bone meet) can prevent successful treatment of the iliopsoas muscles. See an osteopathic doctor or chiropractor. For more information, see chapter 4.

■ Trauma to the muscles, such as from pregnancy, sit-ups, or a fall or other sudden overload.
■ Tightness of the rectus femoris.

Solutions

■ Apply moist heat over the abdomen and upper third of the thigh. Do not do sit-ups. Learn to breathe properly (see chapter 7).
■ See the quadriceps femoris muscle group (65) to treat the rectus femoris. Check the quadratus lumborum muscle (28), since the iliopsoas is rarely involved by itself.

■ Painful menses.

Solutions

■ See an acupuncturist or naturopathic doctor, to treat the cause of painful menses. You may need to see an allopathic health care provider first to rule out serious conditions that require diagnostic tests and surgery.

■ Structural problems such as an anatomically shorter leg or small hemipelvis (either the left or the right half of the pelvic bone).

Solutions

■ See a specialist to be fitted for compensating lifts and pads if you have one leg anatomically shorter than the other, or a small hemipelvis.

Self-Help Techniques

The iliopsoas may be providing "splinting" for other muscles (protecting other weak muscles by contracting), and if this is removed by the iliopsoas being relaxed, it may cause increased tightness and pain from the other muscles. All of the following muscles may need to be checked and treated first *before* treating the iliopsoas, or you may experience soreness and an increase in symptoms.

Check the hamstrings muscle group (56), since shortening of these muscles causes an unnatural tilt to the pelvis that overloads the iliopsoas muscles. Doctors Travell and Simons felt that treating the hamstrings prior to treating the iliopsoas was very important. Also check the gluteus minimus (62), gluteus medius (31), gluteus maximus (30), thoracolumbar paraspinal muscles (18), and posterior neck muscles (9), since trigger points in the iliopsoas can cause and perpetuate trigger points in those other areas.

Applying Pressure

Iliopsoas Pressure

Because these muscles are so deep, it is difficult to access them completely to apply pressure to trigger points. You will not be able to look at what you are doing at the same time as you are applying pressure, since that will cause the muscle you are trying to work on to contract, so you will have to do it by feeling with your fingers. The iliopsoas self-treatment will be difficult if you have long fingernails.

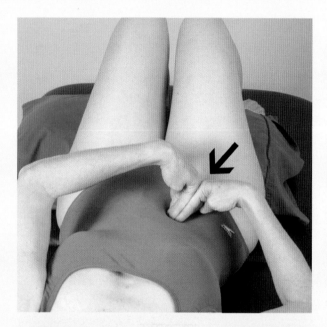 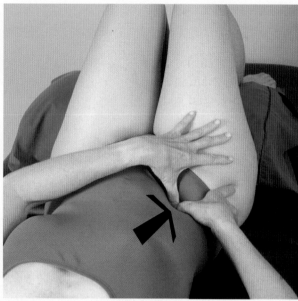

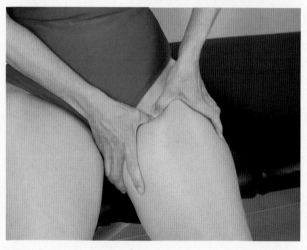

There are three parts of the muscle to test for tenderness and work on. Lie face-up, with something under your knees. Starting four-fingers' width away from the belly button, with your fingers back to back and the knuckles together, first press straight toward your back, then start angling in toward your spine. The position of the fingers and knuckles is very important in being able to apply sufficient pressure. Also do the same technique just above and below your belly button.

Next, hook your thumbs into the front of your pelvis, searching around the rim.

Last, check the front of your thigh, which is a little easier to reach by sitting up with your back supported to take tension off the muscle. This point is a little below the groin and about one third of the way out from the pubic area. This point is difficult to find if it is not tight and tender, but when it *is* part of the problem, a little searching will generally locate it quickly. Be sure not to press too hard in this last area, since there are major nerves and arteries located here.

Stretches

Do not overstretch if you do the In-Bathtub stretch (chapter 17). If you stretch by reaching toward your toes, do not overstretch by forcing it, or you can severely aggravate iliopsoas trigger points.

Abdominal Stretch
See chapter 17.

Hip-Extension Stretch
See chapter 17.

Thigh-Hip Extension Stretch
Grab onto something for support, place one leg stretched out well behind you, and bend the other leg at the knee. Gently extend your pelvis forward.

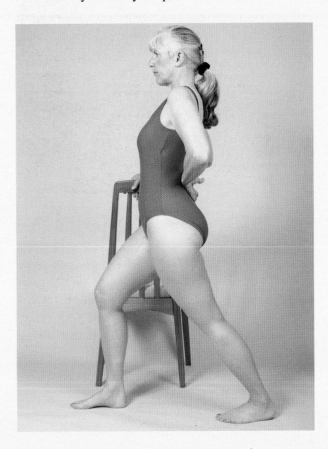 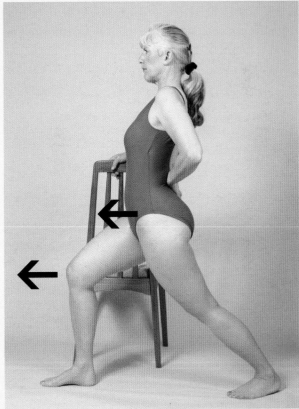

Also Check

For lumbar pain
Quadratus lumborum (28). Abdominal muscles (25, lower portion of rectus abdominis). Thoracolumbar paraspinal muscles (18, longissimus thoracis and multifidi). Gluteus maximus (30). Gluteus medius (31).

For front of the thigh and groin pain
Tensor fascia latae (63). Pectineus (68). Adductor muscles of the hip (67, adductors brevis, longus, and magnus). Quadriceps femoris muscle group (65, rectus femoris, vastus intermedius).

23 Pectoralis Major and Subclavius

The *pectoralis major* muscle covers much of the chest, attaching to the breastbone (*sternum*), to the collarbone (*clavicle*), to most of the ribs, and to the bone in the upper arm (*humerus*). It moves your upper arm and the shoulder girdle, and assists in forced inhalation (as opposed to breathing that you do not have to think about). Tightness can cause your shoulders to be rounded forward in a slumped-looking posture.

Pectoralis major trigger points can mimic the symptoms of a heart attack, but can also be *caused* by a heart attack, so heart and lung problems *must* be ruled out by a health care provider before assuming it is only pain from trigger points. See below for more information.

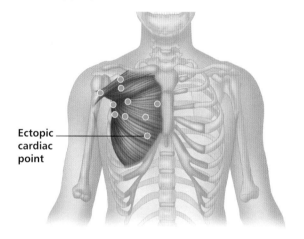

Ectopic cardiac point

Pectoralis major

Subclavius

The *subclavius* muscle lies beneath the clavicle but over the first rib, attaching at the juncture of the first rib and the sternum, and to the clavicle itself. It helps move the shoulder.

Common Symptoms

Pectoralis Major
- Pain referred into the chest, shoulder, breast, and down the inner arm, possibly all the way into the hand. Pain may be severe enough to disturb sleep. Shortening of the pectoralis muscles may cause mid back pain, even if the pectoralis trigger points are latent and not causing referred pain of their own.
- Restricted range of motion and/or chest constriction. The pectoralis major may be involved in a frozen shoulder syndrome. See the subscapularis muscle (37) for a discussion of that condition.

- Breast tenderness, hypersensitivity of the nipple, and/or irritation by clothing on the breast. There may be a feeling of congestion in the breast, a slight enlargement, and a "doughy" feeling caused by impaired lymph drainage.
- Ectopic cardiac arrhythmias such as supraventricular tachycardia, supraventricular premature contractions, or ventricular premature contractions, which are caused by a particular point on the right side of the trunk only, between the fifth and sixth rib, about one to two inches to the left of the nipple.

Subclavius

■ The subclavius can cause pain under the collarbone, down the front upper arm, down the outside of the lower arm, and into the thumb, index, and middle fingers.

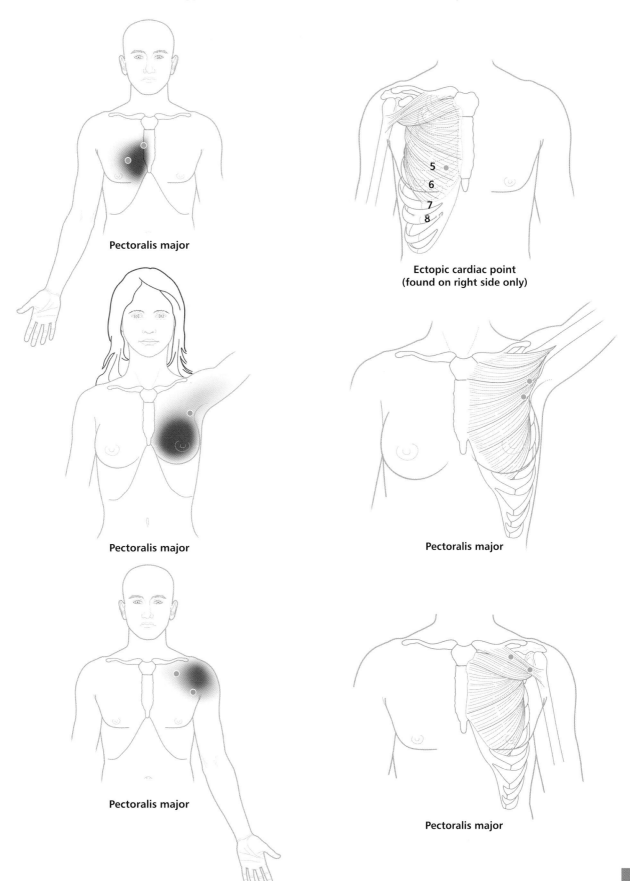

Pectoralis major

Ectopic cardiac point
(found on right side only)

Pectoralis major

Pectoralis major

Pectoralis major

Pectoralis major

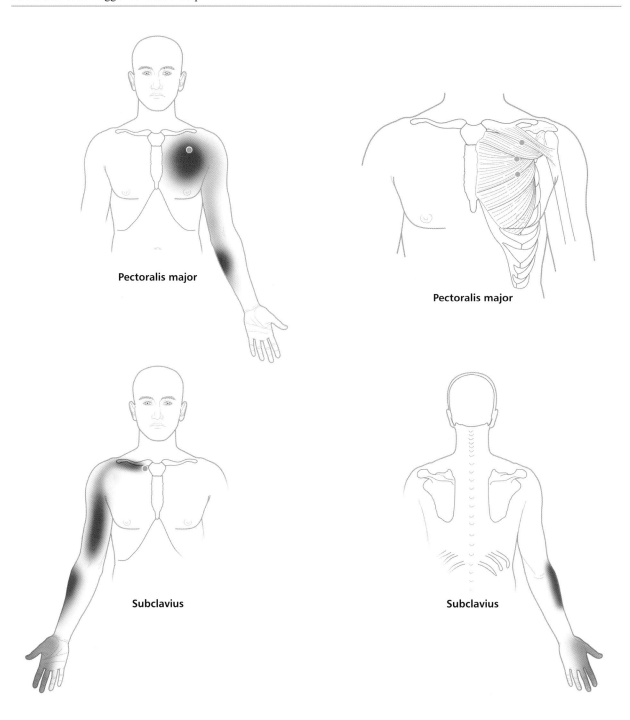

Pectoralis major

Pectoralis major

Subclavius

Subclavius

Causes and Perpetuation of Trigger Points, and Solutions

- Poor posture while sitting, or slouching while standing, allowing your shoulders to round forward.
- Heavy lifting, especially when reaching out, as with a chainsaw. Overuse of the arms where you bring them together repetitively, as in using a pair of bush clippers.
- Exposure to cold air when the muscles are fatigued.
- Immobilization of your arm in a cast or sling.

Solutions

- Get a good pair of custom orthotics that will redistribute your weight slightly to the balls of your feet. This will shift your head back over your shoulders and restore normal cervical and lumbar curves, bring the shoulders back, and open up the chest. See chapter 2, "Footwear."
- Crossing your arms in front of you shortens the pectoralis major muscle, so try to use armrests at the height of your elbows. Get a chair with a good lumbar support. For your car or any seat that does not have adequate lumbar support, use a portable lumbar support. See chapter 2, "Ergonomics," for more information.
- If you must perform work that requires you to lift or hold tools in front of you, take frequent breaks or avoid the activity altogether. Keep your trunk and shoulders warm.
- When lying on your unaffected side, drape your arm over a pillow. When lying on the affected side, tuck a pillow between your arm and chest/belly to keep the arm out at a 90-degree angle.
- If your bras leave indentations on the skin, they are too tight and need to be replaced. See chapter 2, "Clothing."
- If you are in a cast or sling, depending on where the injury is, you may be able to have a practitioner work on this area. Once you are out of the cast or sling, start doing self-help techniques to the extent you are able without causing pain.

- Constant anxiety will probably cause you to hold your breath, and subsequently initiate the formation of trigger points.

Solutions

- See chapter 4 to address emotional factors. See chapter 7 to learn how to breathe properly.

- A heart attack, or open heart surgery where the incision was through the breastbone rather than through the ribs.

Solutions

- Active trigger points in the pectoralis major may cause pain and a feeling of chest constriction that mimics angina. Chest pain is likely to be intermittent and intense when moving the upper arm, and there may also possibly be pain at rest if the trigger points are very active. Pain can disturb sleep. Remember that angina and trigger points can exist concurrently, *so you will still need to undergo cardiac function tests even if you are able to relieve pain with trigger point self-help techniques.* Non-cardiac pain may induce transient T-wave changes in the electrocardiogram, so further tests may be needed. Even with heart disease, pain from trigger points may reflexively diminish the size of the coronary arteries, thereby further increasing myocardial ischemia, so relief of trigger points can increase cardiac circulation as well as relieving discomfort.
- Shortening of the subclavius muscle by trigger points can contribute to vascular thoracic outlet syndrome by causing the clavicle to compress the subclavian artery and vein against the first rib.

Self-Help Techniques

You may also need to work on the anterior deltoid (44), coracobrachialis (45), sternalis (24), sternocleidomastoid (10), scalene (42), trapezius (8), rhomboid (20), and serratus anterior (26) muscles, since they will tend to develop satellite trigger points. The trapezius and rhomboid muscles may become painful after relieving the pectoralis major, so you will probably need to perform self-treatment on them after the pectoralis major muscle.

If you have a frozen shoulder from pectoralis muscle involvement, you may also need to work on the subscapularis (37), infraspinatus (35), teres minor (39), and posterior deltoid (44) muscles. If you have been diagnosed with thoracic outlet syndrome, also check the latissimus dorsi (38), teres major (40), scalene (42), and subscapularis (37) muscles, since trigger points there may mimic thoracic outlet syndrome.

Applying Pressure

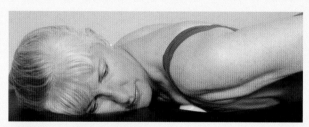

Pectoralis Pressure
Lie face-down with the arm on the side you are treating next to your side. Place a ball above the breast area and be sure to work all the way out to the armpit. You may need to shift your weight a little to the side you are working on as you work out toward the armpit. You may also try hanging your arm over the side of the bed, if it is high enough to allow your arm to dangle. If you are large-breasted, you may find it easier to place the ball on the end of a couch arm or wall and lean into it, but be sure to keep your arm relaxed.

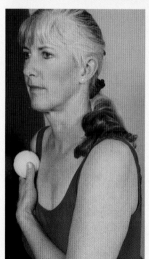

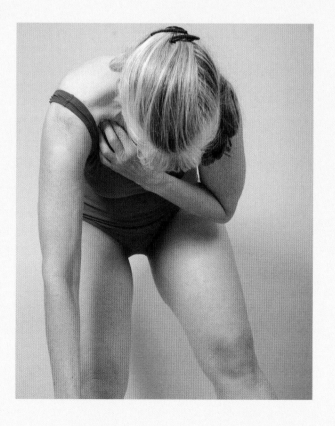

Subclavius Pressure
Much of the subclavius muscle is under the collarbone, so you must lean forward, allowing your arm to dangle, which moves the collarbone away from the trunk. With the opposite hand, press under the collarbone with your fingers, especially working closer to the breastbone.

Stretches

Pectoralis Stretch
See chapter 17.

Also Check

Scalene muscles (42). Thoracolumbar paraspinal muscles (18). Deltoid (44, anterior and posterior portions, satellite trigger points). Coracobrachialis (45, satellite trigger points). Sternalis (24). Sternocleidomastoid (10). Serratus anterior (26). Rhomboid (20). Trapezius (8). Infraspinatus (35). Subscapularis (37). Teres minor (39). Latissimus dorsi (38). Teres major (40).

Differential Diagnosis

If you are unable to relieve your symptoms with trigger point self-help techniques, you may need to see a health care provider to rule out angina, muscle tears, bicipital tendinitis, supraspinatus tendinitis, subacromial bursitis, medial epicondylitis, lateral epicondylitis, C5 to C8 nerve root irritation, intercostal neuritis or radiculopathy, irritation of the bronchi, pleura, or esophagus, a hiatal hernia with reflux, distention of the stomach by gas, mediastinal emphysema, gaseous distention of the splenic flexure of the colon, coronary insufficiency, fibromyalgia, and lung cancer. A sudden, extreme sharp pain during a sudden overload of the muscle may indicate a torn muscle. Skeletal diagnoses that need to be considered include chest wall syndrome, Tietze's syndrome, costochondritis, hypersensitive xiphoid process syndrome, precordial catch syndrome, slipping rib syndrome, and rib-tip syndrome, though many of these may be due either entirely or in part to trigger points.

24 Sternalis

The anatomy of the *sternalis* is highly variable, but this muscle generally overlies the breastbone (*sternum*) and it may be found on only one side of the chest. Only about 5% of the population has a sternalis muscle—its function, if any, is still currently unknown.

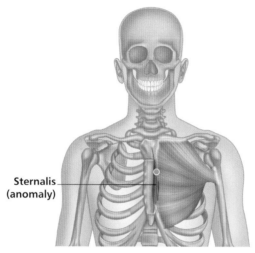

Sternalis (anomaly)

Common Symptoms

■ A deep intense ache under the breastbone that may also extend across the upper chest, into the front of the shoulder, and down the inner upper arm to the elbow. If the referral is on the left side of the body, it may extend past the elbow.

■ Symptoms may be mistaken for a heart attack or angina.

■ A trigger point located around the top of the muscle may be a source of a dry, hacking cough.

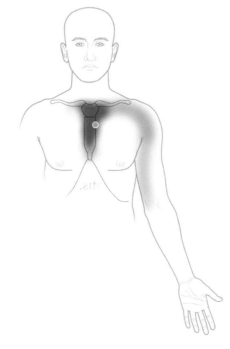

Causes and Perpetuation of Trigger Points, and Solutions

■ Trigger points may develop as satellite trigger points of the sternocleidomastoid muscle (10).
■ A direct trauma to the area, or an acute heart attack or angina.

Solutions
■ Check the sternocleidomastoid muscle (10) for trigger points that may be perpetuating sternalis trigger points. Acupuncture is also helpful for treating pain in the chest area and pain that feels deep to the rib cage.

Self-Help Techniques

Be sure to check the sternocleidomastoid (10) first for trigger points that may be perpetuating sternalis trigger points. Usually trigger points are also found in the pectoralis major muscle (23).

Applying Pressure

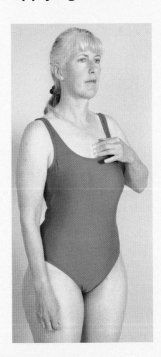

Sternalis Pressure
Trigger points are more common in the upper two-thirds of the muscle, and on the left side of the breastbone (sternum). Use the middle three fingers of one hand to apply pressure. If you need more pressure, place your opposite hand over the one you are using to apply pressure. Follow the treatment with moist heat.

Also Check

Sternocleidomastoid (10). Pectoralis major (23).

Differential Diagnosis
Sternalis pain may be diagnosed as costochondritis, but you should check for trigger points. If you are unable to relieve trigger points with the self-help, you may need to see a health care provider to check for possible gastroesophageal reflux, esophagitis, and C7 nerve root irritation.

25 Abdominal Muscles

Abdominal Oblique, Transversus Abdominis, Rectus Abdominis, Pyramidalis

The abdominal muscles that commonly contain trigger points are the *abdominal oblique, transversus abdominis, rectus abdominis,* and *pyramidalis*. As a group they cover the abdomen, providing a wall for it, and allow you to rotate and bend at the waist.

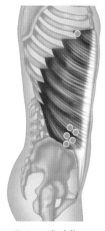

External oblique

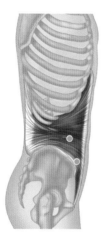

Transversus abdominis

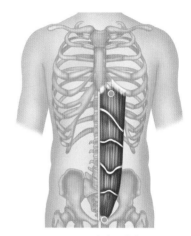

Rectus abdominis

Trigger points in abdominal muscles can cause symptoms such as projectile vomiting, loss of appetite, food intolerance, nausea, belching or burping, heartburn, pain in the bowels, diarrhea, urinary bladder spasms, testicular pain, and painful menses. These symptoms can often be confused with organ problems, but trigger points can be *initiated* by organ diseases and outlast the disease. You need to rule out organ diseases, and any found need to be treated for lasting relief.

Common Symptoms

- See the pictures for all the referral patterns. These pictures show common trigger points, but trigger points located anywhere within the abdominal muscles can refer pain or discomfort to the opposite side of the abdomen and even to the back. Pain may feel like it is in an organ.
- Forceful breathing may increase pain.
- Often symptoms are described as burning, fullness, bloating, swelling, or excessive gas.

Abdominal Oblique and Transversus Abdominis
- The upper trigger points may produce stomach area pain and/or heartburn and other symptoms

commonly associated with a hiatal hernia, but pain is more likely to be continuous, rather than related to the timing of eating or bowel movements. The lower points may produce urinary frequency, retention of urine, bed-wetting, chronic diarrhea, and groin and testicular pain.

- Frequent belching and gas, or projectile vomiting. The trigger point is likely found on the back, at or near the bottom of the rib cage around the end of the twelfth rib, but it may be located elsewhere in one of the abdominal muscles or in the fascia.
- Restricted trunk rotation.

Rectus Abdominis

■ Symptoms of trigger points in the upper portion of the muscle may include pain referred to the mid back that crosses the back in a horizontal band. They can also cause abdominal fullness, heartburn, indigestion, heart-area pain, gall bladder-area pain, peptic ulcer-like pain, gynecological-like pain, and sometimes nausea and vomiting.

■ Trigger points in the area around the belly button are typically aggravated by bending over when lifting and can cause abdominal or intestinal cramping. If your baby is colicky, try gently pressing points around the belly button.

■ Trigger points in the lower third of this muscle can cause referred pain that crosses the low back and sacrum (the triangular bone between the lumbar vertebrae and the tailbone) in a horizontal band, and pain in the penis. They can also cause pain with menses, and pain that *mimics* diverticulitis, kidney stones, and menstrual problems. Other symptoms may include diarrhea, urinary frequency, urinary retention, spasm of the urinary and detrusor sphincter muscles.

■ McBurney's point, usually found on the right side a little way down from the level of the belly button and about three fingers' width away from the midline, can cause symptoms that mimic appendicitis. Pain often occurs premenstrually, or with fatigue or worry. At least 12.4% of appendixes removed are normal and surgery does not solve the pain. In this case, pain is likely due instead to trigger points. However, since a ruptured appendix is life-threatening, you will not have time to rule out trigger points. *With any sudden onset of abdominal pain, go to the emergency room immediately for evaluation, including a blood test for infection.* If you end up having surgery and it did not solve all or part of the problem, search for trigger points.

■ Rectus abdominis syndrome is where an anterior branch of a spinal nerve is entrapped, causing lower abdominal and pelvic pain that simulates gynecological problems in women.

Pyramidalis

■ Pain referred close to the midline, between the belly button and the top of the pubic bone.

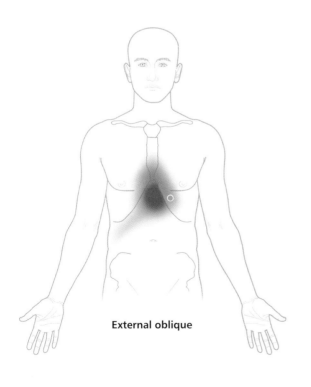

External oblique

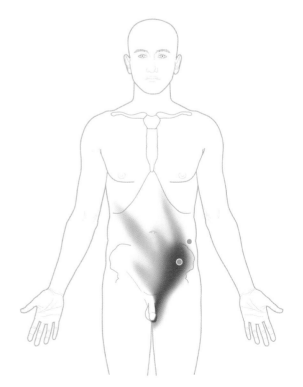

**Lateral abdominals
(oblique and possibly transversus
abdominis muscles)**

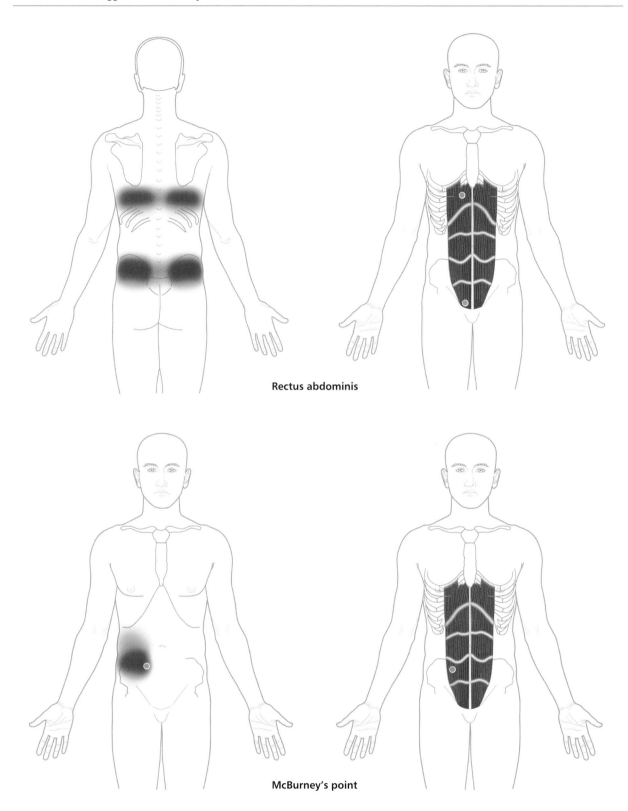

Rectus abdominis

McBurney's point

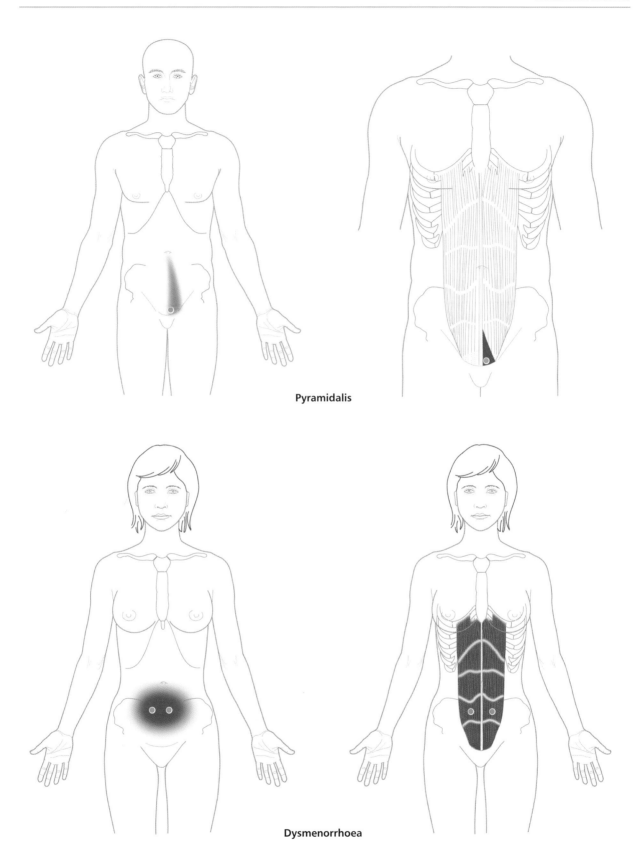

Pyramidalis

Dysmenorrhoea

Causes and Perpetuation of Trigger Points, and Solutions

■ Poor posture such as bending over for long periods of time, situations where your back is not supported, or rotating to one side to see your computer screen. Wearing a tight belt.

Solutions

■ Use a lumbar support everywhere you sit. Modify or replace your misfitting furniture. Take frequent breaks. Make sure your belt, waistband, or pantyhose elastic is not compressing the muscles. See chapter 2 for more information on all of these perpetuating factors. Head-forward posture can be a result of trigger points in the upper rectus abdominis muscle—see chapter 7.

■ Trigger points can be initiated by organ diseases such as peptic ulcers, intestinal parasites (for example *Entamoeba histolytica* and beef or fish tapeworms), dysentery (diarrhea caused most likely by drinking unclean water), diverticulosis, diverticulitis, and gallstones, and may outlast the organ disease even after its resolution. They can also be caused by other medical conditions such as viral infections, or straining due to constipation.

Solutions

■ Treat organ diseases such as ulcers, gallstones, parasites, and diverticulitis to eliminate any perpetuating factors (see chapter 4). Treat the cause of constipation. Try drinking more water and taking calcium/magnesium and folic acid supplements. Acupuncture and herbs are very successful at treating constipation.

■ Direct trauma to the abdominal area, including surgeries such as appendectomies or hysterectomies.

Solutions

■ Scars left from surgeries usually have numerous trigger points, along with associated trigger points in the surrounding tissues. Acupuncture scar treatments are very effective for treating these trigger points, even years after the surgery.

■ Emotional stress or overall fatigue.

Solutions

■ Learn proper breathing techniques (see chapter 7). See chapter 4 to address emotional factors and sleep issues.

■ Tensing up when exposed to cold temperatures.

Solutions

■ Keep your trunk and rest of your body warm.

■ Improper conditioning, for example too many sit-ups too soon or trying to hold your abdomen in continuously.

Solutions

■ Too many sit-ups can not only cause trigger points in the abdominal muscles, but also lead to satellite trigger points in the diaphragm muscle (27). Learn proper conditioning techniques with the help of a physical therapist or other trained specialist who knows how to modify an activity for your set of circumstances. Do not overdo conditioning exercises. You should not do activities that are painful or make you sore afterwards. It is better to add repetitions and increase weights *slowly* so that you make steady progress, rather than hurt yourself and have to stop until you are well again. See chapter 5 for more information.

■ Do not try to hold your abdomen in to make it flat. This actually has the opposite effect, since the chronic tension will form trigger points that cause the muscle fibers to stop their proper contraction function, allowing the abdomen to go slack due to an inability to condition the muscles.

■ Structural imbalances such an anatomically shorter leg or small hemipelvis on one side (either the left or the right half of the pelvic bone).

Solutions

■ See a specialist to get compensating lifts and pads.

Self-Help Techniques

Abdominal pain may be referred from trigger points in the thoracolumbar paraspinal muscles (18), and pain in the back may be referred from trigger points in the abdominal muscles, so you should check both sets of muscles. Gastrointestinal pain and cramping, and nausea and belching, may also be due to trigger points in the thoracolumbar paraspinal muscles. Lower abdominal pain, tenderness, and muscle spasm may also come from trigger points located in the vaginal wall (see pelvic floor muscles, chapter 32). A trigger point high in the adductor muscles of the hip (67) may cause pain referred upward into the groin and lower abdomen.

Applying Pressure

Abdominal Pressure

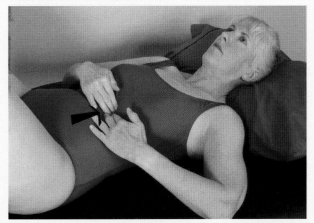

Lying face-up, use your fingers to apply pressure to sensitive points in the entire abdominal area. You may find it easier if you have a pillow under your knees. Be sure to check all the way from the bottom rib to the top of the pubic bone, and out to the sides. When working on the top edge of the pubic bone, press down toward your feet rather than toward your back. You may combine this with applying hot packs or sitting in a warm bath.

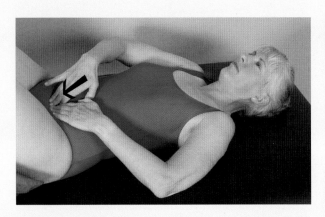
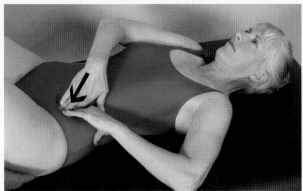

Stretches

Abdominal Stretch

See chapter 17 for this stretch. You may also try the Hip-Extension Stretch in the same chapter as an alternative.

Exercises

Pelvic Tilt Exercise

The pelvic tilt strengthens the rectus abdominis. Once trigger points have been inactivated for a few weeks, you may add this conditioning exercise. With this exercise, be sure to rest between each repetition for an equal amount of time it took to perform the repetition.

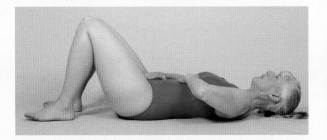
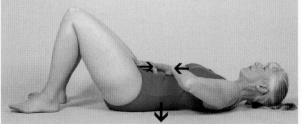
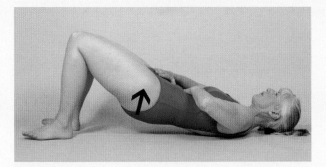

Lie face-up with your knees bent, with one hand over your lower abdomen and one hand above your navel. First flatten out the lumbar area of your back against the floor, which brings the two hands closer together. Then push your butt off the floor so only your feet and mid to upper back are still on the floor—the hands should come even closer together. If your hands get further apart, you are arching your back rather than flattening it correctly. Finally, roll back down to relax on the floor and take a deep breath.

Also Check

Serratus anterior (26). Thoracolumbar paraspinal muscles (18). Intercostals and diaphragm (27, diaphragm). Adductor muscles of the hip (67).

Differential Diagnosis

If you are experiencing sudden abdominal pain, go to the emergency room! Abdominal pain more likely due to trigger points in the rectus abdominis muscle will exhibit palpable nodules and ropiness in the band of muscle down the middle of the abdomen. Abdominal pain more likely due to appendicitis will exhibit a more generalized, board-like rigidity in the entire abdominal musculature. Your health care provider will conduct other tests to evaluate you for appendicitis, including a blood test. I had one patient who suffered from low-grade abdominal pain that was helped minimally by massage and acupuncture. After several months, she had her appendix removed on the advice of a health care provider. Her pain was relieved, and it was determined she had a subclinical chronic irritation of her appendix with fibrous tissues, even though it was not diseased.

Once a health care provider has ruled out appendicitis, you may also need to be evaluated for a peptic ulcer, colitis, painful rib syndrome, urinary tract disease, fibromyalgia, a hiatal hernia, gastric carcinoma, kidney or gallstones, an inguinal hernia, hepatitis, pancreatitis, gynecological disorders, diverticulosis, an umbilical hernia, thoracic or upper lumbar nerve root irritation, costochondritis, ascariasis, epilepsy, and rectus abdominis hematoma. Pain in the upper abdomen may be caused by Tietze's syndrome or slipping rib syndrome. You may need to see a chiropractor or osteopathic physician to be evaluated for pubic and innominate dysfunctions or for vertebral and rib misalignments.

26 Serratus Anterior

The *serratus anterior* muscle has fibers that run from the upper eight or nine ribs to the edge of the shoulder blade (*scapula*) located closest to the spine. It moves the scapula and keeps it from "winging" away from the body.

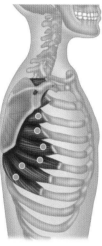

Common Symptoms

■ Pain referred primarily to the side of the chest underneath the armpit and to a spot in the mid back next to the lower end of the shoulder blade, and possibly down the inside of the arm and into the palm and the ring and middle fingers. Possibly breast tenderness.

■ Pain with deep breathing, and shortness of breath to the extent that you may feel you cannot get enough air or finish a sentence without stopping to breathe—you may refer to it as a "stitch" in the side.

■ Difficulty lying on the affected side or getting comfortable at night.

■ "Winging" of the shoulder blade, where the top of the shoulder blade is pulled away from the trunk, and/or your shoulders may be rounded forward.

■ The nerves that supply the serratus anterior can be entrapped by the scalene muscles (42).

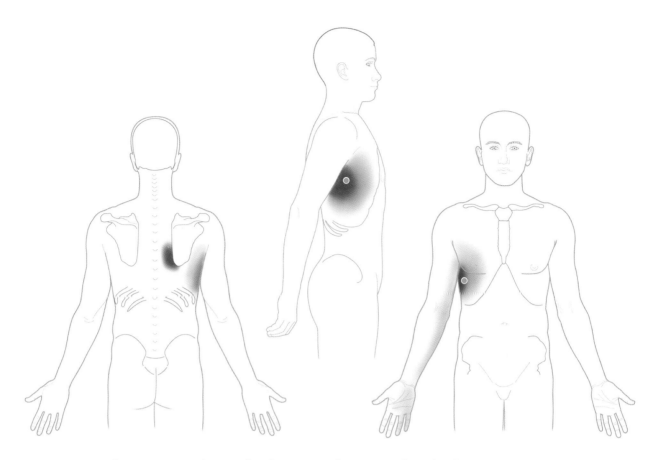

Causes and Perpetuation of Trigger Points, and Solutions

■ Muscle strain from push-ups, running very fast or for long periods, forceful swimming as in the butterfly stroke, or lifting heavy objects overhead.

Solutions

■ Avoid push-ups, chin-ups, and overhead lifting. When sleeping, lie on the unaffected side, and drape the arm of the affected side over a pillow. Learn proper breathing techniques (see chapter 7).

■ Severe coughing.

Solutions

■ If you have a chronic cough, you will need to address the underlying causes (see chapter 4). If you are unable to eliminate the cough, you will need to expel phlegm by clearing the throat and spitting it out, or use a cough suppressant. Acupuncture and herbs are very successful at treating coughs and phlegm.

■ High levels of anxiety.
■ Heart attack.

Solutions

■ Treat anxiety with acupuncture, herbs, homeopathy, and/or counseling. Reduce stressful situations. See chapter 4, "Emotional Factors."

Self-Help Techniques

Also check the trapezius (8), rhomboid (20), and thoracolumbar paraspinal muscles (18) for trigger points, since they can generate similar referral patterns, and/or may contain associated trigger points. The serratus posterior superior (36) may also harbor trigger points simultaneously. Trigger points in the serratus anterior may cause trigger points in the latissimus dorsi (38), scalene (42), and sternocleidomastoid (10), because these muscles are also used for breathing. Other muscles which may harbor trigger points that can cause a stitch in the side are the diaphragm (27) and the external abdominal oblique (25).

Applying Pressure

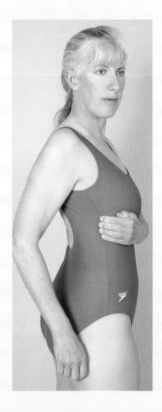

Serratus Anterior Pressure
Lie on the unaffected side and use the fingers of that side to apply pressure to the side of the rib cage below the armpit. It is a fairly large area, so check toward the breast, back toward the shoulder blade, and almost to the bottom of the rib cage.

Stretches

Taking a few *deep* slow breaths may be helpful.

Pectoralis Stretch
This stretch will also benefit the serratus anterior muscle (see chapter 17).

Serratus Anterior Stretch
Hang your arm over the back of a chair and rotate your trunk away from the side you are stretching.

Also Check

Latissimus dorsi (38). Scalene muscles (42). Sternocleidomastoid (10). Thoracolumbar paraspinal muscles (18). Trapezius (8). Rhomboid (20). Serratus posterior superior (36).

Differential Diagnosis
If you are unable to relieve your symptoms with trigger point self-help techniques, you may need to see a health care provider to rule out a rib stress fracture, costochondritis, intercostal nerve entrapment, C7 or C8 nerve root lesions, and herpes zoster. You may need to see a chiropractor or osteopathic physician to be evaluated for mid-thoracic vertebrae that are out of alignment.

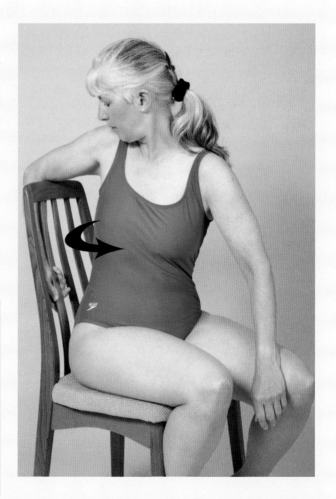

27 Intercostals and Diaphragm

The *intercostal* muscles run between each rib and aid in trunk rotation and breathing. The *diaphragm* bisects the trunk below the rib cage, forming a wall between the abdominal and thoracic cavities, and is used for inhalation.

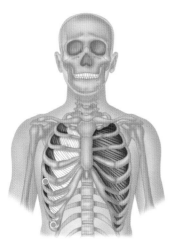

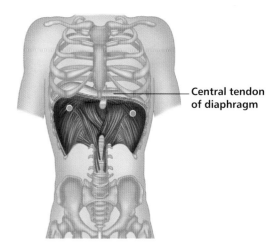

Central tendon of diaphragm

Common Symptoms

Intercostals

■ The intercostal muscles tend to refer aching pain very locally between the adjacent ribs and possibly slightly toward the front of the body. Trigger points that are more active may refer pain to the intercostal space above and below the adjacent rib. The further the trigger point is away from the midline of the body, the more likely it will refer pain toward the midline.

■ Pain is increased when bending the trunk away from the side with the trigger points, and pain is possibly partially relieved when bending toward the affected side. There is likely restricted rotation of the thoracic spine in the mid to upper back in one or both directions.

■ Pain is worse with aerobic exercise, coughing, sneezing, attempting to take a deep breath, or fully exhaling.

■ An inability to raise your arm straight up on the affected side due to pain. If you have been avoiding raising your arm because of the pain, you may be vulnerable to developing a frozen shoulder—see chapter 33 for a discussion of this condition.

■ Possibly an inability to lie on the affected side.

■ Cardiac arrhythmias, including auricular fibrillation, may come from a trigger point in an intercostal muscle on the right side.

Diaphragm

■ The diaphragm causes a "stitch" in the side under the lower border of the rib cage during vigorous exercise and is most intense at the end of a full exhalation. Trigger points in the center of the diaphragm can refer pain to the top of the shoulder on the same side.

■ Chest pain, difficulty breathing, pain with coughing, and an inability to get a full breath, which is possibly accompanied by a fear of dying if breathing is severely impaired.

■ Pain is aggravated by emotional distress.

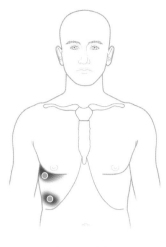

Intercostals

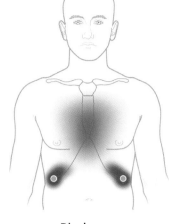

Diaphragm

Causes and Perpetuation of Trigger Points, and Solutions

■ Trauma, especially local trauma such as an impact causing a broken rib, or surgeries such as chest surgery (particularly with the use of chest retractors), or possibly a breast implant.

Solutions
■ If you must wear some kind of brace around the torso after a trauma or surgery, remove it, if possible, for five minutes every three hours, but only after obtaining the approval of your health care provider. Do not wear the brace any longer than necessary. Use gentle trigger point self-pressure as soon as you can comfortably do so without causing damage or additional pain.

■ Medical conditions, such as herpes zoster (shingles) or excessive coughing.

Solutions
■ Trigger points may form in the intercostal muscles as a result of an attack of herpes zoster, and relief of trigger points may be a key factor in relieving post-herpetic pain that is localized, most likely toward the outside and back of the rib cage. Treating shingles with acupuncture, herbs and homeopathy in the initial stages of infection helps prevent the formation of trigger points.
■ If you have a chronic cough, you will need to address the underlying causes. If you are unable to eliminate the cough, you will need to expel phlegm by clearing your throat, or use a cough suppressant. Acupuncture and herbs are very successful at treating coughs and phlegm. See chapter 4 for more information.

■ Medical conditions, such as a pneumothorax (a collapsed lung), pyothorax (an infection in the chest), or a pleural effusion secondary to a tumor (an accumulation of fluid between the membrane lining the lungs and chest cavity) can cause trigger points in the bottom three intercostal muscles, accompanied by pain in the lower part of the chest

Solutions
■ After any of these conditions have been treated, use gentle trigger point self-pressure as soon as you can comfortably do so without causing damage or additional pain.

■ Trigger points in the pectoralis major muscle (23).

Solutions

■ See chapters 23 and 17 to treat the pectoralis major muscle. Restoration of proper posture, especially head positioning, is critical to treating trigger points, since head-forward posture can both cause and perpetuate trigger points in a number of muscles (see chapter 7). Head-forward posture can be aggravated while sitting in a car, at a desk, or in front of a computer, or while eating dinner or watching TV. Using a good lumbar support everywhere you sit will help correct poor sitting posture. Orthotic inserts in your shoes may improve your standing posture. See "Ergonomics" and "Body Mechanics" in chapter 2.

■ Improper breathing.

Solutions

■ See page 55 to retrain yourself in proper breathing techniques.

■ Trigger points in the diaphragm may be caused by aerobic exercise, a persistent cough, or possibly a gastrectomy (removal of part or all of the stomach). Overdoing sit-ups or heavy resistance exercises for the pectoralis and biceps muscles overloads and causes trigger points in the rectus abdominis muscle (25), and may lead to satellite trigger points in the diaphragm.

Solutions

■ Check the other abdominal muscles (25) for trigger points, which may help relieve breathing difficulties. Stop doing excessive aerobic exercise, sit-ups or heavy resistance exercises until trigger points are relieved, and see chapter 5 for information on muscle care. If you have a chronic cough, see chapter 4.

Self-Help Techniques

Also check the serratus anterior muscle (26). Pain while taking a deep breath with the abdomen expanded is more likely to be caused by trigger points in the transversus abdominis muscle (25); pain upon full exhalation with the abdomen pulled in is more likely to be caused by trigger points in the diaphragm.

Applying Pressure

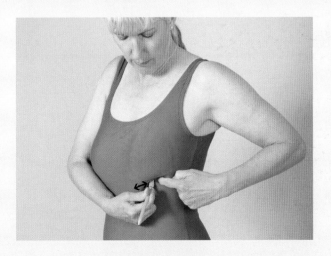

Intercostals Pressure

To apply pressure to the intercostal muscles, buy pencil erasers that fit on the end of a pencil. Using the tip of the eraser, press in between the ribs. Hold the pencil in one hand and use the opposite index finger to help you follow the curve of the space in between the ribs.

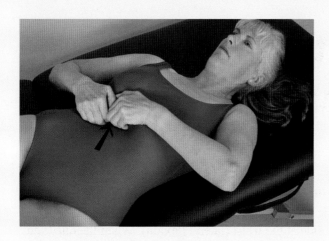

Diaphragm Pressure

To work on the edge of the diaphragm, lie face-up, with your knees bent. Hook the fingers from both hands under the edge of one side of the rib cage, and as you exhale fully, press in and up under the rib cage and pull the ribs outward. Relax and breathe.

Stretches

Triceps Stretch

To stretch the intercostals, do the triceps stretch (41) and focus on feeling the stretch in the rib cage area.

Diaphragm Stretch

To stretch the diaphragm, exhale fully and focus on pushing your belly button out. Inhale fully and focus on sucking in the area just below your rib cage. Do not hold these positions—just do the range of motion rhythmically a couple of times.

Also Check

Serratus anterior (26). Abdominal muscles (25).

Differential Diagnosis

For conditions that mimic pain from intercostal trigger points, or that may be found concurrently, you may need to see a health care provider to rule out heart disease or a heart attack, Tietze's syndrome, thoracic vertebral nerve root irritation, costochondritis, a tumor, pleural effusion, or pyothorax. You may need to see a chiropractor or osteopathic physician to be evaluated for ribs or thoracic vertebrae that are out of alignment. Any of these conditions may be found concurrently with trigger points, so even if you get some relief with trigger point therapy, *you may still need to see a health care provider to ensure that you do not also have a more serious condition.*

For conditions that mimic the pain from diaphragm trigger points, you may need to see a health care provider to rule out a diaphragmatic spasm, a peptic ulcer, gastroesophageal reflux, or gall bladder disease if pain is on the right side only.

28 Quadratus Lumborum and Iliolumbar Ligament

The *quadratus lumborum* muscle attaches to the twelfth rib, to the top of the pelvis, and to the transverse processes of all the lumbar vertebrae. When one side is used alone, it stabilizes the lumbar part of the spine. It can "hike" the hip up, and allow you to bend to the side at the waist (lateral flexion). When the quadratus lumborum muscles on both sides are used together, they allow you to go from a front-bending position to standing up straight and assist with forced breath exhalation, such as when coughing. Trigger points in the quadratus lumborum muscle may be responsible for roughly 30% of sacral-gluteal area pain.

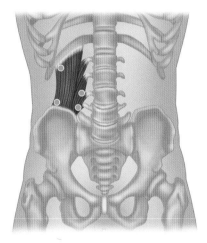

The *iliolumbar ligament* runs from the transverse process of the fifth lumbar vertebra to the pelvis, but some individual variability is noted with an additional attachment to the fourth lumbar vertebra. It serves to stabilize the vertebral spine and can be a major player in lumbar and sacral-gluteal area pain, especially when there is damage to the discs and/or vertebrae in the L4 to L5 to S1 areas.

Do not assume that a finding of bone spurs or narrowing of a lumbar disc space is causing pain, since many people who have these conditions do not have pain, and vice versa. Always assume trigger points are at least a part of the problem. Sometimes people fear that if they have pain in the lumbar region, it indicates they have a kidney infection. However, symptoms of a kidney infection include a high fever and chills. *If you are experiencing these symptoms, go to the emergency room immediately.* Otherwise, check for trigger points and see if you can get relief.

Common Symptoms

- Depending on the location of the trigger points, pain can be referred to various places in the gluteal area, the sacrum, over the hip joint and surrounding area, and even around the front to the groin area, testes, scrotum, and the lower abdomen; see the pictures for the referral patterns. Pain over the sacroiliac joint—where the sacrum and big pelvic bone (*ilium*) meet—and greater trochanter (hip joint) can be mistaken for joint dysfunction.
- Pain is usually deep and aching, but can be sharp or stabbing with movement.
- Pain when climbing stairs, rotating your trunk, or leaning to the opposite side. Range of motion can be restricted when bending forward.

■ Pain can be so intolerable you cannot lie on the affected side, and you may be unable to bear weight on that side. Rolling onto your side, getting up, or getting out of a chair may be extremely painful or impossible. Pain may be unbearable while standing or sitting upright, but you may be able to crawl on your hands and knees. Coughing or sneezing can cause unbearable pain temporarily.

■ Some people may experience a "lightening bolt" of pain down the front of the thigh in a narrow band, or possibly a "heaviness of the hips," calf cramping, and burning sensations in the legs and feet.

■ Pressing on quadratus lumborum trigger points and possibly some gluteus minimus trigger points may reproduce a *sciatica* type of pain distribution, which is more aptly called *pseudo-sciatica*.

■ The iliolumbar ligament can refer pain locally around the fourth and fifth lumbar vertebrae, but can also cause pain that feels like it is deep in the hip joint, in the groin area, or diffuse pain over the front of the thigh.

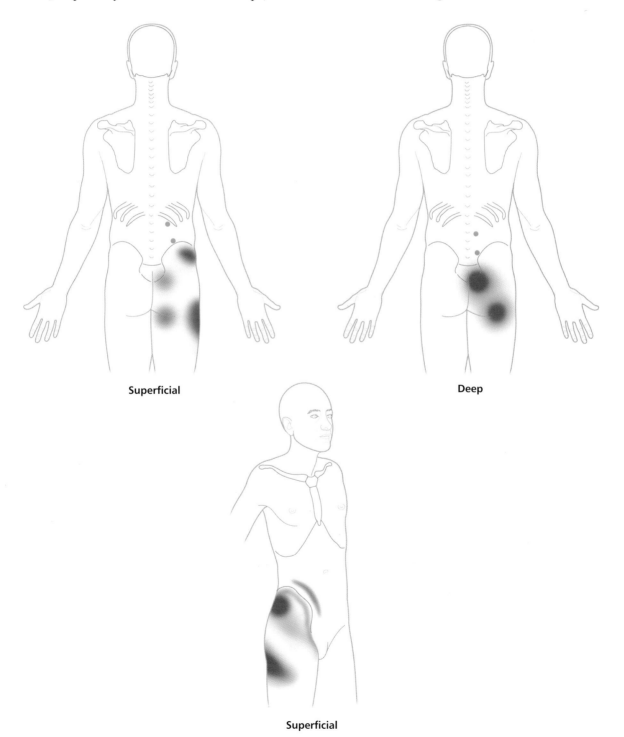

Superficial

Deep

Superficial

Causes and Perpetuation of Trigger Points, and Solutions

■ Awkward movements, such as lifting something heavy (especially when your trunk is rotated at the same time); trying to rise out of a low chair, car, or bed; or attempting to put on pants, socks, and shoes while standing.

Solutions

■ Avoid any heavy lifting, and if you must lift something, be sure to bend at the knees, keep your torso straight, and keep the object close to your body. When standing up from a chair, slide your butt to the front of the chair, turn your entire body a little sideways, put one foot under the front edge of the chair, then stand with the torso erect so that your thighs take the load. You can use your hands to assist you if necessary. Sit down in the opposite sequence. Sit while putting on pants, socks, and shoes. When climbing stairs or a ladder, rotate your entire body 45 degrees and keep your back straight.

■ A repetitive strain from gardening, washing floors, lifting heavy objects, walking in a cast, or walking or running on a slanted surface such as a beach or a road.

Solutions

■ Gardeners should sit on a stool about eight to ten inches high and take frequent breaks. Avoid any heavy lifting, and if you must lift something repetitively, be sure to bend at the knees, keep your torso straight, and keep the object close to your body. If you have to wear a walking cast due to a broken bone, get a shoe for the opposite foot with a sole that matches the height of the bottom of the cast. Walk or run on smooth, level surfaces until trigger points are relieved. Avoid slanted sidewalks, roads, beaches, and running tracks.

■ Sitting with your pelvis tilted by a car or car seat, or sitting with a wallet in your back pocket.

Solutions

■ Always make sure you have proper lumbar support in all sitting locations, including your car. Be sure to slide into the center of your car seat if you have bucket seats. Do not carry a wallet in your back pocket. See chapter 2 for more information on ergonomics and body mechanics.

■ Leaning forward over a desk, sink, or other work surface.

Solutions

■ Stand up straight, rather than bending over sinks and work surfaces. If you must lean over something, keep it brief and support yourself with a free hand. See chapter 2 for more information on ergonomics and body mechanics.

■ Mattresses that are too old or too soft, or sleeping next to someone who is heavier and trying to avoid rolling into them.

Solutions

■ Buy a firm mattress and replace it every five to seven years. You can put plywood between the box springs and mattress to make the surface firmer. See page 16, "Bedtime Furniture," for more information. You may find relief by lying on your back or side. Using a pillow to modify the tilt of your hips or placing it under your knees may be helpful. If you are comfortable lying on your side, place a pillow in front of your legs and put the upper leg on top of it. Make sure your muscles do not get chilled, especially at night.

■ Trauma, such as from an auto accident or a near-fall, where you catch yourself.

Solutions

■ Do the self-help techniques below.

■ Weak abdominal muscles.

Solutions

■ Do the Pelvic Tilt Exercise found in chapter 25. Sit-ups are not a good idea, but you may be able to perform a sit-*back* exercise under the supervision of a physical therapist or other professional.

■ Structural imbalances, such as having one leg anatomically shorter than the other, with as little as $1/8$" difference. Short upper arms can cause you to lean to the side to use armrests, and a small hemipelvis (either the left or the right half of the pelvic bone) tilts your trunk. With either of these structural imbalances, sitting will aggravate the pain.

Solutions

■ See a specialist for compensating lifts and pads. See chapter 4, "Spinal and Skeletal Factors," for more information. If you are getting an anatomical leg-length inequality corrected with lifts, start with a thin lift and gradually use thicker ones until the proper lift height is reached. Work on the thoracolumbar paraspinal muscles (18) during this process to help the back muscles adjust. If you have short upper arms, buy a chair with adjustable arms, or tape sponges or towels to the armrests to increase their height.

Be sure to address any systemic perpetuating factors discussed in chapters 3 and 4 if referred pain from trigger points in the quadratus lumborum muscle has persisted for more than a few weeks or does not respond more than temporarily to trigger point treatment. Particularly examine the sections on vitamin and other nutritional deficiencies, organ dysfunction and disease (especially thyroid inadequacies), acute or chronic viral, bacterial, or parasitic infections, emotional factors, and active allergies that cause a high histamine level in your body.

Self-Help Techniques

Always do the self-treatment on *both* sides! It is rare that only one side is involved, especially in the lumbar and gluteal muscles. Check the gluteus medius muscle (31), since trigger points in that muscle can activate quadratus lumborum trigger points. Trigger points in the gluteus medius and gluteus minimus (62) can cause weakness in the quadratus lumborum. Consider acupuncture for treatment of the quadratus lumborum, since needles are better able to penetrate down to the muscle than massage.

Wrapping your hands around the sides of your waist and pressing downward on the top of your pelvis may give enough temporary relief to allow some movement, as may using your thumbs to apply pressure to the muscle itself.

Applying Pressure

Thoracolumbar Paraspinal Pressure
As part of the quadratus lumborum self-treatment, work on the thoracolumbar paraspinal muscles (18), because most of the time those muscles are also involved to some extent.

Quadratus Lumborum Pressure
When you get to the lumbar area, most people have enough of a curve that they might need to move to the floor and use a tennis ball or baseball, but make sure this is not too hard for you (see the general guidelines in chapter 5). Do not use a softball since it is too large. You may use your hand to move the ball, searching for trigger points in the lumbar area. *Do not press your back onto the ball and if you have been diagnosed with bulging or herniated discs, be very careful not to get too close to the spine!*

Iliolumbar Ligament Pressure
The iliolumbar ligament is in a small dip between the fifth lumbar vertebra and the rim of your pelvis. It is helpful to locate it with your thumb first. Lying face-up with your knees bent, on a hard surface such as a wood or linoleum floor or on a very thin carpet, use a golf ball and your body weight to give you pressure. If this is not enough pressure, put the calf of the same side on top of the opposite knee. You may also wish to continue down a little further onto the top part of the sacrum, in order to get the S1 multifidi (see chapter 18 for a picture of the multifidi muscles).

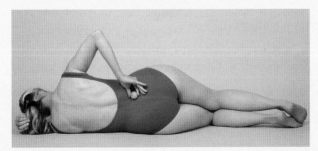 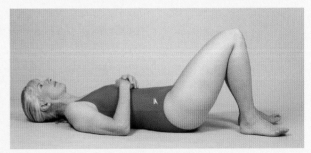

Stretches

Supine Self-Stretch
Lie face-up with your knees bent and with your hands behind your head; if you do not put your hands behind your head, you will not get the stretch. Place one leg over the other knee, and use that leg to gently pull the knee down toward the floor. You should feel the stretch in the lumbar and gluteal areas. Then slip the leg off of the knee, return to neutral position, and repeat on the opposite side. You may repeat this a few times on each side. Follow with the Hip-Hike Stretch below.

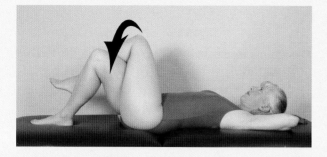

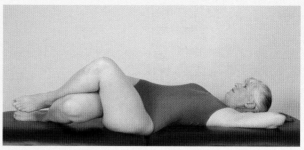

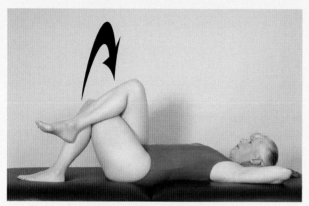

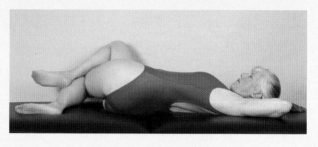

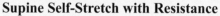

Supine Self-Stretch with Resistance

Once trigger points have been inactivated for a few weeks and are no longer causing referred pain, during the Supine Self-Stretch you may briefly apply resistance to provide an additional stretch. While you are using the left leg to stretch the right side, briefly use the right knee to push up against the left leg, then relax, taking up the slack in the stretch, and repeat. Do the same on the opposite side.

Hip-Hike Stretch

Lie face-up with your legs out straight. Place your hands on your hips, and as you breathe in, stretch one leg down so your pelvis tilts down on that side and you are feeling a stretch in the lumbar area. Exhale as you return to the neutral position. Repeat on the other side.

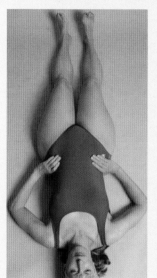

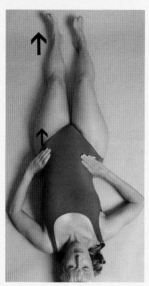

Also Check

Thoracolumbar paraspinal muscles (18). Iliopsoas (22). Abdominal muscles (25). Latissimus dorsi (38). Gluteus medius (31, primary or satellite trigger points). Gluteus minimus (62, satellite trigger points).

Differential Diagnosis

If you are unable to relieve your symptoms with trigger point self-help techniques, you may need to see a health care provider to rule out spinal tumors, myasthenia gravis, gallstones, liver disease, kidney stones, urinary tract problems, intra-abdominal infections, intestinal parasites, diverticulitis, an aortic aneurysm, and multiple sclerosis. See a chiropractor or osteopathic physician for evaluation of vertebrae out of alignment and sacroiliac joint subluxation.

29

Piriformis

Piriformis, Gemelli, Quadratus Femoris, Obturator Internus, and Obturator Externus

The *piriformis* muscle attaches to the inner surface of the sacrum toward the midline of the body, and to the greater trochanter of the femur (upper end of the thigh bone) on the other end. It prevents the thigh from rotating too far in toward the midline when the leg is being used for weight bearing. When the leg is not bearing weight and is straight, the piriformis rotates the thigh toward the outside, but when the hip is flexed to 90 degrees, it helps hold the leg in toward the midline.

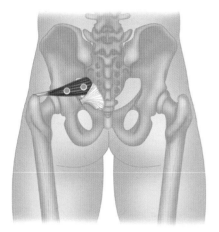

Piriformis

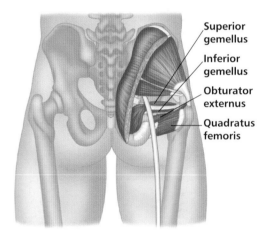

Superior gemellus

Inferior gemellus

Obturator externus

Quadratus femoris

Trigger points in the piriformis are very common and usually involved to some extent anytime there is pain both ocurring locally and radiating from the gluteal/pelvic region. It is commonly called *piriformis syndrome*. Females are affected far more than males, in a ratio of 6:1.

Trigger points in the piriformis muscle can cause pain by nerve entrapment and/or by referral. When the piriformis muscle is enlarged, it easily entraps the sciatic nerve and other major nerves and blood vessels. Even if there is entrapment, there are also likely to be trigger points; these may be part of the cause of the entrapment, since trigger points may cause the muscle to bulge. Even though some or all of the sciatic nerve's fibers pass through the piriformis in approximately 11% of patients, Doctors Travell and Simons speculated that this may actually *prevent* entrapment problems, since in their research of surgeries, no surgeons had reported this nerve-muscle variation in any of their patients being operated on for sciatic nerve entrapment.

There are five other short lateral rotators of the thigh below the piriformis: the *gemelli (superior* and *inferior gemellus), quadratus femoris, obturator internus,* and *obturator externus.* Their referred pain patterns have not been isolated from those of piriformis trigger points. It is always worth considering that the pain may be at least partially coming from one of the other lateral rotators. By performing the pressure techniques on the entire gluteal area, particularly from the middle area on down to the "sit bones" (*ischial tuberosities*), you will likely treat all the trigger points in the short lateral hip rotators.

Common Symptoms

■ Pain referred primarily to the sacroiliac region (the joint where the sacrum and big pelvic bone meet), over the buttock and down the back of the thigh.

■ Pain is worse while sitting and during activity, and you may squirm a lot and shift positions trying to get comfortable. You may have difficulty crossing one leg over the other knee while seated.

■ When lying face-up, your foot will rotate out to the side, rather than being in straight alignment.

■ If the tight or bulging piriformis muscle also entraps the sciatic nerve, the referred pain may extend down all the way to the calf and bottom of the foot, the gluteal muscles may atrophy, the foot may be numb and hard to walk on, and there may be swelling in the leg. Entrapment of the pudendal nerve may cause impotence in males and pain with intercourse in females, as well as pain in the groin or area in front of the anus.

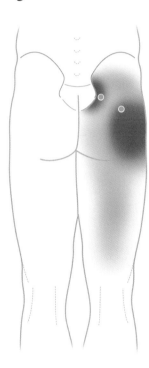

Causes and Perpetuation of Trigger Points, and Solutions

■ Poor sitting posture, such as reading in bed with your knees bent or otherwise sitting so that the majority of your weight is on your buttocks. Sitting on the floor, especially with your knees bent up in front of you, or sitting on your foot. Driving for long periods.

Solutions

■ Do not read in bed, sit on the floor, or sit in any other position that puts most of your weight on your buttocks, and do not sit on your foot. Sit upright with a lumbar support, so that your hamstrings bear some of your weight (see "Ergonomics," page 15). Sitting on a pillow may *temporarily* help ease pain. When sleeping, place a pillow between your legs that goes all the way from the knees to the ankles. Do not bring your legs up to a 90-degree angle. Do not drive for long periods without breaks. You may want to consider having the car fitted with cruise control so you can move your legs periodically.

■ Holding your gluteal area tight.

Solutions

■ As noted above, far more women have piriformis syndrome than men. I have noticed that women often tense their butt muscles when they are suppressing a lot of anger, and these patients tend to be the ones suffering from trigger points in the piriformis. See chapter 4 for a discussion of emotional factors and solutions. You will need to become aware of tightening the gluteals and consciously relax them repeatedly until you retrain yourself not to tense up.

■ Sudden muscle overloads, such as catching yourself from falling, forceful rotation of your body while your weight is on one leg, or twisting sideways while bending and lifting something heavy.
■ Repetitive motion injuries, such as twisting repeatedly while throwing something behind you, running, and, in women, spreading the legs during intercourse.

Solutions

■ Avoid running or playing tennis, soccer, and volleyball until trigger points have been inactivated. Try different positions during intercourse.

■ Injuries, such as a direct blow to the muscle or from car accidents.

Solutions

■ You may need to see a health care provider to rule out a bulging or herniated disc. Even if you do have disc problems, you will likely benefit from trigger point therapy in order to eliminate all the pain. Just do not apply ball-pressure directly on or adjacent to the injured area. Acupuncture works very well on herniated and bulging discs. If you do not have a disc problem, you may perform the self-help techniques without modification.

■ Arthritis of the hip joint or hip replacement surgery, although I believe in many cases the trigger points likely came first and have been left untreated for many years. This causes the joint to jam together, resulting in excessive wear on the ball-and-socket joint.

■ The sacroiliac joint out of alignment.

Solutions

■ Treat trigger points so that you do not end up needing surgical intervention. If you have already had surgery, these techniques will help reduce any remaining pain and prevent further damage to other muscles. If the sacroiliac joint is involved, it must be treated simultaneously with the piriformis muscle. See a chiropractor or osteopathic physician to be evaluated for lumbar and sacroiliac joint dysfunction.

■ If you are being advised to have surgery for piriformis syndrome, be sure to try trigger point therapy and sacroiliac joint release first, as surgery may not be needed if these treatments are successful.

■ Structural imbalances, such as a longer second toe, one leg anatomically shorter than the other, or foot pronation.

■ Over-correcting a shorter leg with a lift that is too high.

Solutions

■ If you have one leg anatomically shorter than the other or a small hemipelvis (either the left or the right half of the pelvic bone), see a specialist for compensating lifts and pads. If your pain started after getting a lift for one side, have it rechecked for proper height. If you have a short big toe and long second toe, get orthotics to prevent pronation. See chapters 2 and 4 for more information.

■ Medical conditions such as chronic pelvic inflammatory disease or infectious sacroiliitis.

Solutions

■ See a health care provider immediately if you suspect you have any kind of infection, especially if accompanied by a feeling of illness and fever.

Self-Help Techniques

If you develop pain deep to the lower edge of the rib cage in the area of the diaphragm after treatment of the piriformis and sacroiliac joint, learn to breathe properly (see chapter 7), and do the self-help techniques for the diaphragm muscle (27).

Applying Pressure*

Thoracolumbar Paraspinal Pressure

As part of the piriformis self-treatment, work on the thoracolumbar paraspinal muscles (18), because most of the time those muscles are also involved to some extent.

---

* A note to massage therapists: Work on the medial external portion of the obturator internus (over the obturator foramen) by moving the patient over to the edge of the table and dropping their leg over the side. Put a chair with a pillow on it under the lower leg so the leg is bent at about 90 degrees. Then treat the obturator internus by pressing in at about a 45-degree angle.

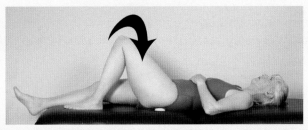

Piriformis Pressure

Lying face-up, use a tennis ball on the bed and search for trigger points in the buttocks area. With your legs bent, work against the edge of the sacrum (the bony triangle between the lumbar spine and the tailbone) and all the way out toward the hip joint in a line about halfway between the top of the pelvis and the bottom curve of the butt. When you are closer to the hip joint (tense your butt muscles and there will be a big dip there), drop your knee out to the side while still keeping your knees bent and you will know when you have located the piriformis if there are trigger points in it.

Stretches

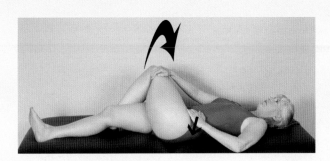

Piriformis Stretch

Lie face-up and cross your left foot over the outside of your right knee. Use your left hand to pull down on the left front of your pelvis. Use your right hand to pull down on the left knee, toward the floor, to assist in a stretch. Inhale and exhale deeply, focusing on relaxing the muscle on the exhale. Repeat on the opposite side.

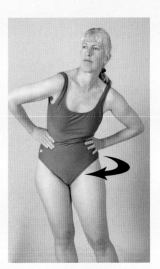

Belly Dancer

While standing, place your hands on your hips and rotate your hips around in as full a circle as is comfortable. Then rotate in the opposite direction.

Also Check

Gluteus minimus (62, posterior portion), Pelvic floor muscles (32, levator ani and coccygeus). Gluteus maximus (30). Gluteus medius (31).

Differential Diagnosis

If you are unable to relieve your symptoms with trigger point self-help techniques, or feel pain on both sides, you will need an MRI to rule out spinal stenosis of the central canal (narrowing of the hole that the spinal cord goes through). Acupuncture can help with the pain, but will not change the spinal stenosis. Surgery may be warranted if the pain is severe enough.

Arthritis in the sacroiliac joint, or other types of arthritis, may cause trigger points to develop in the piriformis and may need to be ruled out.

30 Gluteus Maximus

The *gluteus maximus* muscle attaches to the top of the pelvis, sacrum, and tailbone (*coccyx*) toward the midline of the body, and to the iliotibial band and thigh bone (*femur*) on the other end. It can be more than one inch in thickness. Its large size and fiber orientation is what allows us to stand erect on two legs, and is one of the features that distinguishes humans from other animals, including other primates. The gluteus maximus is a powerful muscle that extends the thigh at the hip and assists in rotation of the thigh away from the midline. It is used for running, jumping, climbing stairs, hiking uphill, swimming, and rising from a seated position.

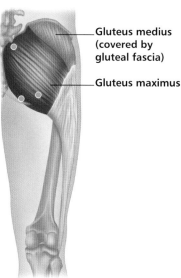

Gluteus medius
(covered by
gluteal fascia)

Gluteus maximus

Common Symptoms

■ Pain referred to the gluteal region, the lower part of the sacrum, sacroiliac joint (where the sacrum and the big pelvic bone meet), and/or tailbone, mostly very close to where the trigger points are located. Pain may feel like it is in the tailbone when sitting, though the trigger point is really off to the side a little.

■ The trigger point along the bottom curve of the butt can refer pain deep within the buttock, or it may feel like a nail pressing on the bone when sitting in a hard seat.

■ Pain is aggravated by walking uphill, especially if you are bent forward, and with swimming, especially in cold water.

■ Restricted range of motion when combined with hamstring tightness.

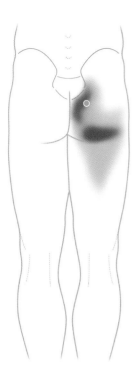 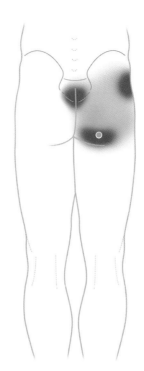 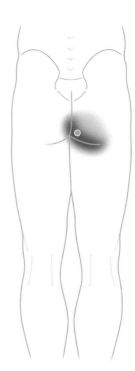

Causes and Perpetuation of Trigger Points, and Solutions

◼ Poor body mechanics, such as walking uphill for a long time while leaning forward, frequently bending over and lifting instead of lifting with your legs, sitting on a wallet in your back pocket, or sitting for too long in one position, particularly if you are reclining and your legs are straight.

Solutions
◼ Leaning forward over work surfaces or sinks and hiking uphill should be limited until trigger points are inactivated. Lifting properly requires bending at the knees, but this places a greater load on the gluteus maximus, so avoid lifting until trigger points are inactivated. If you must lift, bend down on one knee, and then place your hand on your thigh to assist you in rising again. When getting up from a chair, place your hand on your thigh to assist you.
◼ Do not put a wallet in your back pocket. Do not sit for more than 15 to 20 minutes at a time. Walk around briefly before sitting again. Setting a timer placed on the other side of the room will help you to remember to take breaks.

◼ Sleeping on one side with your upper leg pulled up toward your chest and no pillow support underneath it, or sleeping on your back with your legs straight for long periods of time.

Solutions
◼ Place a pillow under your knees if you sleep on your back. When lying on your side, place a pillow between your legs.

◼ Sports activities, such as swimming, especially the crawl stroke and possibly the breaststroke, or leg lifts in either standing or lying positions.

Solutions
◼ If you swim, replace the crawl and breaststroke with the backstroke or sidestroke. Do not do leg lifts.

■ Trauma to the area, such as a direct blow to the muscle, a fall, or a near-fall as your muscles contract to prevent the fall, or receiving intramuscular injections, especially with an irritant medication.

Solutions

■ If you have had an injury, do the self-help techniques below. If you receive intramuscular injections, ask your practitioner if you can switch to the deltoid or thigh muscles. If that is not possible, have the practitioner select sites that are not tender.

■ Structural imbalances, such as the sacroiliac joint being out of alignment, standing with your head too far forward, an anatomical leg-length inequality, or having a big toe that is shorter than the second toe, which causes excessive pronation.

Solutions

■ See a chiropractor or osteopathic physician to see if your sacroiliac joint needs to be adjusted. See chapter 7 for a postural retraining exercise. A true anatomical leg-length inequality of ¼" or more needs to be corrected with a compensating lift. If you have a short big toe and long second toe, wear corrective orthotics to prevent pronation. See chapters 2 and 4 for more information.

Self-Help Techniques

Applying Pressure

Thoracolumbar Paraspinal Pressure
Tightness in the opposite thoracolumbar paraspinal muscles (18) can tilt and rotate the pelvis, causing pain in the hip joint and trigger points in the gluteal muscles. Be sure to work on the thoracolumbar paraspinals first (*both* sides), and then the gluteal muscles on both right *and* left sides.

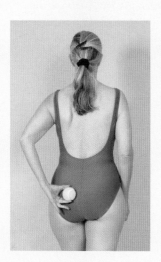
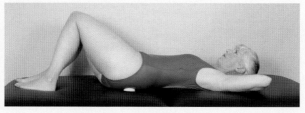
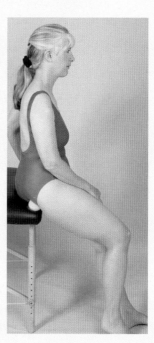

Gluteus Maximus Pressure
Lying face-up, use a tennis ball on the bed to search for trigger points in the gluteal area. In particular, search along the edge of the sacrum (the bony triangle below the spine). Be sure to work toward the bottom of the butt. You may find the lower trigger points are easier to access by leaning against a padded surface such as a couch arm, where you can get pressure on the lower curve of the buttocks and near the tailbone.

Stretches

Low Back Stretching Exercise

See chapter 18 for this stretch, which also benefits the gluteus maximus muscle. Eventually, over time, you should be able to bring your thigh all the way to your chest without pain.

Abdominal Stretch

If the rectus abdominis (25) and iliopsoas (22) muscles contain trigger points, releasing the gluteus maximus can cause them to cramp. If this happens, you will need to stretch those muscles (see chapter 17).

Exercises

The gluteus maximus muscle is not used while riding a stationary bike. It is used only minimally with an increased workload and pedaling rate while bicycling outdoors, or with normal walking. This means that to condition the gluteus maximus once trigger points are inactivated, you must swim, hike uphill, jump, or do some other vigorous activity. Conditioning the gluteus maximus requires that you keep your heart rate within your optimal range for aerobic respiration rather than anaerobic respiration. You can find charts on the internet that will help you determine your optimal range based on your age.

Also Check

Gluteus medius (31). Hamstrings muscle group (56). Thoracolumbar paraspinal muscles (18). Gluteus minimus (62). Iliopsoas (22). Quadriceps femoris muscle group (65, rectus femoris).

31 Gluteus Medius

The *gluteus medius* muscle attaches toward the top of the pelvis on one end, and to the greater trochanter of the thigh bone (*femur*) on the other end. It stabilizes the pelvis when the weight is shifted primarily to the leg on the same side. This muscle is essential for endurance and full strength in walking and other more vigorous activities.

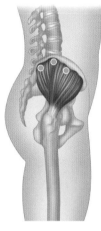

Pain from trigger points in the gluteus medius muscle is frequently referred to as *low back pain*, or *lumbago*, though many people refer to *lumbar* area pain as low back pain. To avoid confusion, I use the terms *lumbar area pain*, *gluteal area pain*, and *sacral area pain*, and avoid the use of the non-specific reference to low back pain.

Common Symptoms

- Pain referred over the sacrum, along the sacroiliac joint (where the sacrum and the big pelvic bone meet), and over the rest of the buttocks, depending on the site of the trigger point. TrP3 is very common in office workers and runners.
- Pain when sitting in a slumped position. Pain while walking, especially if you have a big toe that is shorter than the second toe. Difficulty sleeping on the affected side and possibly on the back.
- Trigger points may contribute to neck pain and headaches.

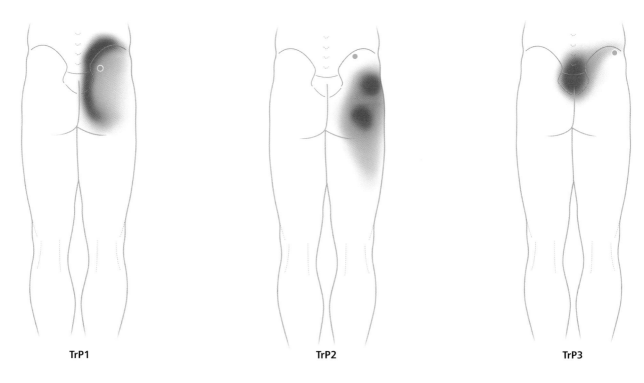

TrP1   TrP2   TrP3

Causes and Perpetuation of Trigger Points, and Solutions

■ Improper body mechanics and ergonomics, such as standing with your weight shifted to one leg for long periods of time, sitting in a chair that is too low, sitting on a wallet in your back pocket, and sleeping in the fetal position.

Solutions
■ Sit down while putting clothing and shoes on your lower body. Avoid sitting for too long in one position and do not cross your legs. Setting a timer placed on the other side of the room ensures that you get up periodically to turn it off. Do not carry a wallet in your back pocket. When sleeping on your side, place a pillow between your knees. The most comfortable position may be lying on the unaffected side, tilted back with your torso supported by a pillow behind you.

■ Sports injuries caused by running, playing long tennis matches, doing aerobic exercises, taking long walks on a sandy beach, or riding an upright bicycle, such as an exercise bike.

Solutions
■ It may be necessary to stop or modify activities that aggravate trigger points until you have inactivated them. You may need to do your self-help techniques before and after the activities.

■ Trauma to the area, such as a direct blow to the muscle, a fall, or a near-fall (as your muscles contract to prevent the fall), or receiving intramuscular injections, especially with an irritant medication.

Solutions
■ If you have had an injury, do the self-help techniques below. If you receive intramuscular injections, ask your practitioner if you can switch to the deltoid or thigh muscles. If that is not possible, have the practitioner select sites that are not tender.

■ Structural imbalances, such as the sacroiliac joint being out of alignment, standing with your head too far forward, an anatomical leg-length inequality, or having a big toe that is shorter than the second toe, which causes excessive pronation.

Solutions
■ See a chiropractor or osteopathic physician to see if your sacroiliac joint needs to be adjusted. See chapter 7 for a postural retraining exercise. A true leg-length inequality of ¼" or more needs to be corrected with a compensating lift. If you have a short big toe and long second toe, wear corrective orthotics to prevent pronation. See chapters 2 and 4.

Self-Help Techniques

If you only get temporary relief with self-treatment, check the quadratus lumborum muscle (28), since trigger points in that muscle can cause and perpetuate trigger points in the gluteus medius. Also check the piriformis muscle (29), since it frequently contains trigger points concurrently with the gluteus medius. If you continue to have pain after a back surgery intended to correct pain, search the entire gluteal area for potential trigger points.

Applying Pressure

Paraspinal Pressure
Tightness in the opposite paraspinal muscles (18) can tilt and rotate the pelvis, causing pain in the hip joint and trigger points in the gluteal muscles. Be sure to work on the paraspinals first (*both* sides), and then the gluteal muscles on both right *and* left sides.

Gluteus Medius Pressure
Common trigger points in the gluteus medius are higher up than most people think, so they are easy to miss. It is also usually tender lower down too, so you may think you have found the muscle, when in fact you have missed it. If you wear briefs or pants that come to your waist, the trigger points are just below your underpants line or your belt, just below the rim of the pelvis. They are also out to the side, so you have to work under the whole rim.

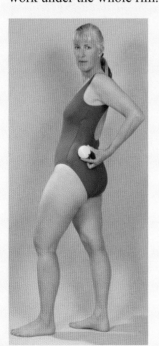

Lie face-up and place a ball close to your sacrum (the bony triangle in between the last lumbar vertebrae and the tailbone). Start working your way outward by moving the ball with your hand, following the rim of the pelvis. Keep going until you get all the way out to the side, to ensure that you have searched the entire muscle.

Stretches

Abductor Stretch

Lie on your bed with the front of your body next to the edge. With the leg on the bed slightly bent, drop the top leg over the edge in front of you, using gravity to give you a stretch.

Then, lying with your back to the edge of the bed, drop the top leg over the edge behind you. With both stretches, use deep breathing to assist in lengthening the stretch.

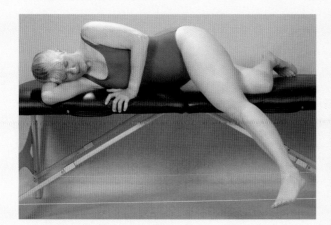 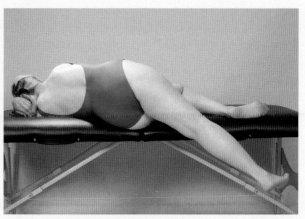

Also Check

Piriformis (29). Gluteus minimus (62). Gluteus maximus (30). Tensor fasciae latae (63). Quadratus lumborum (28).

Differential Diagnosis

If you are unable to relieve your symptoms with trigger point self-help techniques, you may need to see a health care provider to rule out intermittent claudication (narrowing of some of the major arteries) if you or your family has a history of heart or circulatory system problems, since that condition could cause trigger points in the gluteus medius and tensor fasciae latae muscles.

32 Pelvic Floor Muscles

Sphincter Ani, Transversus Perinei, Levator Ani, Coccygeus, Ischiocavernosus, Bulbospongiosus, Obturator Internus

The *pelvic floor muscles* are located, generally, in between the parts of the pelvic bones around the urogenital area. Most of the muscles control functions in the anus, penis, vagina, and urethra, except for the *coccygeus* which acts on the tailbone (*coccyx*) and sacroiliac joint, and the *obturator internus* which acts on the thigh.

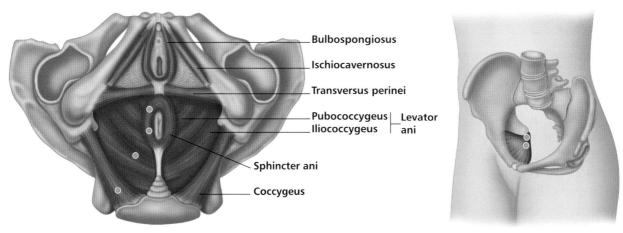

Bulbospongiosus
Ischiocavernosus
Transversus perinei
Pubococcygeus | Levator
Iliococcygeus | ani
Sphincter ani
Coccygeus

Obturator internus

Eighty-three percent of patients affected by trigger points in the pelvic floor muscles are female. Because the symptoms can be so distressing and so poorly diagnosed in relation to trigger points, I am including a chapter so that you can find a professional who can evaluate the presence of trigger points and their perpetuating factors. Although there is little you can do for self-help pressure and stretching techniques to treat trigger points, you can still address some of the potential perpetuating factors yourself.

Common Symptoms

Sphincter Ani

■ The area of referred pain includes the tailbone and often includes the anal area and the lower part of the sacrum (the triangular bone between the lumbar vertebrae and the tailbone), and may cause painful bowel movements. It is hard for the patient to explain exactly where the pain is and they usually describe it as tailbone, hip, or back pain.

Transversus Perinei

■ The area of referred pain includes the tailbone and often includes the anal area and the lower part of the sacrum. It is hard for the patient to explain exactly where the pain is and they usually describe it as tailbone, hip, or back pain.

Levator Ani (includes the *pubococcygeus* and *iliococcygeus* muscles)

■ The area of referred pain includes the tailbone and often includes the anal area and the lower part of the sacrum. It is hard for the patient to explain exactly where the pain is and they usually describe it as tailbone, hip, or back pain.

■ Trigger points may cause vaginal pain, especially during intercourse, or rectal pain or pain inside the pelvis. Sitting may be uncomfortable and pain may be aggravated by lying on the back or by having a bowel movement.

■ There may possibly be a relationship with constipation or frequent bowel movements.

■ Pain may be diagnosed as *coccygodynia*, although the tailbone itself is usually normal and not tender. Pain may also be diagnosed as *levator ani syndrome* or other similar terms.

Coccygeus

■ The area of referred pain includes the tailbone and often includes the anal area and the lower part of the sacrum. It is hard for the patient to explain exactly where the pain is and they usually describe it as tailbone, hip, or back pain.

■ Sitting may be painful.

■ Trigger points are likely to be a cause myofascial backache late in pregnancy and early on in labor.

■ Pain may be diagnosed as *coccygodynia*, although the tailbone itself is usually normal and not tender.

Ischiocavernosus

■ Trigger points are likely to refer pain to the genital area, such as the vagina and the base of the penis beneath the scrotum, or the area between the scrotum or vagina and the anus.

Bulbospongiosus

■ Trigger points are likely to refer pain to the genital area, such as the vagina and the base of the penis beneath the scrotum.

■ Trigger points may possibly cause aching pain in women in the area between the vagina and the anus, and possibly pain with intercourse, particularly during entry.

■ Trigger points may possibly cause pain in men in the region of the back of the scrotum, discomfort sitting erect, and sometimes a degree of impotence.

Obturator Internus (intrapelvic portion)

■ Trigger points may cause vaginal pain and also pain referred to the anal and tailbone areas and to the upper back of the thigh; there may be referred pain and a feeling of fullness in the rectum.

Post-Surgical Vaginal Wall Trigger Points

■ After a hysterectomy, trigger points may form in the vaginal wall, which can refer pain to the lower abdomen and uterine paracervical area. The patient usually describes the pain in what are familiar terms to them: *ovarian pain, menstrual cramps,* or *bladder spasms*; pressure on the vaginal trigger points reproduces the symptoms.

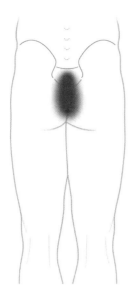 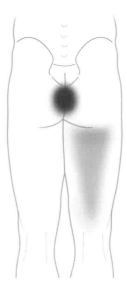

Causes and Perpetuation of Trigger Points, and Solutions

- Muscle spasm and tenderness can be caused by articular dysfunction at the sacroiliac junction (the slightly moveable joint where the sacrum and the big pelvic bone meet is not moving properly). Also, trigger points in the pelvic floor muscles that attach to the sacrum can destabilize the sacroiliac joint.
- Trigger points in the pelvic region can be activated by a severe fall, an auto accident, or surgery in that area.

Solutions

- See a chiropractor or osteopathic physician to identify and treat dysfunctions of the lumbrosacral, sacroiliac, and sacrococcygeal joints. Some physical therapists specialize in treating pelvic muscles and use a variety of techniques, including strengthening programs.

- Most of the time it is impossible for the person to identify a particular event that triggered the pain. In these cases, nutritional or other systemic perpetuating factors need to be identified and addressed.

Solutions

- See chapters 3 and 4.

- Levator ani trigger points can be activated by sitting with a slumped posture for long periods.

Solutions

- Sit upright with proper lumbar support (see chapter 2).

- Chronic inflammation such as hemorrhoids, endometriosis, chronic salpingo-oophoritis, chronic prostatovesiculitis, and interstitial cystitis have been associated with levator ani syndrome.

Solutions

- See a health care provider to diagnose and treat any chronic inflammation.

Treatment Techniques (for Practitioners)

Applying Pressure

The coccygeal region and the coccygeus muscle are more difficult to palpate from the vagina than the rectum because of the two layers of rectal mucosa and one layer of vaginal mucosa. For this reason, *a good exam and treatment must include both rectal and vaginal exams.*

The sphincter ani, levator ani, coccygeus, obturator internus, and sacrococcygeus ventralis muscles are best examined and treated through the rectum. First check for hemorrhoids, since they can make examination painful and be a cause of trigger points. If the anal sphincter has trigger points, this can also cause a great deal of pain, so the solution is to have the patient bear down to enhance relaxation as the practitioner slowly inserts a finger. If this is still too painful, try a vaginal exam.

In women, the bulbospongiosus muscle can only be examined vaginally. Parts of the coccygeus and obturator internus can be better examined vaginally. The transversus perinei, ischiocavernosus, and bulbospongiosus are examined externally in men, and the first two examined externally in women.

A detailed explanation of the examination of pelvic floor muscles is found in *Myofascial Pain and Dysfunction: The Trigger Point Manual,* Vol. 2, *The Lower Extremities* (Travell and Simons 1992, pp. 110–29).

Also Check

Gluteus maximus (30). Piriformis (29).

33 Shoulder, Upper Arm, and Elbow Pain

Many common conditions affecting the shoulder, upper arm, and elbow can be caused entirely or in part by trigger points, including *frozen shoulder, tennis elbow, and thoracic outlet syndrome.* Rotator cuff injuries can be caused by sudden stress on muscles that are already tight from trigger point contractions, and trigger points will form after the injury and prevent proper healing.

Frozen Shoulder

Trigger points in the subscapularis muscle (37) primarily cause severe painful restriction of motion, and the diagnosis of *frozen shoulder, adhesive capsulitis,* or *hemiplegia* is often used. These are general terms used to describe shoulder pain and restriction of movement, and are usually not a specific diagnosis of what is actually going on physiologically in the shoulder girdle. As symptoms get worse, the patient cannot lift their arm above shoulder level and cannot reach across their chest. Pain is constant whether using or resting the arm, but is worse with movement and at night. As trigger points in other muscles become involved, they each add their own pain patterns and restriction of movement.

Sometimes thickened tissues are found in the shoulder girdle area in the muscles, the synovial capsule, bursa, or ligaments, but the problem still likely began with trigger points in the subscapularis. In fact, trigger points in the subscapularis muscle can cause blood vessels to constrict, decreasing the amount of oxygen reaching the muscle cells, and can subsequently actually *form* fibrous, or thickened, tissues in adjacent muscles and lead to *true* adhesive capsulitis. Subscapularis trigger points and any trigger points in the surrounding affected muscles must be treated in order for therapy to be effective. The other muscles that typically get involved with the subscapularis in a frozen shoulder are the pectoralis major (23), latissimus dorsi (38), supraspinatus (34), and teres major (40).

Travell and Simons, in *Myofascial Pain and Dysfunction: The Trigger Point Manual, Vol. 1, The Upper Half of the Body* (1999, chapters 18 and 26), give a lengthy discussion of the use of the term frozen shoulder and treatment for the shoulder girdle area; I strongly encourage you to read this if your practitioner has used the diagnoses of adhesive capsulitis, *frozen shoulder,* or hemiplegia, and perhaps share the information with them. Often this condition is treated too aggressively in the initial stages, causing increased pain and involvement of additional muscles.

If you do the self-help for all of the muscles in this section, you will likely get a great deal of relief, or complete relief. Acupuncture is also very effective in treating pain and restricted range of motion in the shoulder area, usually coupled with use of a special "TDP" heating lamp and/or use of Moxa—a herb burned or sprayed over the local area. Chinese herbs may be prescribed. I definitely recommend trying other techniques before considering surgery, unless an MRI has determined that muscles, tendons, or ligaments are seriously torn or detached, in which case surgery is necessary.

Rotator Cuff Injuries

The subscapularis (37), supraspinatus (34), infraspinatus (35), and teres minor (39) are the four muscles that form the *rotator cuff*. Unfortunately, all too often, pain felt in the shoulder area is diagnosed as a rotator cuff injury without investigating the cause of the pain. A rotator cuff tear must be diagnosed by an MRI, and it is helpful to know which muscle or muscles contain the tear. Pain is more often due to trigger points in one of those areas. Even if a tear is confirmed, trigger points may also be present, especially if tightness in the muscle contributed to the overload that led to the tear.

Thoracic Outlet Syndrome

Thoracic outlet syndrome is a collection of symptoms rather than a specific disease, though it is often represented by health care providers as though it were a particular condition. There is wide disagreement and confusion in most medical literature about what symptoms define the condition and what causes it. Trigger points are frequently overlooked as a cause of abnormal tension in the scalene muscles, and are mostly likely a major cause of thoracic outlet syndrome, though it might more aptly be called *pseudo-thoracic outlet syndrome.*

Travell and Simons (1999, chapter 20, "Scalene Muscles") provide a lengthy discussion of the use of the term thoracic outlet syndrome, and I highly recommend that you read it if your health care provider has used this diagnosis, and share the information with them. It is definitely worth having a trained practitioner check all of the muscles listed below to see if you may be harboring trigger points, especially if you are considering surgery. Surgery has a less than 50% success rate for thoracic outlet syndrome, most likely because trigger points have not been considered or relieved. Additional problems often develop subsequent to the unsuccessful surgeries. There may be a few patients with anatomical abnormalities that require surgical correction for complete relief, but the majority of patients will have a higher success rate with non-surgical intervention.

Trigger points in the scalene (42), pectoralis major (23), latissimus dorsi (38), teres major (40), and subscapularis (37) muscles can all refer pain in patterns that mimic *thoracic outlet syndrome symptoms,* and are particularly confusing if more than one muscle develops trigger points, so be sure to check all of those muscles. The trapezius (8), pectoralis minor (43), and levator scapula (19) can also refer pain that gets diagnosed as thoracic outlet syndrome. The subclavius muscle (23) can become enlarged and may cause the first rib to be elevated and compress the subclavian vein, so check for trigger points in that muscle too, and see a chiropractor or osteopathic physician to determine if the first rib needs to be adjusted. Also check the supraspinatus (34), infraspinatus (35), sternocleidomastoid (10), and splenius capitis (9) for associated trigger points. Satellite trigger points tend to develop in the triceps (41), deltoid (44), pectoralis (23 and 43), and forearm (48) muscles.

Tennis Elbow

Muscle pain on the outside of the elbow is usually labeled *tennis elbow*. The trigger points that cause pain in that area are likely to develop in the following order: supinator (49); brachioradialis (48); extensor carpi radialis longus (48); extensor digitorum (48); triceps (41); anconeus (41); and the biceps (46) and brachialis (52) together. Check those muscle chapters and see if you can relieve your tennis elbow.

Solutions
Nighttime Lying Posture
With any shoulder, upper arm, or elbow problems, you may find it helpful to lie in one of the positions shown in these photos to reduce pain and other symptoms at night.

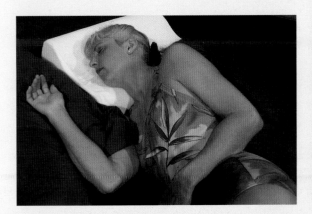 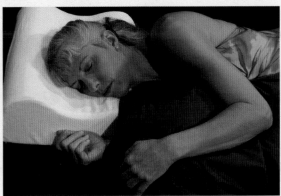

Each muscle chapter in this section will contain additional solutions for these conditions and others affecting this part of the body.

34 Supraspinatus

The *supraspinatus* is one of the muscles forming the *rotator cuff*, along with the infraspinatus, teres minor, and subscapularis muscles. It attaches to the top of the shoulder blade (*scapula*) and to the bone in the upper arm (*humerus*). It stabilizes the humerus and moves the arm away from the body.

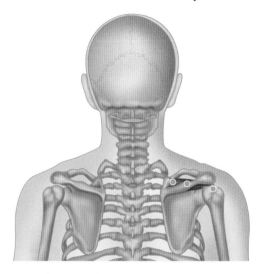

Pain felt in the shoulder area may often be diagnosed as a rotator cuff injury (see chapter 33) without investigating the cause of the pain, and it may actually be from trigger point referral instead. Pain from supraspinatus trigger points may also be misdiagnosed as subdeltoid bursitis, though both bursitis and trigger points may be present concurrently.

Common Symptoms

▥ A deep ache in the shoulder area, mainly around the outside of the upper end of the upper arm, and it may also be felt strongly in the elbow and/or run down the outside of the arm, sometimes all the way to the wrist. Pain is more of a dull ache while resting the arm, but more intense when lifting the arm.

▥ An inability to reach behind your back and touch the opposite shoulder blade with your fingers. A moderately restricted range of motion is also noticeable when reaching toward the head or participating in sports.

▥ The shoulder may make clicking or snapping sounds, probably due to the tight muscle interfering with the normal glide of the shoulder joint.

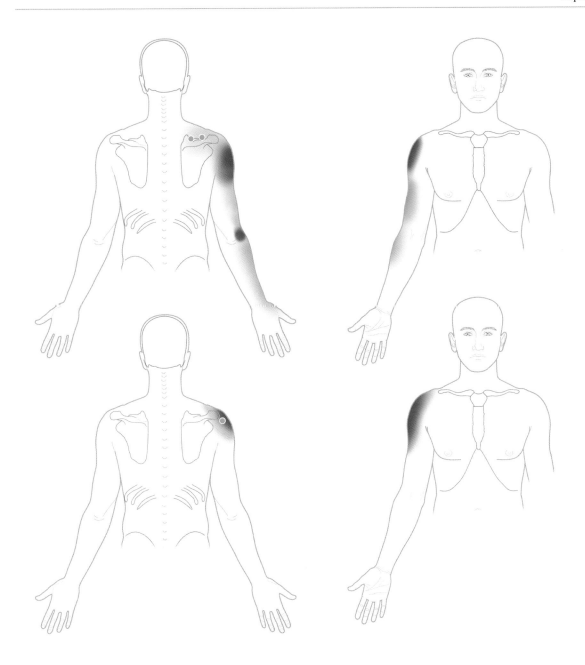

Causes and Perpetuation of Trigger Points, and Solutions

▨ Carrying heavy objects with your arm at your side (e.g. heavy purse, laptop, briefcase, or luggage), or lifting a heavy object to or above shoulder height.

Solutions
▨ Purchase luggage with wheels or ask for help with carrying it. Use a daypack instead of a briefcase or heavy purse, or use a shoulder strap that you can wear diagonally across your torso. Do not lift items overhead or hold your arms out or up continuously.

▨ Walking a dog that pulls at the leash.

Solutions
▨ Get a head halter for a dog that pulls—it will prevent most breeds from pulling.

Self-Help Techniques

Be sure to also check the infraspinatus (35) and trapezius (8) muscles, since they are nearly always involved as well. Work on the deltoid muscle (44) *after* these muscles, since it tends to develop satellite trigger points. You may also need to work the latissimus dorsi muscle (38).

Applying Pressure

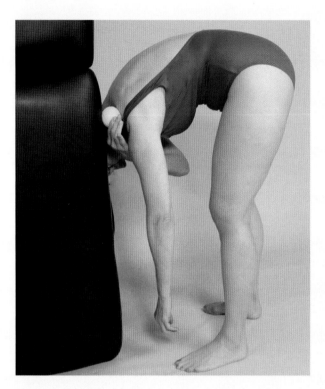

Supraspinatus Pressure

Stand in a doorway and place a tennis ball in the groove in the doorjamb, and continue to hold onto the ball with your opposite hand. Bend over at about 90 degrees *and be sure to let your head go completely limp!* Lean into the ball with however much pressure you want to apply. Still holding onto the ball with your opposite hand and continuing to keep your head fully relaxed, work spots across the top of the shoulder.

Stretches

Infraspinatus Stretch

The infraspinatus stretch will also benefit the supraspinatus (see chapter 35). If there is any suspicion of a tear in one of the rotator cuff muscles, *do not stretch this muscle until a tear is ruled out by an MRI. Prior to getting an MRI, or if a tear is confirmed, only do the pressure technique above.*

Also Check

Infraspinatus (35). Trapezius (8). Deltoid (44, satellite trigger points). Latissimus dorsi (38). Subscapularis (37). Teres minor (39).

Differential Diagnosis

If you are unable to relieve your symptoms with trigger point self-help techniques, you may need to see a health care provider to rule out cervical arthritis or spurs with nerve root irritation, entrapment of the suprascapular nerve, or a brachial plexus injury. Subdeltoid bursitis, rotator cuff tears, and supraspinatus trigger points may all cause tenderness where the tendons of the rotator cuff muscles attach at the shoulder joint, but only trigger points will cause spot tenderness in the mid portion of the supraspinatus muscle. A rotator cuff tear causes severe pain and usually exhibits a limited arc of motion, and must be diagnosed by an MRI. You may need to see a chiropractor or osteopathic physician to be evaluated for a C5 or C6 vertebra out of alignment.

35 Infraspinatus

The *infraspinatus* muscle lies over the back of the shoulder blade (*scapula*) and attaches to the bone of the upper arm (*humerus*). It stabilizes that end of the humerus and rotates the upper arm. Trigger points in this area are becoming increasingly common as people spend more time on computers, especially on the side used as the "mouse arm."

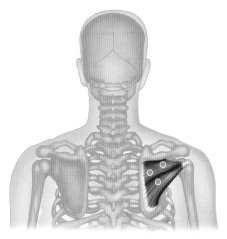

The infraspinatus is one of the four muscles comprising the *rotator cuff*; the other three are the supraspinatus, teres minor, and subscapularis. Unfortunately, pain felt in the shoulder area is often misdiagnosed as a rotator cuff injury (see chapter 33) without investigating the cause of the pain, and it may actually be from trigger point referral instead.

Common Symptoms

▦ Referred pain on the front of the shoulder and deep within the joint. Pain may also refer into the forearm and occasionally the fingers, or into the base of the skull. Occasionally, pain will refer to the mid back area over the rhomboid muscles and sometimes this will activate and perpetuate the lower trapezius trigger points, which must be inactivated before infraspinatus trigger points can be inactivated.

▦ Possibly referred pain when sleeping on either the affected or the opposite side at night, which then disrupts sleep.

▦ The arm may "fall asleep" at night and sometimes even during the day.

▦ Loss of mobility, including difficulty reaching behind the back or sometimes raising the arm to the head in front.

▦ Shoulder girdle fatigue, weakness of grip, and lack of power with tennis strokes.

▦ Hyperhydrosis in the area of pain referral (excessive sweating at times that you would not normally sweat, i.e. not due to exercising or extreme heat).

▦ Entrapment of the suprascapular nerve by concurrently tight infraspinatus and supraspinatus muscles can cause shoulder pain and atrophy of the infraspinatus muscle.

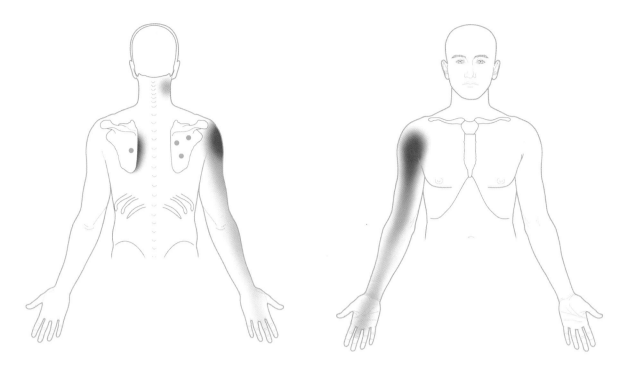

Causes and Perpetuation of Trigger Points, and Solutions

■ Anything that requires you to hold your arms out in front of you or above your head for extended periods of time with your arms not well supported, such as computer use (especially your "mouse arm"), kayaking, driving, or tennis.

■ Pulling a sled, wagon, or person behind you, or reaching behind you to get something off a night stand.

■ A sudden overload of the muscle by catching yourself while attempting to prevent a fall, or trying to hold onto something heavy.

Solutions

■ Modify or replace your misfitting furniture and pay attention to your body mechanics. See chapter 2 for more information, especially the section on your computer workstation. If you cannot avoid doing activities that require you to hold your arms out in front for extended periods, take frequent breaks or switch arms periodically. Do not lift heavy objects until your trigger points are inactivated. You will need to use something similar to a shopping cart instead of a wagon or sled for moving objects, since you will need to push rather than pull.

■ Apply heat packs to the muscle at bedtime for 15 to 20 minutes. As always with the application of heat, be sure to rest the pack on the muscle, rather than lying on the heat pack, which can cut off needed circulation and cause burns. Lie on the side that is not bothering you and drape the affected arm over a pillow for support.

■ Hard tennis serves or pushing yourself with ski poles.

Solutions

■ You will have to stop or modify these activities—try changing arms with your tennis serve or serving more gently, and skate with your skis rather than pushing with your poles.

Self-Help Techniques

Also check the teres minor (39), supraspinatus (34), deltoid (44), biceps (46), teres major (40), pectoralis major (23), subscapularis (37), and latissimus dorsi (38) for trigger points, since some of these muscles are usually also involved.

Applying Pressure

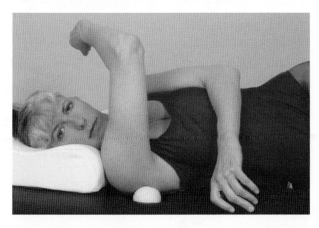

Infraspinatus Pressure

This is one of the more challenging muscles to teach, as patients nearly always initially work in the rhomboid area, thinking they have succeeded in finding the infraspinatus since the rhomboid area is almost always tender as well. Lie on the affected side, with your arm out at an angle of approximately 90 degrees, and thoroughly search the back of your shoulder blade. If you are lying on your back, you are probably getting too far in toward the spine. I find it is helpful to have the patient reach under their arm and locate the muscle with their fingertips first, as with most people this is where their fingers will reach. Be sure to work all the way out to the armpit and then you will know you are treating the correct area. Most people will need to do this on the bed with a fairly soft ball, since this muscle is usually quite tender.

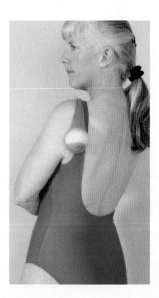
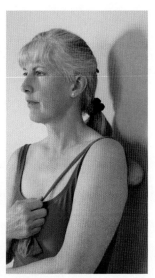

If lying on the affected side is too painful, an alternative is to put a ball in a long sock, dangle the sock over your shoulder, and lean against a wall or couch with however much pressure is comfortable. Remember you will need to angle your body out a little bit from the wall or couch, otherwise you will get in too close to the spine and miss the infraspinatus muscle. The affected arm should be totally relaxed. When the tenderness decreases, start performing your self-treatment on the bed, since this is the preferred position.

Stretches

Infraspinatus Stretch
Stretch by grasping the affected arm above the elbow and bring your arm across your chest.

Then put your affected arm behind your back, use the opposite hand to grasp at the wrist, and gently pull on the arm. You can do this in a shower to help facilitate the stretch.

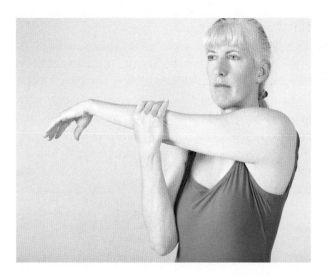
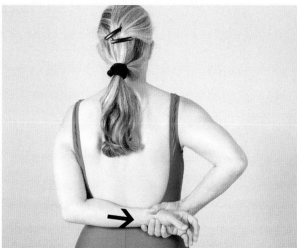

Also Check

Supraspinatus (34). Teres minor (39). Deltoid (44, anterior and posterior portions, satellite trigger points). Biceps brachii (46). Pectoralis major (23). Teres major (40). Latissimus dorsi (38). Subscapularis (37).

Differential Diagnosis
If you are unable to relieve your symptoms with trigger point self-help techniques, you may need to see a health care provider to rule out entrapment of the suprascapular nerve at the spinoglenoid notch where it passes from the supraspinatus to the infraspinatus muscle. This can be diagnosed by a test for prolonged nerve conduction latency and/or atrophy of the infraspinatus, and the abnormality causing it confirmed by an MRI or ultrasound. Arthritis in the shoulder joint can also cause a similar pain pattern.

Since infraspinatus trigger point pain referral patterns are the same as those of C5, C6 and C7 nerve root irritation due to disc problems, the latter needs to be confirmed by considering additional neurological problems and electromyographic findings. If you have been unsuccessfully treated for bicipital tendonitis or scapulohumeral syndrome, check the infraspinatus, biceps, pectoralis major, and pectoralis minor for trigger points. A rotator cuff tear causes severe pain and usually exhibits a limited arc of motion, and must be confirmed by an MRI.

36 Serratus Posterior Superior

The *serratus posterior superior* muscle attaches to *fascia* (connective tissue) which attaches to vertebrae C6 through T2 at the midline, and to the second through fifth ribs underneath the shoulder blade (*scapula*). Trigger points located underneath the scapula can be particularly aggravated by pressure from the scapula.

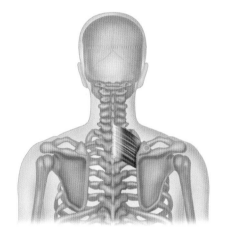

Trigger point under scapula (shoulder blade)

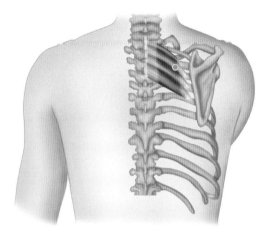

Trigger point palpable with the shoulder blade and arm moved forward

This muscle frequently contains trigger points and often gets missed by practitioners because the shoulder blade needs to be moved out of the way in order to access the most common trigger point. Placing the arm over the side of the massage table moves the shoulder blade forward and exposes the trigger point.

Common Symptoms

- Pain referred over the shoulder blade (often a deep ache), down the back of the arm and into the little finger. Pain may be increased by lifting objects out in front of you and by lying on the affected side, due to the shoulder blade pressing on the trigger points.
- Occasionally pain may be felt in the upper chest area.
- There may be referred numbness into the hand.

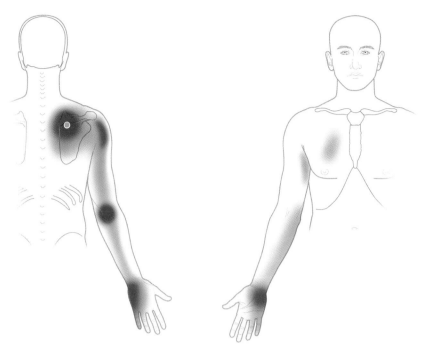

Trigger point is under the shoulder blade

Causes and Perpetuation of Trigger Points, and Solutions

▦ Writing at a high desk or table, or frequently reaching far forward.

Solutions

▦ Use a lumbar support at work, at home, and while traveling. See page 15, "Ergonomics," for a proper workstation setup. Modify your workstation so that everything is easily accessible, in order to avoid reaching forward frequently.

▦ Coughing, asthma, emphysema, and improper breathing techniques.

Solutions

▦ See page 34 for solutions to resolve a chronic cough. See page 55 to learn proper breathing techniques.

▦ Severe scoliosis.

Solutions

▦ Some scoliosis will be corrected with trigger point pressure self-treatment. You may also need to see a chiropractor or osteopathic physician. If you have an anatomically shorter leg or a small hemipelvis (either the left or the right half of the pelvic bone), be sure to see a specialist to be fitted for compensating lifts and pads. See page 30, "Spinal and Skeletal Factors," for more information.

▦ The shoulder blade compressing the muscle against the underlying rib when lying down.

Solutions

▦ Lie on the side that is not bothering you and drape the affected arm over a pillow for support.

Self-Help Techniques

Also check the scalene muscles (42), since trigger points in those muscles may cause trigger points in the serratus posterior superior, or occasionally vice versa. The rhomboid muscle (20) and the iliocostalis thoracis, longissimus thoracis, and multifidi muscles (18) may contain related trigger points.

Applying Pressure

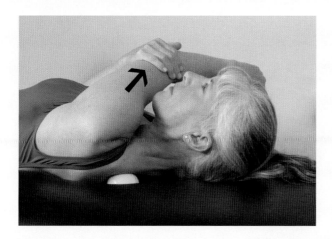

Serratus Posterior Superior Pressure

This one is a little tricky to get with the ball. You must hold your arm across your chest while lying on the ball, and be sure to get all the way up next to the top of the inner edge of the shoulder blade. It will also likely be tender lower, so you may think you have treated the trigger point, but have actually missed it. If you do not hold your arm across your chest, your arm will drop down a little bit and the shoulder blade will cover the trigger point. You may want to seek the help of a massage therapist to make sure you are finding this trigger point.

Also Check

Scalene muscles (42). Rhomboid (20). Thoracolumbar paraspinal muscles (18).

Differential Diagnosis

If you are unable to relieve your symptoms with trigger point self-help techniques, you may need to see a health care provider to be evaluated for thoracic outlet syndrome, a C7/C8 nerve root irritation, olecranon bursitis, and ulnar neuropathy. Referred numbness from serratus posterior superior trigger points into the C8/T1 distribution of the hand may be mistaken for a nerve root irritation, so be sure to check for trigger points if you have been given this diagnosis. You may need to see a chiropractor or osteopathic physician for evaluation of a T1 vertebra out of alignment. There will usually be tenderness over the vertebrae if this is the case.

37 Subscapularis

The *subscapularis* muscle attaches to the anterior (front) surface of the shoulder blade (*scapula*), between the shoulder blade and the rib cage, making it difficult to access more than just a small portion of the muscle with finger pressure. It also attaches to the bone in the upper arm (*humerus*) and keeps this bone in the shoulder joint during arm movement while also helping to move the upper arm.

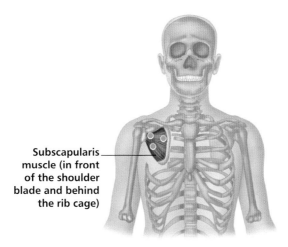

Subscapularis muscle (in front of the shoulder blade and behind the rib cage)

The subscapularis is one of the muscles of the *rotator cuff* and can be the primary muscle involved in a frozen shoulder. Referred pain from the subscapularis, latissimus dorsi (38), teres major (40), scalene (42), and pectoralis major (23) muscles can be misdiagnosed as thoracic outlet syndrome. See chapter 33 for a discussion of both of these conditions.

Common Symptoms

▥ Severe pain referred primarily over the back of the deltoid area, with possibly some referral over the shoulder blade, down the triceps area, and possibly a strap-like area of referred pain and tenderness around the wrist, which is worse on the back side.

▥ Restricted range of motion, often severely limited as the condition progresses, including an inability to reach backward with the arm at shoulder level, as when throwing a ball.

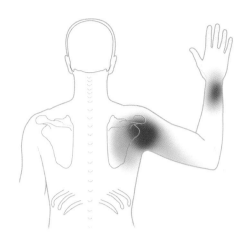 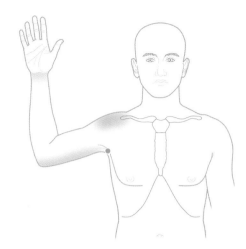

Causes and Perpetuation of Trigger Points, and Solutions

■ Overuse of muscles that are not accustomed to repetitive motions, such as the crawl stroke or pitching a ball, or repeated forceful overhead lifting, as when swinging a child up and down.
■ Slumped posture.

Solutions
■ See chapter 2, "Ergonomics" and "Body Mechanics," to correct sitting and work postures. See chapter 7 for an exercise to restore proper posture. You will need to stop doing any of the repetitive motions mentioned above until trigger points are relieved.
■ When you sleep on the affected side or on your back, use a pillow between your trunk and upper arm to keep your arm out at a 90-degree angle. When the affected side is toward the ceiling, drape your arm over a pillow. When sitting, move your arm frequently, resting it on the back of the couch or car seat, or on an armrest. When standing, hook your thumb in your belt.

■ Sudden trauma, such as reaching back to stop yourself from falling, catching an object from falling, dislocating your shoulder, breaking the upper arm, or tearing the shoulder joint capsule.
■ Long-term immobilization, such as in a cast or a shoulder splint.

Solutions
■ Treat all of the muscles listed below, in addition to reviewing chapter 33.

Self-Help Techniques

Related trigger points may also be found in the teres major (40), latissimus dorsi (38), pectoralis major (23), infraspinatus (35), and teres minor (39), so be sure to also check those muscles.

Applying Pressure

Treating this muscle will require the assistance of a therapist of some kind, as the subscapularis is difficult to access on your own for applying pressure.

Stretches

Pectoralis Stretch

Stretching the pectoralis muscles will help treat the subscapularis muscle. After application of heat over the shoulder blade and pectoralis major areas, do the stretch in chapter 17.

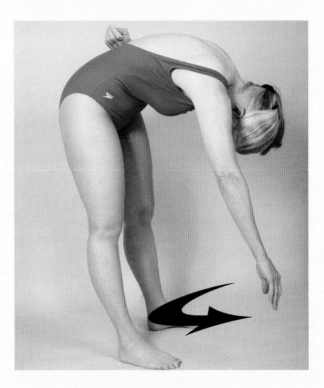

Subscapularis Stretch

Lean over with your arm hanging down and swing your arm in a wide circle in a clockwise direction for the left arm and a counter clockwise direction for the right arm. Be sure to keep your head totally relaxed.

You may also stretch this muscle by resting your arm across the back of a car seat or couch, by reaching your arm up and behind your head, or by reaching toward the ceiling.

Also Check

Pectoralis major (23). Teres major (40). Latissimus dorsi (38). Triceps brachii (41, satellite trigger points). Deltoid (44, satellite trigger points). Supraspinatus (34). Infraspinatus (35). Teres minor (39).

Differential Diagnosis

Pain from subscapularis trigger points can either mimic or occur concurrently with rotator cuff tears, adhesive capsulitis, a C7 nerve root irritation, a true thoracic outlet syndrome, or a nerve impingement, so you may need to see a health care provider and undergo an MRI or other diagnostic tests to check for those conditions. In true adhesive capsulitis, an arthrogram contrast medium shows that the normally rounded outline of the capsule is replaced by a squat, square contracted patch, along with restrictions of the joint volume, serration of the bursal attachments, failure to fill the biceps tendon sheath, and partial obliteration of subscapular and axillary recesses. Adhesive capsulitis exhibits less pain and more rigidity than that caused by trigger points, and often requires short-term oral steroids. A rotator cuff tear causes severe pain and usually exhibits a limited arc of motion.

38 Latissimus Dorsi

The *latissimus dorsi* muscle attaches at the body's midline to vertebrae T7 through L5 and the sacrum, out along the top edge of the pelvis, and to the last three or four ribs. The fibers gather together at the back wall of the armpit to attach to the bone of the upper arm (*humerus*). It moves the arm in various directions and can be used to bring the shoulder girdle in a downward direction.

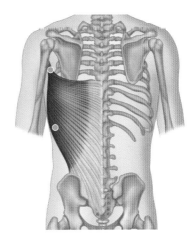

This muscle is an often-overlooked source of trigger point referral, primarily because there are many other muscles that cause symptom referral in the same area. If you have pain in this area and treating other muscles has given none or only temporary relief, be sure to check the latissimus dorsi for tenderness. If you are unable to identify any particular activity that aggravates mid back pain, this muscle may be the culprit.

The latissimus dorsi may be involved in a frozen shoulder, and referred pain from this muscle and other muscles can be misdiagnosed as thoracic outlet syndrome. See chapter 33 for a discussion of these conditions and the other muscles that may be involved.

Common Symptoms

▨ The main referral is a constant, dull ache under and adjacent to the bottom of the shoulder blade. Pain can sometimes travel down the arm and into the ring and little fingers.

▨ The upper trigger point is more common. There is a less common trigger point on the side above the waist that refers pain to the front of the shoulder and sometimes just above the hip area.

▨ Initially pain may *only* be caused by lifting a heavy object in front of you and not felt at rest. It is difficult to obtain relief by moving around, and pain will be worse as you reach up and out with a heavy object in your hands.

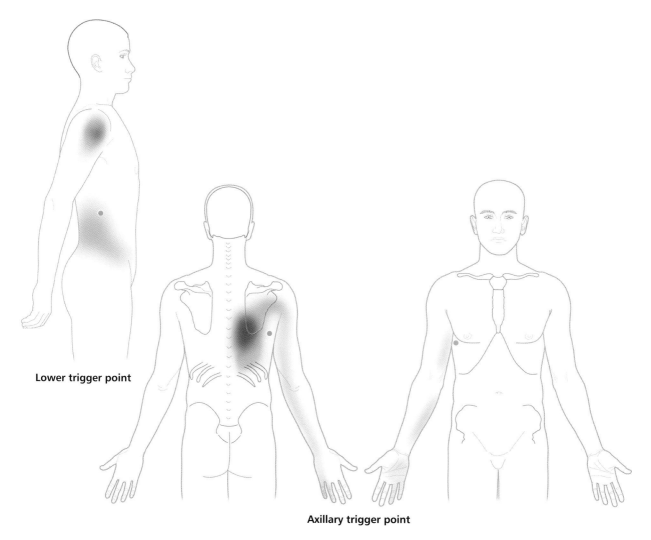

Lower trigger point

Axillary trigger point

Causes of and Perpetuation of Trigger Points, and Solutions

■ Carrying boxes or other heavy objects in front of you, or working with a heavy chainsaw or other tool at shoulder level.
■ Activities such as weight lifting or pulling weights down overhead, hanging from a swing or rope, aggressively swimming the butterfly stroke, throwing a baseball, throwing heavy bags of laundry or other objects repeatedly, or weeding a garden.

Solutions

■ Avoid reaching up and above to hold or retrieve objects. Use a foot stool or stepladder if necessary. If you must pull down on something, keep your upper arm at your side. Modify or cease any aggravating activities.
■ At night, avoid drawing your arm tightly into your body. Instead, try to keep your elbow out away from your body—you may try putting a pillow next to your trunk to help with this.

■ A tight bra strap around your chest.

Solutions

■ Wear bras that fit properly. If you see elastic marks on your skin after you take your bra off, the straps are too tight. See page 19, "Clothing," for more information.

Self-Help Techniques

Check the serratus posterior superior (36), since pain referral from that muscle can cause trigger points in the latissimus dorsi. Also check the teres major (40) and triceps (41), since these muscles will often concurrently develop trigger points with the latissimus dorsi.

Applying Pressure

Latissimus Dorsi Pressure
With the arm of the affected side resting on the back of a couch, use the opposite hand to reach under the armpit and pinch an area about one inch below the armpit. Be sure to pinch as close to the rib cage as possible, rather than just pinching a fold of skin. Pressing with the fingers may be more effective for some people and will

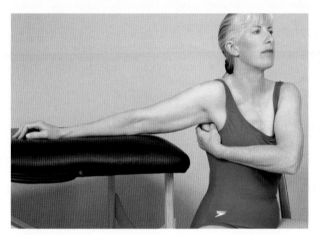 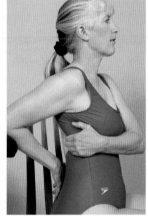

be effective for reaching the lower trigger points too.

You may also try lying on a tennis or racquet ball if the muscle is not too tender. Lie on the bed, with your arm out straight above your head—the tender spot will likely be just below the armpit.

Stretches

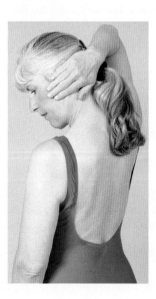 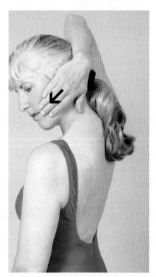

Latissimus Dorsi Stretch
Wrap the hand of the affected side behind your head and, if possible, touch your fingers to your opposite ear. Reach even further forward if you are not forcing the stretch. Ideally you will eventually be able to reach all the way to the corner of your mouth.

Pectoralis Stretch
Stretching the pectoralis muscles will help treat the latissimus dorsi muscle (see chapter 17).

Follow both stretches with a hot pack applied for 15 to 20 minutes. Lay the hot pack on you, rather than lying on the hot pack, which can cut off needed circulation and cause burns.

Also Check

Teres major (40). Triceps brachii (41, satellite trigger points). Abdominal muscles (25, rectus abdominis, upper portion). Subscapularis (37). Thoracolumbar paraspinal muscles (18, iliocostalis thoracis, satellite trigger points). Serratus anterior (26). Serratus posterior superior (36). Serratus posterior inferior (21). Hand and finger flexors (51, satellite trigger points). Trapezius (8, lower portion, satellite trigger points).

Differential Diagnosis

If you are unable to relieve your symptoms with trigger point self-help techniques, you may need to see a health care provider to rule out entrapment of the suprascapular nerve at the spine of the scapula, a C7 nerve root irritation, or an ulnar neuropathy, all diagnosed through electrodiagnostic examinations. Bicipital tendonitis may be caused by trigger points in the biceps muscle. You may need to see a chiropractor or osteopathic physician to be evaluated for innominate dysfunction or misalignment of any of the vertebrae between and including T7 to L4. The head of the humerus (upper arm bone) may need to be checked for its position in the shoulder joint.

39

Teres Minor

The *teres minor* muscle attaches near the outer edge of the shoulder blade (*scapula*) and to the bone in the upper arm (*humerus*). It helps stabilize the humerus while the arm is being moved and rotates the upper arm at the shoulder joint.

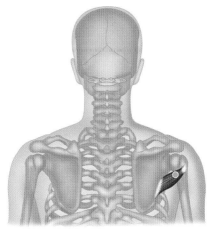

The teres minor is one of the four muscles forming the *rotator cuff*, along with the infraspinatus, supraspinatus, and subscapularis, and usually only harbors trigger points if the infraspinatus is also involved. Unfortunately, pain felt in the shoulder area is often misdiagnosed as a rotator cuff injury (see chapter 33) without investigating the cause of the pain, and it may actually be from trigger point referral instead.

Common Symptoms

- Localized referred pain deep in the posterior deltoid, which is likely only noticeable after infraspinatus trigger points have been inactivated.

- Possibly numbness and tingling of the ring and little fingers, which is aggravated by reaching above shoulder height or behind the body.

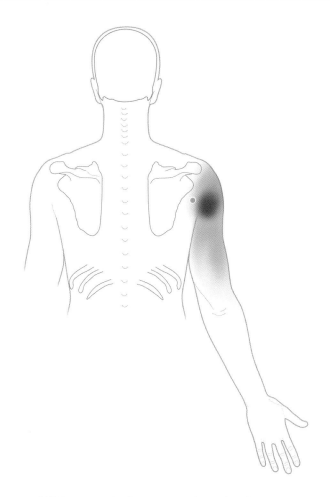

Causes and Perpetuation of Trigger Points, and Solutions

▪ A sudden overload of the muscle by catching yourself while attempting to prevent a fall, holding onto something such as the steering wheel during an auto accident, or trying to hold onto something heavy.

▪ Anything that requires you to hold your arms out in front of or above you for extended periods of time with the arms not well supported, such as computer use (especially your "mouse arm"), kayaking, driving, or tennis. Repetitively reaching for something behind you.

Solutions

▪ Modify or replace your misfitting furniture and pay attention to your body mechanics. See chapter 2 for more information, especially the section on your computer station. If you cannot avoid doing activities that require you to hold your arms out in front for extended periods, take frequent breaks or switch arms periodically. Do not lift heavy objects until your trigger points are inactivated.

▪ Apply heat packs to the muscle at bedtime for 15 to 20 minutes. As always with the application of heat, be sure to rest the pack on the muscle, rather than lying on the heat pack, which can cut off needed circulation and cause burns. Sleep with your arm out at a 90-degree angle and put a pillow between your upper arm and trunk if necessary.

Self-Help Techniques

Applying Pressure

Infraspinatus Pressure
Read the infraspinatus muscle chapter (35) and be sure to perform the self-help on that muscle first before working on the teres minor.

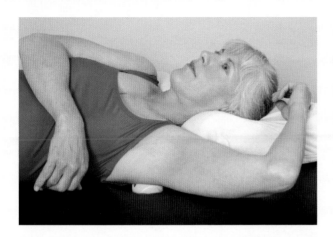

Teres Minor Pressure
After working on the infraspinatus, continue with the ball out toward the upper arm. The muscle is in the dip between the trunk and upper arm, behind the back wall of the armpit. Lie on your side with your arm extended up a little bit toward your head. If you want less pressure, put your head on a pillow *behind* the upper arm. If you want more pressure, rest your head *on* your upper arm. Using a tennis or racquet ball, work all the way from the outer edge of the shoulder blade to about a quarter of the way down your upper arm.

Stretches

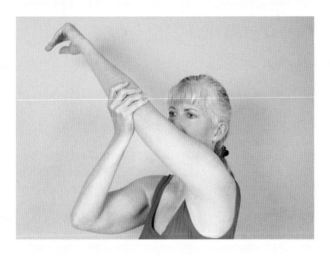

Teres Minor Stretch
Stretch by grasping the affected arm above the elbow and bring your arm up and across your face.

Also Check

Infraspinatus (35).

Differential Diagnosis
If you are unable to relieve your symptoms with trigger point self-help techniques, you may need to see a health care provider for further diagnostic testing. Symptoms of quadrilateral space syndrome include shoulder pain and selective atrophy of the teres minor muscle due to compression of the axillary nerve by fibrous bands as it passes through the quadrilateral space, and can be diagnosed by an MRI. Numbness and tingling of the ring and little fingers can be confused with ulnar neuropathy or C8 nerve root irritation, and can be diagnosed by an electrodiagnostic evaluation. Subdeltoid bursitis can cause symptoms similar to pain referred from teres minor trigger points. If there has been an impactful injury, an acromioclavicular separation may need to be ruled out. A rotator cuff tear causes severe pain and usually exhibits a limited arc of motion, and must be confirmed by an MRI.

40 Teres Major

The *teres major* muscle attaches near the bottom of the shoulder blade (*scapula*) and to the bone in the upper arm (*humerus*). Along with the latissimus dorsi, it forms the back "wall" of the armpit. It moves the upper arm in various directions.

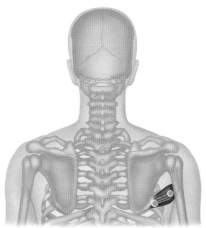

Referred pain from the teres major can be misdiagnosed as thoracic outlet syndrome. See chapter 33 for a discussion of that condition and the other muscles that may be involved.

Common Symptoms

Pain referred primarily to the outside and back of the shoulder and over the back of the upper arm, and sometimes over the back of the forearm. Usually pain is felt when using the arm out in front or when reaching forward and up.

A slight restriction in range of motion when reaching overhead, but for most people not usually by a noticeable amount. If the posterior deltoid, teres minor, and subscapularis also develop trigger points, range of motion can be greatly restricted and the shoulder area can become very painful, resulting in a frozen shoulder—see chapter 33 for a discussion of that condition.

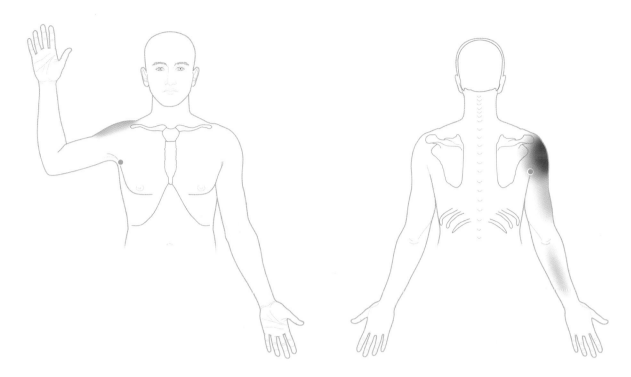

Causes and Perpetuation of Trigger Points, and Solutions

- Any activity that requires sustained resistance, such as driving a car that is hard to steer or lifting weights overhead.
- Dancing with someone who forces their partner's arms into position.

Solutions

- Avoid strenuous activities that aggravate trigger points in the teres major, such as lifting weights overhead, until self-help techniques have lessened the pain substantially. Be sure that your car is easy to steer or that any activity you perform on a regular basis is modified until it no longer causes trigger point activation. Drape the affected arm over a pillow at night.

Self-Help Techniques

Trigger points will also usually be found in the latissimus dorsi (38) and triceps (41). If the posterior deltoid (44), teres minor (39), and subscapularis (37) muscles also become involved and result in a painful frozen shoulder, then you will need to check and work on those muscles too.

Relieving teres major trigger points may release tightness in the rhomboid muscle (20), which may develop trigger points as a result of a tight teres major pulling on the mid back area.

Applying Pressure

Teres Major Pressure
Lie on your side and extend your arm so that it is sticking straight up above your head. Remember, the teres major forms the back wall of the armpit, so be sure you are working on that area.

You may also rest the arm on the back of a couch or adjacent chair and "pinch" the muscle in between your thumb and fingers.

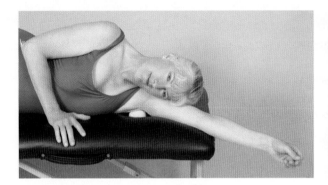
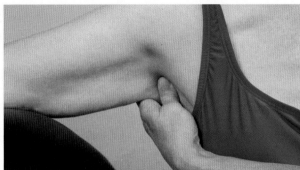

Stretches

Triceps Stretch
The stretch for the triceps also benefits the teres major (see chapter 41).

Also Check

Latissimus dorsi (38). Triceps brachii (41). Deltoid (44, posterior portion). Teres minor (39). Subscapularis (37).

> **Differential Diagnosis**
> If you are unable to relieve your symptoms with trigger point self-help techniques, you may need to see a health care provider to be evaluated for subacromial or subdeltoid bursitis, supraspinatus tendonitis, C6 or C7 nerve root irritation, and true thoracic outlet syndrome, any of which can cause similar pain patterns.

41 Triceps Brachii and Anconeus

The *triceps brachii* muscle has three attachments on the upper end: two of the heads attach to the bone in the upper arm (*humerus*) and cross one joint; the third attaches to the shoulder blade (*scapula*) and crosses two joints. At the other end, all three heads attach to the two bones in the lower arm (ulna and radius) just below the elbow joint. The *anconeus* is a small muscle that barely spans the elbow joint, attaching to the ends of the bones on either side. The anconeus and all the heads of the triceps brachii are used to straighten the arm at the elbow. The head of the triceps that crosses the shoulder joint is also used to move the upper arm.

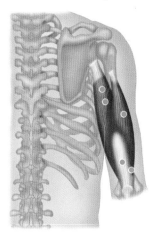

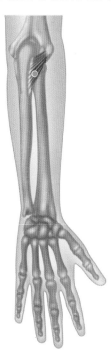

Trigger points in these muscles are very common and, unfortunately, are also commonly overlooked by practitioners. They play a major role in elbow pain; see chapter 33 for a discussion of tennis elbow.

Common Symptoms

- See the pictures for all the various pain referral patterns. Pain around the elbow is one of the most common referral patterns and often causes and perpetuates trigger points in adjacent muscles. Pressing or tapping on one of the bony parts of the elbow may be painful.

- Pain from some trigger points may only be activated during certain sports that require full forceful extension at the elbow, such as tennis and golf.
- If the triceps entraps the radial nerve, you may get tingling and numbness over the back of the lower forearm, wrist, and hand to the middle finger.

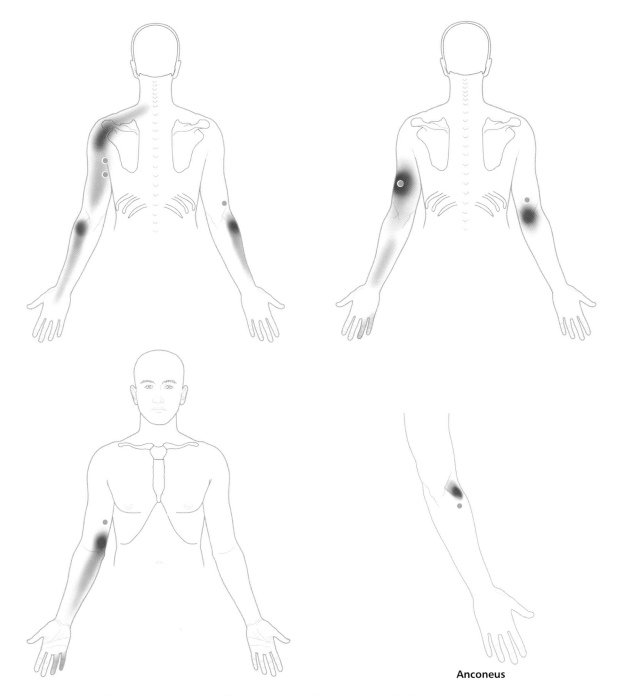

Anconeus

Causes and Perpetuation of Trigger Points, and Solutions

- Poor body mechanics, such as driving for long periods (especially excessive manual gear shifting), hand-sewing without elbow support, or using a computer without proper arm supports.
- A profession that requires a lot of pressure with the arms, such as massage therapy.

Solutions

- Keep your upper arms by your sides as much as possible when typing, writing, reading, and sewing. Use armrests of a proper height whenever possible. You shouldn't have to lean to the side; the arms should be at the height of your elbow. See chapter 2 for more information.

■ Sports strains sustained during activities such as tennis, golf, or excessive conditioning (e.g. push-ups, chin-ups).

Solutions
■ Use a lighter tennis racquet or shorten the grip. Avoid chin-ups and push-ups.

■ Using forearm crutches or a cane that is too long.

Solutions
■ Start using forearm crutches gradually, if possible. Make sure your cane is not hiking up your shoulder or forcing your triceps to bear much of your weight.

■ Short upper arms.

Solutions
■ See page 15, "Ergonomics," and page 31, "Skeletal Asymmetries," for solutions to compensate for short upper arms.

Self-Help Techniques

You may also need to work on the latissimus dorsi (38), teres major (40), teres minor (39), supinator (49), extensor carpi radialis longus (48), brachioradialis (48), and serratus posterior superior (36) muscles to obtain complete relief.

Applying Pressure

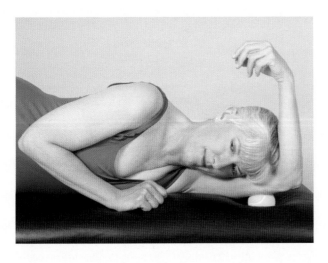

Triceps Pressure

Lie on your side with your arm extended above your head. If you want less pressure, put your head on a pillow *behind* the upper arm. If you want more pressure, rest your head *on* your upper arm. Using a tennis or racquet ball, rest your upper arm on the ball, working all the way from the back of your shoulder down to your elbow. Be sure to treat the front and back edges of the muscle too, by rotating the arm a little in both directions, since this muscle covers the entire back of the upper arm and trigger points can be found throughout the muscle. You may also pinch this muscle.

Stretches

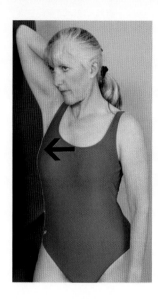

Triceps Stretch

Standing sideways to the wall, place your elbow on the wall above your head, with your forearm bent and your hand behind your head. Lean slightly into the wall to get a gentle stretch.

Also Check

Biceps brachii (46). Brachialis (52). Latissimus dorsi (38). Teres major (40). Teres minor (39). Supinator (49). Hand extensors and brachioradialis (48, extensor carpi radialis longus, brachioradialis). Serratus posterior superior (36).

Differential Diagnosis

Referred pain from triceps trigger points may be misdiagnosed as tennis elbow, tendonitis, lateral or medial epicondylitis, olecranon bursitis, thoracic outlet syndrome, arthritis, or a C7 nerve root irritation, though these may occur concurrently. If trigger point self-help techniques do not relieve your pain, you may need to see a health care provider to rule out these conditions.

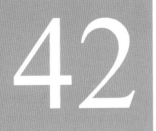

Scalene Muscles

The *scalene* group is comprised of three pairs of muscles: the *scalenus anterior, medius,* and *posterior*. Fifty percent or more of the population also have a *scalenus minimus* on at least one side of the body. The muscle parts attach above to the cervical vertebrae and below to the first and second ribs, and sometimes the scalenus posterior also attaches to the third rib. The scalene group stabilizes the cervical spine and elevates the first and second ribs during inhalation.

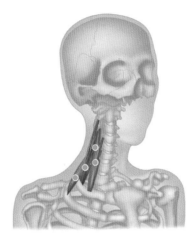

Scalene muscle trigger points are a major contributor to back, shoulder, and arm pain, and are commonly overlooked by practitioners. They also contribute to headaches when combined with trigger points in the neck and chewing muscles. Referred pain on the left side of the chest may be mistaken for angina.

See chapter 33 for a discussion of thoracic outlet syndrome, and chapter 47 for a discussion of carpal tunnel syndrome. Scalene muscle trigger points can be responsible for many symptoms that are attributed to both those conditions, in addition to their referred pain patterns.

Because these muscles are located in the front of the neck, I do not teach pressure techniques due to the risk of injury. It is important to see a trained practitioner to check the scalene muscles for trigger points and to treat them. You may still do the stretches below and remedy any perpetuating factors to resolve trigger point activation and perpetuation.

Common Symptoms

- Pain referred to the chest, mid back, and/or over the outside, back, and front of the arm and into the wrist and hand. You may be able to reproduce pain by turning your head to the side and then putting your chin down toward your shoulder. You may be able to relieve pain by putting the back of your forearm across your forehead and moving your elbow forward, which moves the collarbone away from the scalene muscles.
- Pain may disturb sleep, but it can be relieved by sleeping sitting or propped up.
- There may be minimal restriction of range of motion when rotating the head, but greater restriction when bending it to the side.

- Tight scalene muscles may elevate the first rib, leading to compressed nerves, arteries, veins, and lymph ducts, causing numbness, tingling, and loss of sensation in the fourth and fifth fingers and side of the hand, and stiffness and swelling in the fingers and back of the hand, which is worse in the morning.
- There may be a perceived (but not actual) numbness of the thumb and tingling.
- Possibly finger stiffness and/or tendency to drop items unexpectedly.
- Phantom limb pain in amputees.

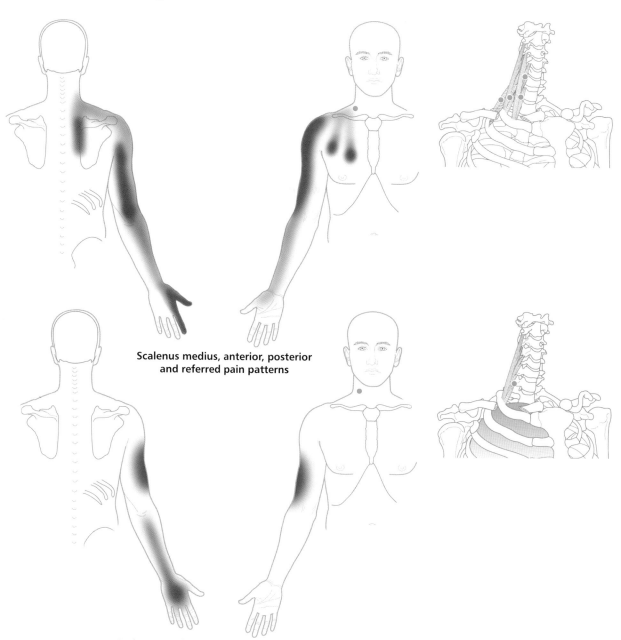

Scalenus medius, anterior, posterior and referred pain patterns

Scalenus medius and referred pain patterns

Causes and Perpetuation of Trigger Points, and Solutions

- Muscle overloads during activities such as pulling or lifting (especially with your hands at waist level), horse-handling or riding, playing tug-of-war, hauling ropes while sailing, or competitive swimming.
- Poor ergonomics or body mechanics such as when carrying awkwardly large objects, playing some musical instruments, having an armrest too high or too low, or sleeping with your head and neck lower than the rest of your body, as when the bed is tilted.
- Injuries such as whiplash from a car accident or falling on your head, or pain from a bulging or herniated cervical disc, which may linger even after surgery. Limping after an injury.
- Trigger points in the sternocleidomastoid (10) or levator scapula (19).
- Surgical removal of a heavy breast.

Solutions

- Avoid activities that aggravate scalene trigger points until they are inactivated. Resolve the source of limping, if at all possible, and treat all associated trigger points. Avoid carrying packages in front of your body or pulling hard on anything. Keep cold drafts off of your neck by using a scarf or neck gaiter.
- When seated, make sure you have good lighting from behind when you read, so your head is not turned to the side. Rest your elbow on an armrest or other surface and sit straight rather than tilted to the side, no matter what your activity. Use a headset for the phone, rather than holding it to your ear or cradling it between your ear and shoulder. When using a computer, ensure that the monitor is straight ahead and at eye level, and that your elbows rest comfortably on the chair armrests set at the proper height. If you have difficulty hearing and tend to turn to one side to hear better, turn your entire body to the side, or get a hearing aid if possible. See chapter 2 for more information.
- Do not read in bed. Elevate the head of your bed 3–3½" to provide mild traction at night. Multiple pillows will not provide the same effect and will probably cause more pain. You should get a good non-springy pillow that provides support for the cervical spine and keeps the spine in alignment. A chiropractor's office will usually stock well-designed pillows. Apply heat to the front of your neck before bedtime. When getting up from a lying position, roll onto your side first, and when rolling over in bed, keep your head on the pillow rather than lifting it.
- Acupuncture may successfully treat herniated and bulging discs with plum blossom and cupping techniques, though surgery may be necessary. If you have had surgery, seek the help of a physical therapist, acupuncturist, or massage therapist to help treat your trigger points.

- Improper breathing techniques, or coughing due to an acute or chronic illness.

Solutions

- Learn to breathe properly (see chapter 7). Eliminate causes of coughing by treating the underlying illness as quickly as possible; see the information on acute and chronic infections in chapter 4.

Asymmetries, such as a shorter leg or small hemipelvis (either the left or the right half of the pelvic bone), spinal scoliosis (the spine is not straight), an extra rib at the top (a cervical rib), or loss of an arm.

Solutions

If you have a short leg or small hemipelvis, even as little as $^3/_8$" or less, you will need to get fitted by a specialist for lifts to compensate, or it is unlikely you will be able to resolve scalene trigger points. Some scoliosis will be corrected with the trigger point pressure self-treatment. See page 30, "Spinal and Skeletal Factors," for more information. Even if you have an extra cervical rib, relieving the scalene trigger points may be enough to eliminate symptoms.

Self-Help Techniques

Check the sternocleidomastoid (10) and levator scapula (19) first, since these muscles can activate and perpetuate scalene trigger points.

Trigger points in the pectoralis major (23), latissimus dorsi (38), teres major (40), and subscapularis (37) can all refer pain in patterns that mimic thoracic outlet syndrome symptoms. It can be particularly confusing if more than one muscle develops trigger points, so be sure to check all of those muscles. The trapezius (8), pectoralis minor (43), and levator scapula (19) can also refer pain that may be diagnosed as thoracic outlet syndrome. The subclavius muscle (23) can get enlarged and may cause the first rib to be elevated and compress the subclavian vein, so check for trigger points in that muscle too, and see a chiropractor or osteopathic physician to determine if the first rib needs to be adjusted.

Applying Pressure

I do not teach self-help pressure to this muscle due to all the major nerves and arteries in the front of the neck. You will need to go to a trained practitioner such as a physical therapist or a massage therapist.

Stretches

If you are doing the pectoralis stretch (17), only do the top two positions and not the bottom one until the scalene muscles have improved. If you have an extra cervical rib, only do the top position.

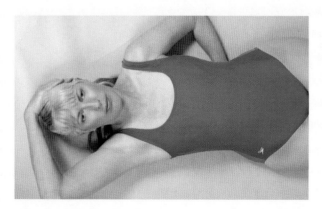

Put your opposite hand over the top of your head and, looking straight at the ceiling, pull your head gently toward your shoulder, then release and take a deep breath.

Side-Bending Neck Stretch

You may wish to apply heat prior to this stretch. Lie face-up, with the hand of the side you are stretching pinned under your butt.

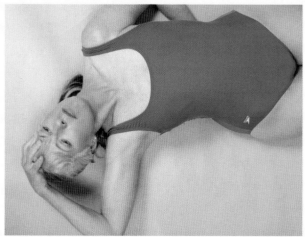

Repeat with your head turned slightly toward the left, and again with your head turned slightly toward the right. This will stretch different parts of the muscle.

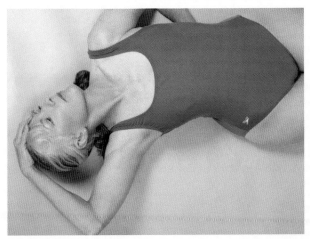 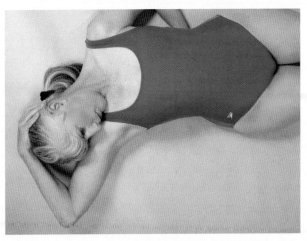

Stretch the opposite side following the same sequence. You may repeat the stretches for each side a few more times.

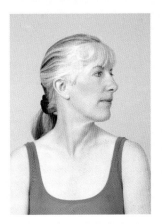 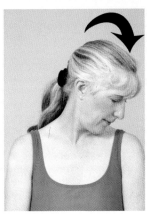

Scalene Stretch
While sitting up, rotate your head all the way to one side and then bring your chin down. Return to the forward position and take a deep breath. Repeat on the opposite side. You may do this up to four times in each direction.

Also Check

Sternocleidomastoid (10). Levator scapula (19). Trapezius (8, upper portion). Posterior neck muscles (9, splenius capitis). Pectoralis major and subclavius (23, both muscles). Pectoralis minor (43). Latissimus dorsi (38). Teres major (40). Subscapularis (37). Triceps brachii (41, satellite trigger points). Deltoid (44, satellite trigger points). Brachialis (52). Hand extensors (extensors carpi radialis, extensor carpi ulnaris, and extensor digitorum) and brachioradialis (48).

Differential Diagnosis
If you are unable to relieve your symptoms with trigger point self-help techniques, you may need to see a health care provider to rule out a C5 to C6 nerve root irritation. The pain pattern can be very similar to scalene trigger points, or both may be present. You may need to see a chiropractor or osteopathic physician to be evaluated for T1, C4, C5, and C6 vertebral misalignments, or for elevation of the first rib.

43 Pectoralis Minor

The *pectoralis minor* muscle attaches to the top outer corner of the shoulder blade (the *coracoid process* of the *scapula*) and to the third, fourth, and fifth ribs. It may also attach as high as the first rib and as low as the sixth rib. It pulls the scapula and shoulder girdle down and forward, and assists the muscles in the upper chest with forced inhalation.

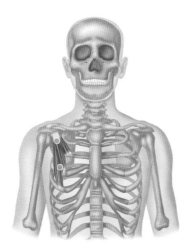

Trigger points are common in the pectoralis minor muscle, and pain referral frequently gets misdiagnosed as carpal tunnel syndrome. A pectoralis minor *entrapment*, where the muscle is chronically tight from trigger points or other causes and its tendon pinches the axillary artery and the brachial plexus nerve, can also be misdiagnosed as carpal tunnel syndrome. Entrapment of the brachial plexus nerve causes numbness and uncomfortable sensations in the ring and little fingers, back of the hand, outside of the forearm, and palm side of the thumb, index, and middle fingers. Pain referral and other symptoms caused by muscle tightness and trigger points are more aptly called *pseudo* carpal tunnel syndrome, and surgery on the carpal tunnel will not resolve the problem. See chapter 47 for an additional discussion of carpal tunnel syndrome.

Common Symptoms

▥ Pain referred mainly over the front of the shoulder and sometimes over the chest and/or down the inside of the arm into the middle, ring, and little fingers, which can mimic pain from angina.

▥ Shoulders are typically rounded forward and there may be difficulty in taking a deep breath.

▥ Range of motion is restricted when reaching forward and upward, or reaching backward with the arm at shoulder level.

▥ Shortening of the pectoralis minor muscle fibers as a result of trigger points may lead to arm pain, coracoid pressure syndrome (arm pain caused by muscles compressing the brachial plexus nerve fibers), and weakness of muscles in the mid back in the areas of the lower portion of the trapezius and rhomboid muscles.

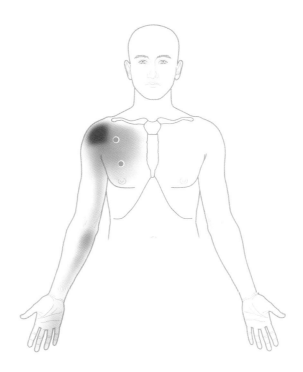

Causes and Perpetuation of Trigger Points, and Solutions

■ Poor ergonomics and posture, especially when seated.

Solutions
■ Modify or replace your misfitting furniture. See chapter 2 for a discussion of proper ergonomics and body mechanics.

■ Carrying a daypack or backpack without a chest strap, allowing the shoulder straps to compress the muscle, or wearing bras with shoulder straps that are too tight.
■ Using crutches with your weight supported by your armpits.
■ Gardening, such as digging with a hand tool.

Solutions
■ Be sure to use a pack with both proper shoulder padding and a chest strap to distribute weight away from the armpit area. Avoid bras that compress the pectoralis minor muscle; try to find one with a wider shoulder strap or a padded strap. Use crutches properly by supporting your weight on your hands, not your armpits. Gardening activities that aggravate your pain may need to be avoided until trigger points are relieved.

■ Scalene or pectoralis major trigger points, and/or weakness of the lower portion of the trapezius muscle.

Solutions
■ Check for trigger points in the pectoralis major (23) and scalene (42) muscles, since they will keep trigger points in the pectoralis minor activated. If trigger point self-help techniques do not relieve your pain, you may need to see a physical therapist to see if you would benefit from strengthening the trapezius muscle.

■ Trauma, such as fractured ribs, firing a rifle with the butt on your chest instead of the front of your shoulder, a whiplash injury, or open heart surgery that was performed through the breastbone (sternum) instead of through the ribs.

Solutions

■ Check all the muscles around the torso, shoulder girdle, and neck areas for trigger points.

■ Coughing or improper breathing, since the pectoralis minor is used for breathing.

Solutions

■ Address the causes of an acute or chronic cough (see chapter 4). Learn to breathe properly (see chapter 7).

■ While pectoralis minor trigger points can mimic angina pain, it is possible for pain from *true* angina to cause and perpetuate pectoralis minor trigger points.

Solutions

■ Treat the underlying cause of angina by following advice from your health care provider, along with treating the related trigger points.

Self-Help Techniques

Check for trigger points in the pectoralis major (23) and scalene (42) muscles, since they will keep trigger points in the pectoralis minor activated. Also, check the sternocleidomastoid (10) and anterior deltoid (44) muscles.

Applying Pressure

Pectoralis Major Pressure
The pectoralis major pressure (23) will also treat the underlying pectoralis minor.

Stretches

Pectoralis Stretch
See chapter 17.

Also Check

Pectoralis major (23). Scalene muscles (42). Deltoid (44, anterior portion). Sternocleidomastoid (10). Sternalis (24).

Differential Diagnosis
If you are unable to relieve your symptoms with trigger point self-help techniques, you may need to see a health care provider to rule out *true* thoracic outlet syndrome, C7 and C8 nerve root irritation, supraspinatus tendonitis, bicipital tendonitis, and medial epicondylitis. You may need to see a chiropractor or osteopathic physician to be evaluated for elevation of the third, fourth, and fifth ribs.

44 Deltoid

The *deltoid* muscle attaches near the shoulder joint and covers the top end of the upper arm on the front, side, and back. It comes to a point in about the middle of the outside upper arm. The various fibers move the upper arm in a variety of directions.

Trigger points in the deltoid are common and frequently develop as satellite trigger points from pain referral from other muscles.

Common Symptoms

■ Pain is usually localized in the deltoid area. Pain is worse with the arm in motion, with deep, less intense pain at rest.

■ Restricted range of motion, most often having difficulty raising the arm more than 90 degrees to the front or sides, though it can be less than 90 degrees in severe cases. This may be accompanied by a loss of strength.

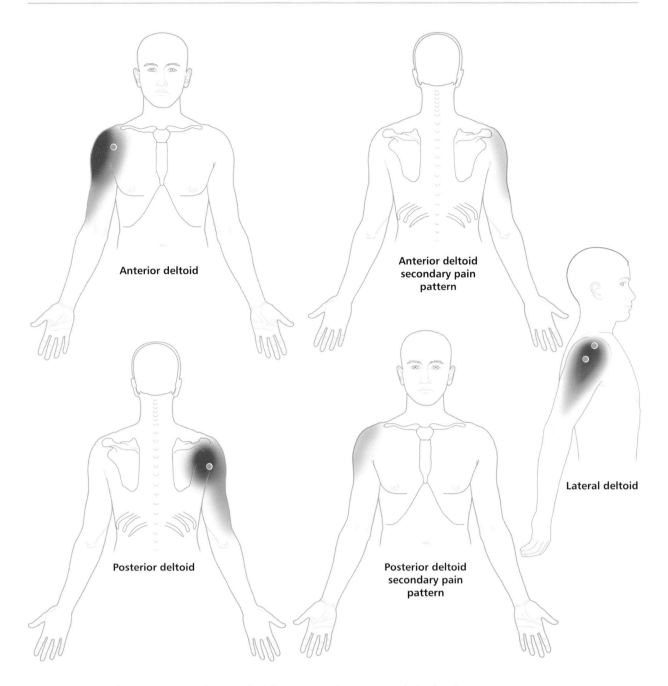

Anterior deltoid

Anterior deltoid
secondary pain
pattern

Lateral deltoid

Posterior deltoid

Posterior deltoid
secondary pain
pattern

Causes and Perpetuation of Trigger Points, and Solutions

- Vigorous, jerky, repetitive movements, such as when reeling in big fish or pushing yourself with ski poles.
- A direct blow or sudden strain to the area, as with a rifle recoil, sports injury, or catching yourself from a fall.
- Holding something, such as a power tool, at shoulder level or above for a long time.

Solutions

- Avoid lifting heavy objects on the affected side and modify or cease any aggravating activities until trigger points have been inactivated. If you are firing a rifle, place a pad between the butt of the gun and your shoulder.
- Be careful going down stairs, to prevent a near-fall. Hold onto the railing and watch your feet placement carefully.

Injections such as vaccines, vitamins, or antibiotics into the deltoid muscle can activate latent trigger points.

Solutions
If you receive intramuscular injections, check with your health care provider to see if you can inject into a different muscle.

Self-Help Techniques

Be sure to check the supraspinatus (34), infraspinatus (35), and scalene (42) muscles for trigger points that could be causing referral to and activation of satellite trigger points in the deltoid muscle. These will need to be inactivated first in order to provide lasting relief of symptoms from deltoid trigger points.

If you find trigger points in the front of the deltoid, check the pectoralis major muscle (23) close to the armpit, the biceps muscle (46), and the back part of the deltoid. If you find trigger points in the back of the deltoid, check the triceps (41), latissimus dorsi (38), and teres major (40) muscles.

Applying Pressure

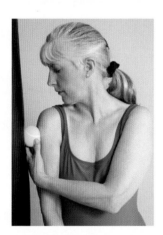

Deltoid Pressure
Use a tennis ball in a doorjamb. Place the ball in a lip of the doorjamb to help stabilize the ball, and keep holding the ball in your opposite hand so the ball does not slip away from you as you search for trigger points. Be sure to work the front, side, and back of the muscle, and from the top to bottom, to apply pressure to the entire deltoid.

Stretches

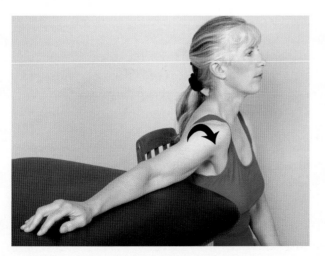

Couch Stretch
Stretch the front part of the muscle by placing your arm over the back of a couch and rotating your shoulder forward.

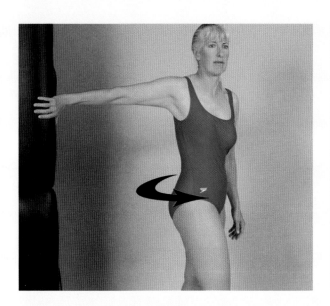
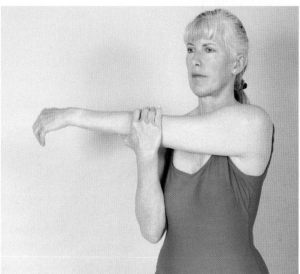

Against-Doorjamb Stretch

Stand in a doorway with your arm straightened at or slightly higher than 90 degrees, with your palm on the doorjamb and your thumb pointing down. Put the foot of the same side as your arm about one step in front of you, and rotate your body gently away from your hand. As you rotate your shoulder forward and down, you will feel the stretch move into the front portion of the deltoid, the coracobrachialis, and the biceps muscles.

Posterior Deltoid Stretch

For the posterior portion of the deltoid muscle, pull your arm across your chest, using the opposite hand to grasp your arm near the elbow.

Pectoralis Stretch

Perform the middle and lower positions of the pectoralis stretch, which will also help treat the deltoid muscle (see chapter 17).

Also Check

Pectoralis major (23). Biceps brachii (46). Triceps brachii (41). Latissimus dorsi (38). Teres major (40). Infraspinatus (35). Supraspinatus (34). Scalene muscles (42).

Differential Diagnosis

Trigger points in the deltoid muscle are commonly misdiagnosed as rotator cuff tears, bicipital tendonitis, subdeltoid bursitis, glenohumeral joint arthritis, a nerve impingement, or a C5 nerve root irritation. If you are unable to relieve your pain with the trigger point self-help, you may need to see a health care provider for an MRI, x-ray, or other diagnostic test to confirm or rule out the above diagnoses. Even if you do have one of these conditions, it is likely there are also trigger points involved.

If the shoulder joint is sprained, dislocated, separated, or out of alignment, there will be localized tenderness only over the joint rather than in the deltoid muscle, unless you also have trigger points that were present prior to the acute injury which also cause tenderness.

45 Coracobrachialis

The *coracobrachialis* muscle is on the front of the shoulder, in the crease between the trunk and the upper arm. It attaches to the top outer corner of the shoulder blade (the *coracoid process* of the *scapula*) and to the bone in the upper arm (*humerus*). It helps move the upper arm at the shoulder joint, but not everyone has this muscle.

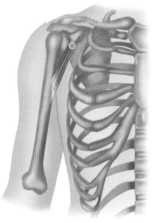

If you have already checked and inactivated trigger points in the deltoid, pectoralis major, latissimus dorsi, teres major, supraspinatus, triceps, and biceps muscles and still have some symptoms, check the coracobrachialis muscle for trigger points. It rarely develops trigger points on its own; they more likely develop secondary as satellite trigger points.

Common Symptoms

- Pain referred to the anterior deltoid, over the triceps on the back of the upper arm, down the back of the lower arm, and sometimes into the back of the hand and middle finger.
- If only coracobrachialis trigger points are involved, pain is felt when reaching forward and up above past the ear when the arm is straight, and range of motion is restricted. If additional trigger points are involved, this will cause pain with movement in other directions too.

- When placing the affected arm in the small of your back, it is difficult to get your hand past the spine without pain, whereas normally you should be able to touch the other arm with your fingers.
- An entrapment of the musculocutaneous nerve may cause atrophy of the biceps muscle and reduced sensation on the back of the lower arm.

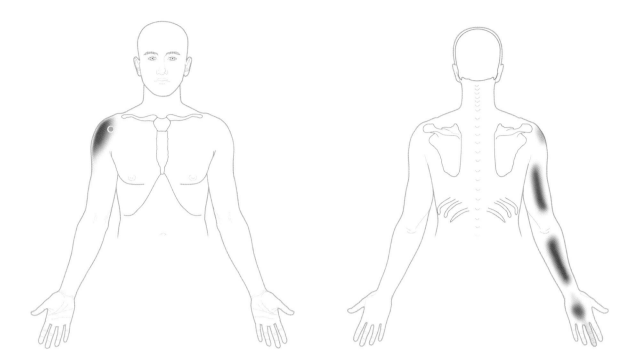

Causes and Perpetuation of Trigger Points, and Solutions

▦ Activation and perpetuation of trigger points in the coracobrachialis muscle likely occur only as satellite trigger points of the muscles listed under "Also Check".

Solutions
▦ In order to obtain lasting relief from symptoms caused by trigger points in the coracobrachialis muscle, first work on trigger points in the other muscles.
▦ When lifting, hold objects close to your body, with your palms face-up, as much as possible.

Self-Help Techniques

Check the deltoid (44), triceps (41), pectoralis major (23), latissimus dorsi (38), supraspinatus (34), teres major (40), and biceps (46) muscles first, and relieve any trigger points as needed.

Applying Pressure

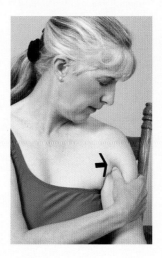

Coracobrachialis Pressure
Using the hand of the unaffected side, wrap your fingers around the deltoid. With your thumb knuckle bent, dig the end of your thumb into the front of the shoulder on the outside of the crease, pressing toward the bone in the upper arm. Some of my patients have found they prefer to use something like a pressure gadget of some kind; these are often sold in massage stores or catalogs, or see www.pressurepositive.com.

Stretches

Warm the area on the front of your shoulder/crease with moist heat before performing these stretches.

Pectoralis Stretch
Use the pectoralis stretch, lower hand position (see chapter 17).

Couch Stretch
See chapter 44.

Against-Doorjamb Stretch
See chapter 44 for this stretch. As you rotate your shoulder forward and down, you will feel the stretch move into the front portion of the deltoid and the coracobrachialis.

Also Check

Supraspinatus (34). Deltoid (44). Triceps brachii (41). Biceps brachii (46). Pectoralis major (23). Teres major (40). Latissimus dorsi (38).

Differential Diagnosis
Symptoms from trigger points in the coracobrachialis muscle can be similar to C7 nerve root irritation, carpal tunnel syndrome, subacromial bursitis, supraspinatus tendonitis, and acromioclavicular joint dysfunction. If you are unable to relieve your symptoms with trigger point self-help, you may need to see a health care provider for an MRI, x-ray, or other diagnostic test to confirm or rule out one of those diagnoses.

46 Biceps Brachii

The *biceps brachii* muscle is located on the front of the upper arm. There are two attachments on the shoulder blade (*scapula*) and one on the *radius*, the larger of the two bones of the lower arm. Because this muscle crosses the elbow joint as well as the shoulder joint, it moves both the upper arm and the lower arm, including rotation of the lower arm.

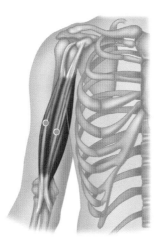

Common Symptoms

■ Trigger points in the biceps are typically found in the mid to lower part of the muscle and refer superficial achy pain over the front of the upper arm and front of the shoulder, and possibly cause an ache or soreness over the upper trapezius (top of the shoulder) or the crease of the elbow.

■ Weakness and pain when raising the hand above the head while the elbow is bent.

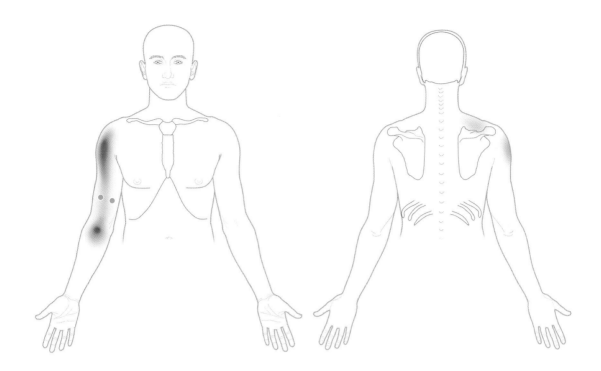

Causes and Perpetuation of Trigger Points, and Solutions

■ Repetitive motion injuries, such as during sports (throwing a ball, or playing basketball or tennis), writing (either with a pen or using a keyboard), playing the violin or guitar, using a screwdriver for a long period, shoveling snow, or lifting heavy objects with your palms facing upward and/or with your arms extended forward.
■ Trying to catch yourself from falling.

Solutions
■ You may need to modify or stop any aggravating activities until the trigger points are inactivated. Carry items either in a daypack, or with your palms face-down.
■ At night, be sure not to draw your arm tightly into your body. Instead, try to keep the elbow out from the body—you may try putting a pillow next to your trunk to help with this.

■ Trigger points in the infraspinatus can cause satellite trigger points to form in the biceps brachii.

Solutions
■ Check the infraspinatus muscle (35) for trigger points.

Self-Help Techniques

Trigger points in the brachialis (52), supinator (49), triceps (41), deltoid (44, front portion), supraspinatus (34), trapezius (8, upper portion), and coracobrachialis (45) muscles usually develop concurrently or within a few weeks' time of biceps trigger points, so you should also check those muscles.

Applying Pressure

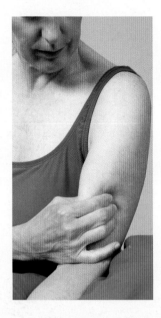

Biceps Brachii Pressure
With the opposite hand, either pinch the biceps between the thumb and next two fingers or just use your thumb to apply pressure.

Stretches

Against-Doorjamb Stretch
The against-doorjamb stretch (44) will help treat the biceps muscle.

Also Check

Infraspinatus (35). Brachialis (52). Supinator (49). Triceps brachii (41). Deltoid (44, front portion). Supraspinatus (34). Trapezius (8, upper portion). Coracobrachialis (45).

Differential Diagnosis
If you are unable to relieve your symptoms with trigger point self-help techniques, you may need to see a health care provider for an MRI, x-ray, or other test to rule out or confirm a diagnosis of bicipital tendonitis, subdeltoid bursitis, C5 nerve root irritation, bicipital bursitis, and glenohumeral arthritis.

47 Forearm, Wrist, and Hand Pain

The use of computers has caused a huge increase in the number of patients with referred pain from trigger points in the forearm muscles. Often patients will complain of pain over the outside of the elbow or the back of the wrist, and subsequently may have been misdiagnosed with *tennis elbow, tendonitis, or carpal tunnel syndrome*. They are often given a brace to wear, which may afford some relief but does not solve a trigger point-caused problem.

For a discussion of tennis elbow, see chapter 33.

Carpal Tunnel Syndrome

Carpal tunnel syndrome may occur in conjunction with thoracic outlet syndrome (discussed in chapter 33), or the symptoms of carpal tunnel syndrome may be mimicked by trigger points and more aptly called *pseudo-carpal tunnel syndrome*. The carpal tunnel consists of the transverse carpal ligament located on the palm side of the hand just below the wrist, and the eight wrist bones which form the other three sides of the tunnel. When one of the nine long flexor tendons passing through it swells or degenerates, or something causes the tunnel to get smaller, the narrowing of the canal can result in compression or entrapment of the median nerve. This causes burning, numbness, tingling, weakness, or muscle damage in the hand and fingers.

True carpal tunnel syndrome is likely caused by using tools that vibrate or by prior injuries, such as a broken or sprained wrist that caused swelling. Some people have a smaller carpal tunnel and are more predisposed to having problems as a result. There are several systemic predisposing factors which may play a part, such as an overactive pituitary gland, hypothyroidism, rheumatoid arthritis, or fluid retention during pregnancy or menopause.

In fact, the majority of carpal tunnel syndrome diagnoses are in fact *mis*diagnoses and are really symptoms caused by trigger points. If you have been diagnosed with carpal tunnel syndrome, it is worth checking for trigger points in the scalene muscles (42), pectoralis minor (43), biceps (46), brachialis (52), coracobrachialis (45), hand and finger extensors and brachioradialis (48), hand and finger flexors/pronator teres (51), palmaris longus (50), and adductor/opponens pollicis (53).

If you are considering surgery, be sure to treat the trigger points yourself and, ideally, get the assistance of a trained practitioner to ensure your success. Surgery has a poor rate of success, likely due to referred symptoms from trigger points not being considered as the cause. I have even had a patient who tested positive for carpal tunnel syndrome using a nerve conduction test, and after one treatment on her forearms, her symptoms disappeared. When I ran into her a couple of years later, her symptoms had still not returned.

Pectoralis Minor Entrapment

A pectoralis minor entrapment, where the muscle is chronically tight from trigger points or other causes and its tendon pinches the axillary artery and the brachial plexus nerve, can be misdiagnosed as carpal tunnel syndrome and will not be resolved by surgery on the carpal tunnel. Entrapment of the brachial plexus nerve causes numbness and uncomfortable sensations of the ring and little fingers, back of the hand, outside of the forearm, and palm side of the thumb, index, and middle fingers. Check the pectoralis minor (43) and also the biceps (46), coracobrachialis (45), and trapezius (8) muscles for associated trigger points.

Solutions

Artisan's Stretch

Put your hands out in front of you, palms face-down and fingers spread. At the same time as you slowly rotate your hands to palms face-up, start making a fist, starting with your little finger. By the time your hand is fully rotated, the fist is complete and you also bend at the wrist.

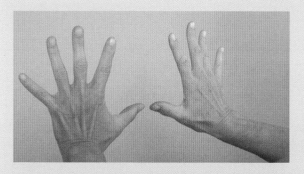
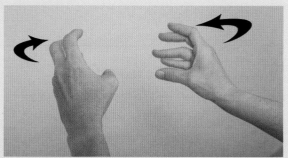

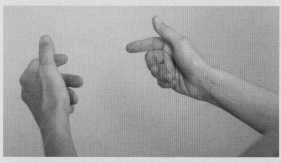
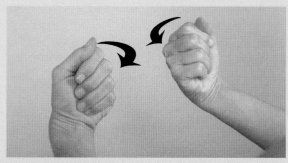

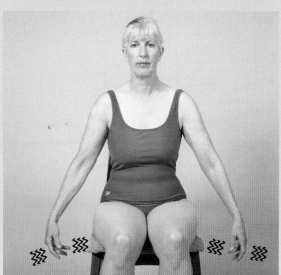

Finger Flutter Exercise

Put your arms at your sides and shake your hands, keeping your wrist and fingers loose so the lower arm gets the benefit too.

Each chapter in this section will contain additional solutions.

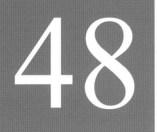

48 Hand Extensors, Brachioradialis, and Finger Extensors

Extensor Carpi Radialis Longus, Extensor Carpi Radialis Brevis, Extensor Carpi Ulnaris, Extensor Digitorum, Extensor Indicis, Extensor Digiti Minimi

The *hand extensors* attach to the humerus bone of the upper arm around the elbow area, and via tendons to the metacarpal bones of the hand. They move the hand at the wrist and also stabilize the wrist while the fingers are being used for grasping.

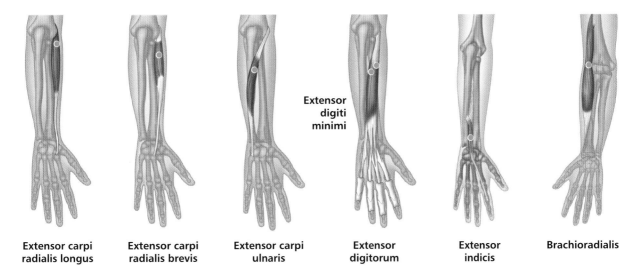

Extensor digiti minimi

| Extensor carpi radialis longus | Extensor carpi radialis brevis | Extensor carpi ulnaris | Extensor digitorum | Extensor indicis | Brachioradialis |

The anatomy of the *finger extensors* is very complicated, but the combined attachment for the *extensors digitorum* and *digiti minimi* at their uppermost end is on the humerus bone of the upper arm at the elbow, and tendons attach to the bones in the fingers on the other end. The *extensor indicis* attaches to the ulna bone of the lower arm above the wrist, and to the index finger via a tendon. The finger extensors move the hand at the wrist, and move the fingers either together or separately.

The *brachioradialis* attaches to the humerus bone above the elbow and to the radius bone of the lower arm near the wrist. It moves the lower arm at the elbow joint.

Usually trigger points will form in more than one of the above-listed muscles but the self-help treatment is the same, so for the purpose of a self-help book, they have been listed together in one chapter.

Common Symptoms

■ See the pictures for the various pain referral patterns, and consider that it is likely that more than one of these muscles is involved, causing a composite pain pattern rather than one of these individual patterns.

■ Pain is worse when shaking hands, turning a doorknob, using a screwdriver, or performing any similar motions. Pain may be enough to wake you at night.

■ Trigger points in the finger extensors will cause finger stiffness, pain into the back of the forearm, hand, fingers, and possibly the elbow area, and arthritis-like pain in the finger joints. With the hand extensors and brachioradialis muscle, pain is likely to first appear on the outside of the elbow and then spread to the wrist and hand.

■ Weakness of grip that causes you to unexpectedly drop items or spill when pouring or drinking; the larger the item, the more severe the problem. There may be a loss of coordination and increased muscle fatigability during repetitive movements.

■ Entrapment of the radial nerve may cause weakness of the back of the forearm muscles and/or numbness and tingling over the back of the hand.

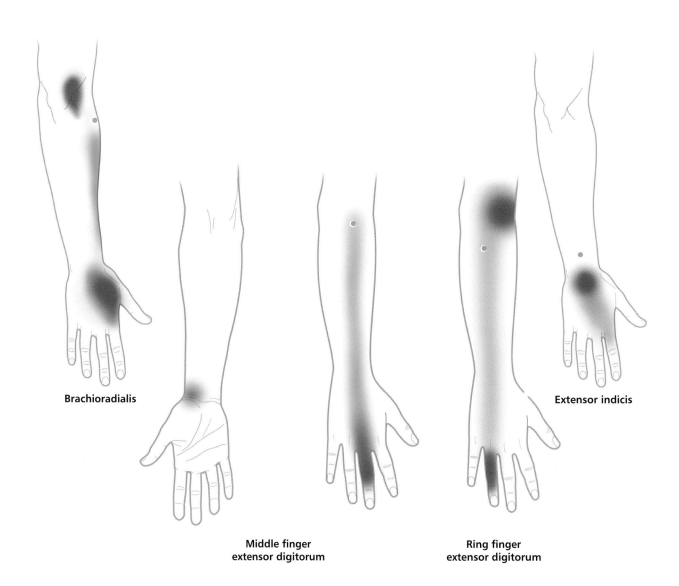

Brachioradialis

**Middle finger
extensor digitorum**

**Ring finger
extensor digitorum**

Extensor indicis

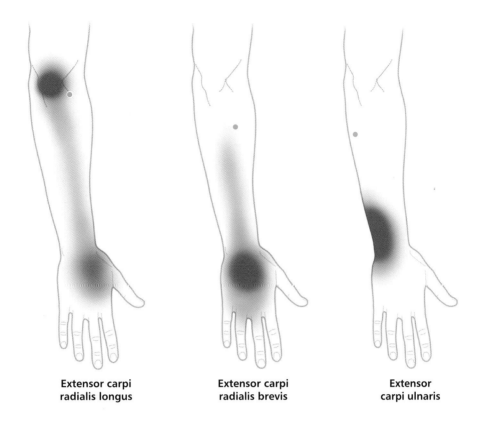

| Extensor carpi radialis longus | Extensor carpi radialis brevis | Extensor carpi ulnaris |

Causes and Perpetuation of Trigger Points, and Solutions

■ Gripping an object forcefully and/or repetitively—the larger the item, the more severe the problem. Examples are writing, weeding, waxing a car, shaking hands, using tools, ironing, throwing a Frisbee, kayaking, scraping ice off a windshield, or giving massages. Repetitive arm/hand motions such as computer use (especially the "mouse arm"), playing a violin or guitar, or using an adding machine.

■ The extensor carpi ulnaris is more likely to develop trigger points after trauma such as a broken arm, or after surgery or trauma in the shoulder joint or elbow.

■ The finger extensors are likely to develop trigger points from repetitive finger movements, such as when playing the piano, doing carpentry or mechanical repairs, and playing with finger beads or rubber bands.

Solutions

■ Avoid motions that require twisting the forearm and/or grasping repeatedly over long periods until trigger points are inactivated. Learn to alternate hands; for example, learn to use your computer mouse with both hands. Buy a keyboard that is ergonomically correct.

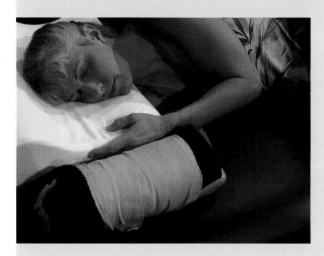

■ If you tend to curl your fist up under your chin in bed, prevent this by making a soft splint. Use an ace-bandage to strap a rolled towel over your forearm, wrist, and palm. A wrist brace can be worn temporarily until trigger points are relieved, but should not be considered a long-term solution.

■ Referral from trigger points in the scalene muscles (42) can cause trigger points to form in the extensors carpi radialis or ulnaris, or the extensor digitorum. Referral from trigger points in the supraspinatus muscle (34) can cause trigger points to form in the extensor carpi radialis. Referral from trigger points in the serratus posterior superior muscle (36) can cause trigger points to form in the extensor carpi ulnaris. Trigger points in the supinator (49) and brachioradialis muscles usually form concurrently.

Solutions

■ Check the above-listed muscles for potential primary trigger points.

Self-Help Techniques

Applying Pressure

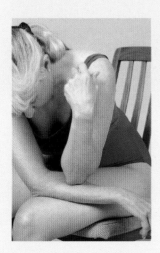

Hand and Finger Extensors Pressure
Place your forearm across your lap. If you have large breasts, you may need to rest your arm on a table in front of you. Using your other elbow, apply pressure to the muscles on the outside and back of the forearm. Push the muscle on the thumb side (the brachioradialis) out of the way toward your trunk to also access the extensor carpi radialis longus underneath it, which is a very important muscle to work on.

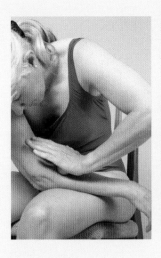
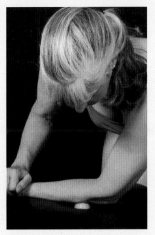

Alternatively, using a golf ball cradled in the palm of your hand, rotate the elbow of that hand out in front of you so that you do not stress the forearm muscles in that arm, and press the golf ball into tender points.

To treat points that your elbow cannot reach, with your forearm on a flat surface and your palm face-up, use the opposite hand to help press your forearm onto the golf ball. Be careful not to hurt your back if you do this last part.

Stretches

Artisan's Stretch
See chapter 47.

Finger Flutter Exercise
See chapter 47.

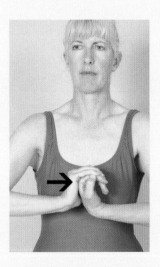

Finger Extensor Stretch
To stretch the finger extensors, put your forearm in front of your lower chest with the elbow bent at about 90 degrees, palm face-up, and the hand bent upward at the wrist and into a fist. Use the opposite hand to assist in a gentle stretch.

Also Check

Triceps brachii (41). Biceps brachii (46). Supinator (49). Brachialis (52). Scalene muscles (42). Serratus posterior superior (36). Supraspinatus (34).

Differential Diagnosis
If you are unable to relieve your symptoms with trigger point self-help techniques, you may need to see a health care provider to be evaluated for lateral epicondylitis, a C5 to C8 nerve root irritation, carpal tunnel syndrome, de Quervain's disease, or arthritis. You may need to see a chiropractor or osteopathic physician to check for volar subluxation of the wrist bones or distal radioulnar joint dysfunction.

49 Supinator

The *supinator* muscle attaches to both the ulna and the radius bones of the lower arm, just below the elbow. Because it wraps around the radius, its prime function is to rotate the forearm so that the thumb is pointing away from the midline of the body. It also assists in flexing the forearm at the elbow, bringing the hand toward the shoulder.

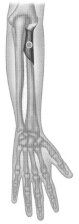

Back of forearm

Pain from trigger points in the supinator is frequently diagnosed as *tennis elbow*, though there is usually lack of recognition by many practitioners that trigger points are the causative factor. The hand and finger extensors are commonly also involved. Surgery is probably unnecessary, so try the trigger point self-help techniques first.

Common Symptoms

■ Aching pain referred to the outside of the elbow and web of the thumb, and possibly to the back of the forearm, which may continue even after the aggravating activity is stopped.

■ Tenderness when tapping on the outside of the elbow.

■ Trigger points may possibly cause entrapment of the radial nerve, which leads to weakness when opening the hand and uncomfortable sensations on the back of the wrist and forearm.

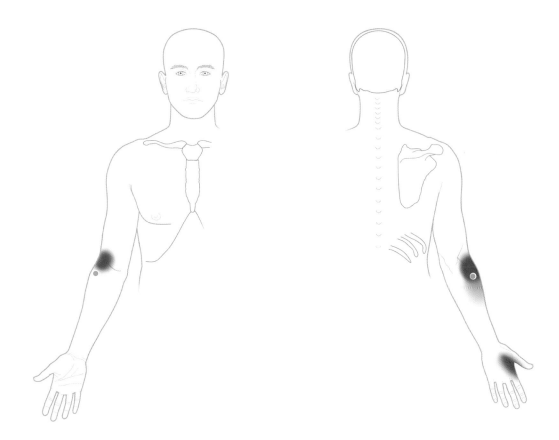

Causes and Perpetuation of Trigger Points, and Solutions

■ Repetitive motions with the arm held straight, for example playing tennis or walking a dog on a leash. Carrying a heavy briefcase with the arm straight or hoisting a briefcase onto a desk into the ready-to-open position.

■ Repetitive grasping movements, such as wringing clothes, turning stiff doorknobs, unscrewing a tight jar lid, shaking hands, washing walls, raking leaves, waxing a car, giving massages, or ironing.

■ A sudden strain on the muscle.

Solutions

■ If you play tennis, keep your elbow slightly bent and the head of the racquet slightly up. A lighter racquet and a smaller handle will also be helpful. Do not play every day, in order to give your muscles a chance to recuperate.

■ Train your dog not to pull on the leash, switch hands, or get a head halter so the dog is not able to pull so much. Purchase a briefcase with a shoulder strap that can be worn diagonally across your torso, rather than carrying it hanging from one hand. Lift the briefcase onto a table with both hands rather than swinging it up with one hand. When shaking hands, try to alternate hands and offer the palm face-up. Do not rake leaves. Carry packages with your palms face-up.

■ An elastic support with a hole for the point of the elbow may be worn during activities that aggravate the supinator, but this should only be worn for short time periods, because it will reduce circulation to the muscles.

Self-Help Techniques

Trigger points are also often found concurrently in the triceps (41) and finger extensors and brachioradialis (48), so you will want to also check those muscles. The brachialis (52), biceps (46), and sometimes palmaris longus (50) may also get involved.

Applying Pressure

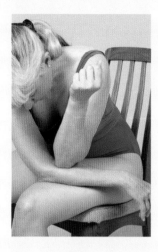

Supinator Pressure

Place your forearm across your lap with your palm face-up. If you have large breasts, you may need to rest your arm on a table in front of you. Using your opposite elbow, apply pressure to the muscles on the upper front third of the forearm, particularly close to the elbow crease and from the middle to the outside of the forearm.

Alternatively, use a golf ball cradled in the palm of your hand, rotate the elbow of that hand out in front of you so you do not stress the forearm muscles in *that* arm, and press the golf ball into tender points. See chapter 48 for an example of using the golf ball on the forearm.

Also Check

Triceps brachii (41). Hand and finger extensors and brachioradialis (48). Brachialis (52). Biceps brachii (46). Palmaris longus (50).

Differential Diagnosis

If you are unable to relieve your symptoms with trigger point self-help techniques, you may need to see a health care provider to rule out lateral epicondylitis, entrapment of the posterior interosseous nerve, a C5 to C6 nerve root irritation, de Quervain's disease, or possibly arthritis. You may need to see a chiropractor or osteopathic physician for evaluation of articular dysfunction of the distal radioulnar joint.

50 Palmaris Longus

The *palmaris longus* muscle may be absent or variable in its location along the forearm. If present, it generally runs from the humerus bone of the upper arm at the elbow, to connective tissue called the *palmar aponeurosis,* which covers most of the palm below the skin. Its main function is to cup the palm, but it also assists in movement of the hand at the wrist.

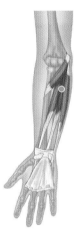

Due to the tenderness and the wrist and hand pain associated with trigger points in the palmaris longus muscle, symptoms may be mistaken for carpal tunnel syndrome. However, because of the variable location of this muscle, if it extends under the carpal ligament, it may cause *true* carpal tunnel syndrome. Trigger points in the muscle would increase tension in the tendon and would aggravate carpal tunnel symptoms, and self-help would likely only partially relieve symptoms. See chapter 47 for more information on carpal tunnel syndrome.

Untreated trigger points and tightness in the palmaris longus will eventually affect the cutaneous tissue in the palm, and can be a factor in the development of the nodules, fibrous bands, and pain of "Dupuytren's contracture." Dupuytren's contracture is more common in men and in people with alcoholism, diabetes, and epilepsy, and tends to develop mostly in the 40s age range. Trigger point self-help techniques may possibly help stop the progression of nodule-formation and Dupuytren's contracture. Acupuncture may also help, especially plum blossom technique over the nodules, in addition to needles inserted into the palmaris longus and other hand and finger flexors. Current medical surgical guidelines are that if you can still lay the hand palm-down flat on a surface, surgery is not indicated. If the condition has progressed to the point that it is interfering with your activities, and you are not able to get enough relief with self-help techniques and/or trigger point needling, then consult with a surgeon.

Common Symptoms

- Referred pain that is superficial and feels like pricking by a needle, and is felt in the palm and possibly in the front of the forearm.
- Difficulty in using tools due to tenderness in the palm.

- Variable palmaris longus muscle configurations and attachments may cause pain in the back of the lower arm, compression neuropathy, or a "dead feeling" in the forearms.
- In advanced cases of Dupuytren's contracture, the palm is contracted and there is an inability to lay the hand flat on a surface.

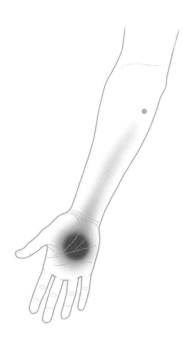

Causes and Perpetuation of Trigger Points, and Solutions

- Referred pain from the middle head of the triceps muscle near the elbow will cause satellite trigger points in the palmaris longus.

Solutions
- Be sure check for trigger points in the triceps muscle (41) and work on them first.

- Direct trauma, such as falling on your outstretched hand, pressure from tools being held improperly and digging forcibly into the palm, or using a racquet with the handle end pressed into the palm.

Solutions
- Do not use any tool or sports equipment that digs into your palm.

Self-Help Techniques

Applying Pressure

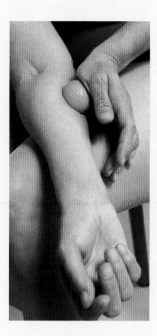

Palmaris Longus Pressure
Place your forearm across your lap. If you have large breasts, you may need to rest your arm on a table in front of you. Press a golf ball or other pressure device cradled in the palm of your hand into tender points.

Alternatively, using your opposite elbow, apply pressure to the muscles on the front of the forearm, particularly close to the elbow crease. See chapter 51 for an example of using your elbow on the forearm.

Stretches

Anterior Forearm Stretch
See chapter 51.

Also Check

Hand and finger flexors (51).

51 Hand and Finger Flexors

Flexor Carpi Radialis and Ulnaris, Flexors Digitorum Superficialis and Profundus, Flexor Pollicis Longus, and Pronator Teres

The *hand and finger flexors*, depending on the individual muscle, attach above either to the humerus bone of the upper arm or to the radius or ulna bones of the lower arm, close to or at the elbow. Most of these muscles attach to the bones in the thumb and fingers via tendons, though the pronator teres attaches to the radius bone in the middle of the lower arm, and the flexor carpi ulnaris attaches to the pisiform bone in the wrist, via their respective tendons. The hand flexors move the hand at the wrist; the finger flexors help move the hand at the wrist, and some of them also move the fingers.

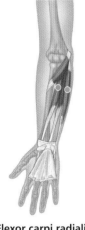

Flexor carpi radialis and ulnaris

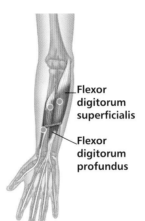

Flexor digitorum superficialis

Flexor digitorum profundus

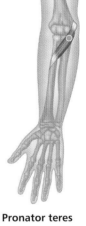

Pronator teres

Common Symptoms

■ Pain refers in various patterns over the front of the forearm, the front of the wrist, the palm, and the fingers and thumb. Pain can feel like it is projecting off the ends of the thumb and fingers, like a "bolt of lightening." See the pictures for the most common pain referral patterns.

■ Finger stiffness and painful cramping. Difficulty in using scissors, one-handed garden clippers, or tin shears, or putting curlers, bobby pins, or clips in your hair. An inability to cup your hand while your palm is face-up, as when brushing something off of a counter into your cupped hand.

■ Symptoms are aggravated by stress, cold drafts, and loud noises.

■ "Trigger finger," where the finger gets stuck in the fist-closed position, is caused by a constriction of a tendon in the palm, about one-thumb's width above the crease between the palm and the finger

■ Entrapment of the ulnar nerve at the elbow can cause uncomfortable sensations, burning pain, numbness, and loss of sensation in the fourth and fifth fingers, and may lead to clumsiness and grip weakness.

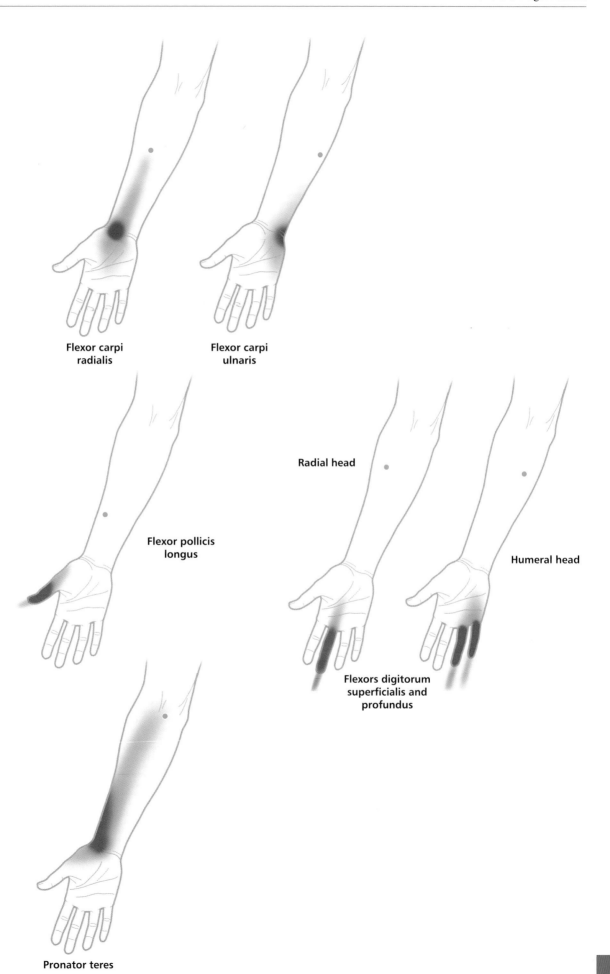

Flexor carpi
radialis

Flexor carpi
ulnaris

Flexor pollicis
longus

Radial head

Humeral head

Flexors digitorum
superficialis and
profundus

Pronator teres

233

Causes and Perpetuation of Trigger Points, and Solutions

- Repetitive gripping of small-handled tools or a racquet or paddle, such as a kayak or canoe paddle. Gripping a steering wheel or ski poles too firmly. Punching holes with a one-handed hole punch repetitively, as when punching tickets or receipts at events or store entrances. Giving massages.
- Weeding a garden can cause trigger points in the flexor pollicis longus.
- A fracture at the wrist or elbow can cause trigger points in the pronator teres.

Solutions
- Stretch your fingers frequently. Keep your hand and forearm supported when sitting.
- When using small-handled tools, rest and stretch regularly, and change activities frequently if possible. Avoid repeatedly pressing anything into your palm. If using a one-handed hole punch, switch hands often and trade off frequently with other personnel if possible.
- If you are rowing, uncurl your fingers as the oar sweeps back. When kayaking, "feathering" your paddle may help. Learn to relax your grip when steering or skiing, and hold onto the sides of the steering wheel. Racquets should be held slightly up rather than tilted down.

- Primary trigger points in the scalene muscles (42), pectoralis minor (43), pectoralis major and subclavius (23), serratus anterior (26), supraspinatus (34), infraspinatus (35), latissimus dorsi (38), serratus posterior superior (36), triceps (41), hand extensors and brachioradialis (48), palmaris longus (50), and/or adductor and opponens pollicis (53) can cause satellite trigger points to develop in the hand and finger flexors.

Solutions
- Check these muscles for primary trigger points.

- The cause of trigger finger is unclear, but may possibly be caused by pressing something relatively pointy repeatedly into the palm.

Solutions
- Trigger finger may be relieved either by acupuncture needling or possibly by applying pressure to a tender spot in the palm fairly close to the affected finger, approximately opposite the knuckle when you look at the hand from the side.

Self-Help Techniques

It is a good idea to work both the front *and* the back of the forearm (48), since relief of trigger points on the front can reactivate trigger points on the back.

Applying Pressure

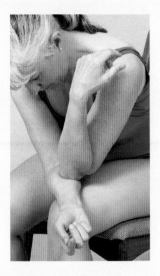

Hand and Finger Flexors Pressure
Place your forearm across your lap with your palm face-up. If you have large breasts, you may need to try resting your arm on a table in front of you. Using your other elbow, apply pressure to the muscles on the front upper two-thirds of the forearm.

Alternatively, use a golf ball cradled in the palm of your hand, rotate the elbow of that side out in front of you so you do not stress the forearm muscles in *that* arm, and press the ball into tender points. See chapter 50 for an example of using the golf ball on the forearm.

Stretches

Stretch the muscles frequently.

Artisan's Stretch
See chapter 47.

Finger Flutter Exercise
See chapter 47.

Hand Interosseous Muscles Stretch
See chapter 54.

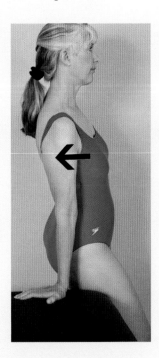

Anterior Forearm Stretch
Find a surface about the height of your palm. Point your fingers backward and, keeping your arm straight, press your palm into the surface so that you are getting a stretch on the front of the forearm. You may lean back just a little bit to get an additional gentle stretch as the muscles loosen up.

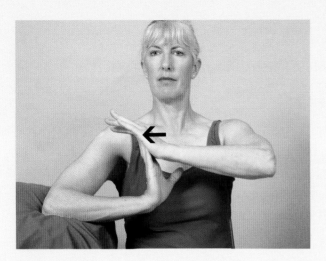

Finger Extension Stretch
Support your elbow on the side to be stretched. Using the palm of the opposite side, gently stretch your fingers back until you feel a stretch in your fingers, palm, and forearm.

Also Check

Scalene muscles (42). Pectoralis minor (43). Pectoralis major and subclavius (23). Serratus anterior (26). Supraspinatus (34). Infraspinatus (35). Latissimus dorsi (38). Serratus posterior superior (36). Triceps brachii (41). Hand extensors and brachioradialis (48). Palmaris longus (50). Adductor and opponens pollicis (53).

Differential Diagnosis

If you are unable to relieve your symptoms with trigger point self-help techniques, you may need to see a health care provider to rule out medial epicondylitis, ulnar neuropathy, osteoarthritis of the wrist, C5, C7, C8, or T1 nerve root irritation, or carpal tunnel syndrome. Carpal tunnel syndrome must be confirmed by a median nerve conduction study. Referral from trigger points in the hand and finger flexors may get misdiagnosed as thoracic outlet syndrome. You may need to see a chiropractor or osteopathic physician to be evaluated for a distal radiocarpal dysfunction and/or a dorsal misalignment of the wrist bones.

52 Brachialis

The *brachialis* muscle attaches to the lower half of the humerus bone of the upper arm, and to the ulna bone in the lower arm, near the elbow. Its function is to bring the forearm toward the shoulder, but it can also bring the upper arm toward the lower arm, as when doing chin-ups. Trigger points are commonly caused by acute overload and repetitive stress.

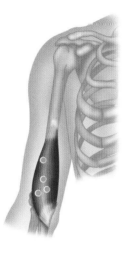

Common Symptoms

■ Pain or tenderness referred around the base of the thumb and the thumb pad. Some pain may be present at the elbow crease and perhaps over the front of the upper arm.

■ There may be loss of sensation and tingling and numbness on the back of the thumb if the radial nerve is entrapped by trigger points in the brachialis muscle.

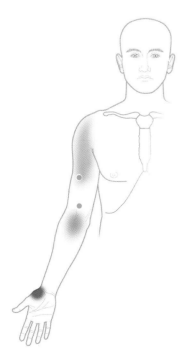

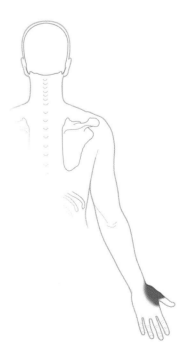

Causes and Perpetuation of Trigger Points, and Solutions

■ Stressors on the muscle such as heavy lifting, holding a power tool, carrying groceries or a purse, playing a guitar or violin, holding a phone to your ear, or meticulous ironing.
■ Using crutches.

Solutions
■ Avoid lifting heavy items, and when you lift lighter items, keep your palms face-up. When playing an instrument, stretch your arm out whenever possible. Avoid carrying groceries for very far as much as possible. Buy a purse with a long strap that can be worn diagonally across your torso, rather than carrying one in your hand. Use a headset or speaker phone when talking on the phone, or use the opposite arm to hold a phone to your ear.
■ At night, be sure not to draw your arm tightly into your body. Instead, try to keep the elbow out from the body—you may try putting a pillow next to your trunk to help with this.

■ Primary trigger points in the supinator muscle can cause satellite trigger points in the brachialis and biceps muscles.

Solutions
■ Check the supinator muscle (49) for primary trigger points.

Self-Help Techniques

Applying Pressure

Brachialis Pressure

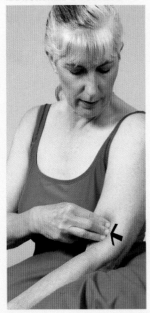

Using your opposite hand, hook your thumb around the inside of your upper arm, and use your finger to move the biceps toward your thumb and torso while at the same time pressing into the muscle underneath. The area extends from about the middle of the upper arm, almost down to the elbow crease.

Stretches

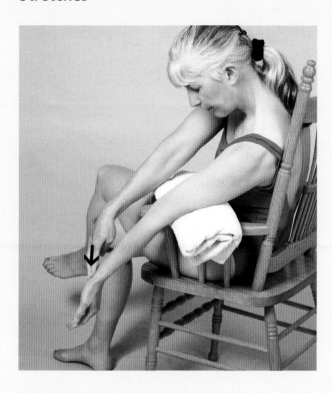

Brachialis Stretch
While supporting your upper arm just above the elbow on a chair or couch arm with the palm face-up, use the opposite hand to push down gently on the inside of the wrist.

Also Check

Biceps brachii (46). Brachioradialis (48). Supinator (49). Adductor and opponens pollicis (53, adductor pollicis).

Differential Diagnosis
Symptoms from trigger points in the brachialis muscle are similar to those of C5 and C6 nerve root irritation, bicipital tendonitis, supraspinatus tendonitis, and possibly carpal tunnel syndrome. If you are not able to get pain relief from trigger point self-help techniques, you may need to see a health care provider for an MRI to rule out other causes.

53

Adductor and Opponens Pollicis

The *adductor pollicis* muscle attaches to the metacarpal bones of the index and middle fingers, and to the thumb, spanning the web between the index finger and the thumb. The *opponens pollicis* muscle attaches to the trapezium bone of the wrist, and to connective tissue over the wrist bones called the *flexor retinaculum*. The adductor pollicis brings the thumb toward the index finger, while the opponens pollicis brings the thumb across the palm to touch the ring and little fingers.

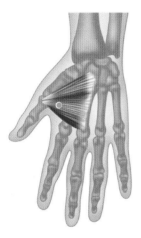

Adductor pollicis

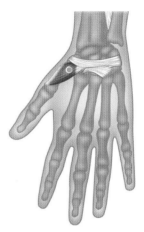

Opponens pollicis

Common Symptoms

■ Aching pain referred over the thumb pad, into the thumb, and over part of the wrist. Referred pain can be erroneously attributed to a joint problem, and people will frequently self-diagnose as having arthritis.

■ Weakness and difficulty with any fine motor movements that require the thumb to grasp, such as sewing, buttoning a shirt, writing, or holding onto items.

■ "Trigger thumb," where the thumb locks in the closed position, can be caused by a tender spot in or near one of the forearm flexor tendons located under the thumb pad or in the web between the thumb and first finger.

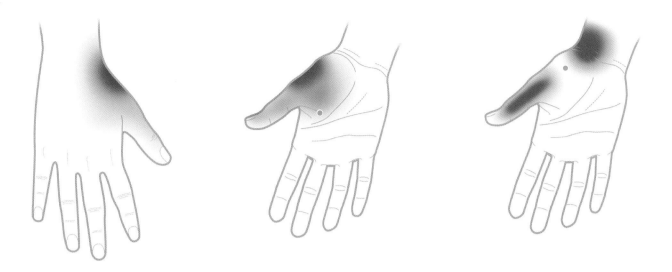

Causes and Perpetuation of Trigger Points, and Solutions

■ Grasping things with your thumb and fingers, such as weeding a garden (particularly with difficult-to-pull weeds), using small paint brushes for artwork, sewing, handwriting, crocheting or knitting, and giving massages.
■ Residual pain from a fracture.

Solutions

■ When weeding, loosen the dirt with a spade first, weed for short periods, and alternate hands. Take frequent breaks when sewing, crocheting, knitting, writing, and painting.

Self-Help Techniques

Also check the scalene (42), brachialis (52), supinator (49), and extensor carpi radialis longus and brachioradialis (48) muscles, since they can also refer pain to this area and should be treated prior to the thumb muscles if they contain primary trigger points. Active trigger points are almost always also found concurrently in the hand interosseous muscles (54) between the thumb and first finger.

Applying Pressure

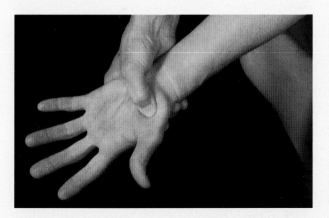

Pollicis Pressure
If your opposite thumb is unaffected, you may use that to apply pressure all over and around the thumb pad on the affected side. If both thumbs are affected, use the eraser on the end of a pencil to apply pressure. Some massage stores sell pressure devices that are easily held in the palm of the hand, or see www.pressurepositive.com. Just be sure to use a pressure tip that is not much bigger than the eraser on the top of a pencil, or you will not get enough focused pressure for the trigger points.

Stretches

Artisan's Stretch
See chapter 47.

Finger Flutter Exercise
See chapter 47.

Hand Interosseous Muscles Stretch
See chapter 54.

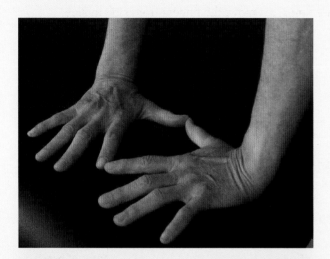

Adductor Pollicis Stretch
Place both hands, palms down flat, on a surface in front of you, with index finger to index finger and thumb to thumb, and the thumbs pointing back toward you. You may also do this in warm water.

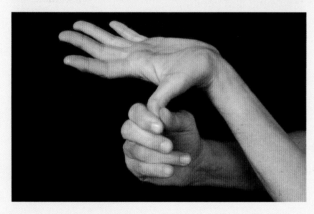

Opponens Pollicis Stretch
With your palm face-up, use your opposite hand to reach underneath the hand you are treating and pull down gently on the thumb.

Anterior Forearm Stretch
See chapter 51.

Also Check

Scalene muscles (42). Brachialis (52). Supinator (49). Hand and finger extensors and brachioradialis (48, extensor carpi radialis longus, brachioradialis). Hand interosseous muscles (54).

Differential Diagnosis
If you are unable to relieve your symptoms with trigger point self-help techniques, you may need to see a health care provider to rule out carpal tunnel syndrome, de Quervain's disease, and osteoarthritis. If you have a flexor pollicis longus muscle (not everyone does), it may cause compression neuropathy of the anterior interosseous nerve. You may need to see a chiropractor or osteopathic physician to be evaluated for misalignments of a metacarpal or carpal bone, especially at the thumb carpometacarpal joint.

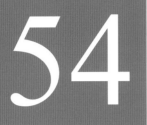

54 Hand Interosseous Muscles and Abductor Digiti Minimi

The *hand interosseous* muscles are located between carpal bones in the hand. The *abductor digiti minimi* muscle is located on the outside of the ring finger. These muscles move the fingers from side to side.

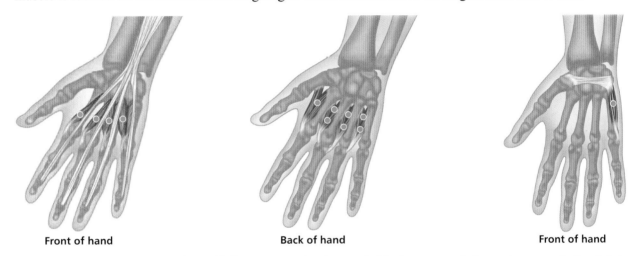

Front of hand   Back of hand   Front of hand

People frequently erroneously self-diagnose as having arthritis because of the pain around the joint. Inactivating trigger points in the interosseous muscles and resolving any applicable perpetuating factors may help delay or stop the progression of some types of osteoarthritis.

Trigger points in the hand interosseous muscles may possibly contribute to the formation of "Heberden's nodes"—hard bumps which are initially tender and about the size of a pea on one side of the joint closest to the fingertip. Heberden's nodes are more common in women and often appear within three years after menopause. If you have Heberden's nodes, look for trigger points in the interosseous muscles. Once the trigger points are inactivated, tenderness should disappear immediately, and over time the node itself will probably disappear.

Common Symptoms

■ Pain referred on the back and palm of the hand, and down one or more fingers. Pain is usually worse on one side of the joint and slightly closer toward the fingertip.

■ Finger stiffness that interferes with fine motor movements, such as buttoning, writing, and grasping objects, and difficulty in bringing the fingers together or making a fist.

■ A tight interosseous muscle or trigger point may entrap a finger nerve, causing superficial numbness on one side of the finger.

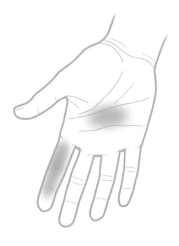 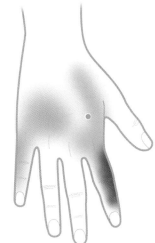

First dorsal interosseous

**Note: These are sample referral patterns.
Trigger points in any of these muscles will cause referral
into the corresponding fingers.**

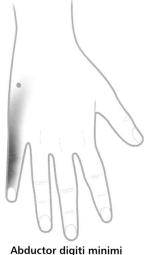 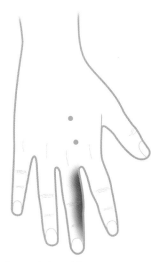

Abductor digiti minimi　　　　　　**Second dorsal interosseous**

Causes and Perpetuation of Trigger Points, and Solutions

■ Repetitive grasping with the fingers pinched together, for example using small tools, paintbrushes, and needles, pulling weeds, gripping golf clubs tightly, or giving massages.

Solutions
■ Learn not to grasp items tightly, and take frequent breaks. Limit the amount of time for any given activity.

Self-Help Techniques

Also check for trigger points in the adductor and opponens pollicis (53), hand and finger flexors (51), hand and finger extensors (48), latissimus dorsi (38), pectoralis major (23), pectoralis minor (43), scalene (42), and triceps (41) muscles.

Applying Pressure

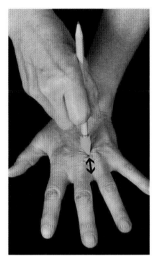 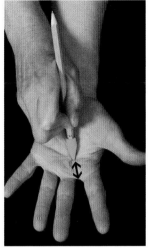 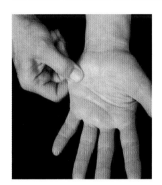

Hand Interosseous Muscles Pressure
Buy pencil erasers that fit on the end of a pencil. Using the tip of the eraser, press in between the bones of the hand on both the back side and the palm side. You may also rub with the eraser back and forth.

Use your opposite thumb to work on the outside edge of the hand, or pinch the muscle in between your opposite thumb and fingers.

Stretches

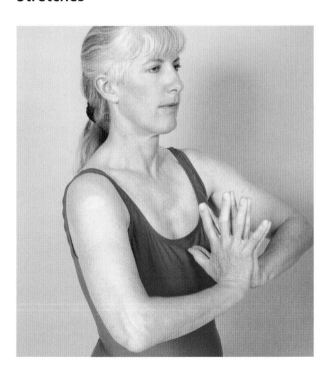

Hand Interosseous Muscles Stretch
With your forearms in front of your chest, hands palm to palm and fingers to fingers, separate your fingers and press your palms against each other with the fingers pointed upward, so your fingers and the front of your forearms are getting a good stretch.

Artisan's Stretch
See chapter 47.

Finger Flutter Exercise
See chapter 47.

Anterior Forearm Stretch
See chapter 51.

Adductor Pollicis Stretch
See chapter 53.

Also Check

Adductor and opponens pollicis (53). Hand and finger flexors (51). Hand and finger extensors and brachioradialis (48). Latissimus dorsi (38). Pectoralis major (23). Pectoralis minor (43). Scalene muscles (42). Triceps brachii (41).

Differential Diagnosis
Pain from trigger points in these muscles may be misdiagnosed as a C6, C8, or T1 nerve root irritation, ulnar neuropathy, or thoracic outlet syndrome. Finger pain and numbness can be due to nerve entrapment of the brachial plexus by the scalene or pectoralis minor muscles. You may need to see a chiropractor or osteopathic physician to be evaluated for misalignment of bones in the hand.

55 Leg, Knee, and Foot Pain

Several conditions can be caused by trigger points and will benefit from self-help techniques, including plantar fasciitis, hallux valgus and associated bunions, shin splints (properly called periosteal irritation), and compartment syndromes.

Plantar Fasciitis

Contrary to its suffix "-itis" and what was originally thought, plantar fasciitis is not an inflammatory process, but rather is caused by tension overload on the plantar aponeurosis, a fascial attachment on the big bone in the heel (calcaneus). It is caused by tightness in the gastrocnemius (58), soleus (59), abductor hallucis, flexor digitorum brevis and/or abductor digiti minimi (71) muscles. The quadratus plantae muscle (72) may also be involved.

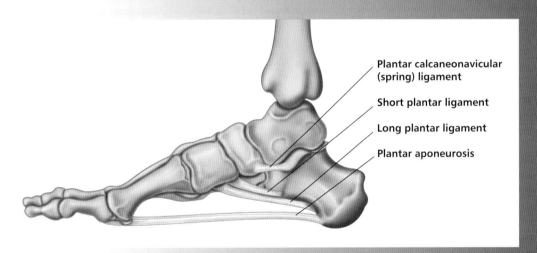

Plantar calcaneonavicular (spring) ligament

Short plantar ligament

Long plantar ligament

Plantar aponeurosis

Treating trigger points and getting good orthotics with arch supports and deep heel cups are effective therapies. You will need to avoid running, jumping, and possibly walking, until symptoms have decreased. You may need to lose weight, if necessary, since additional weight puts a lot of stress on the lower leg and foot structures. Numerous repeated injections of steroids can lead to rupture of the plantar aponeurosis, so you should try the treatments listed above first. The longer the condition goes on and the more you limp, the more muscles get involved, all the way up through the back and neck, so you should start self-treatment immediately.

Hallux Valgus and Bunions

Hallux valgus is a painful condition where the big toe spreads out to the side at the joint closest to the foot, and becomes deformed. Tightness and trigger points in the flexor hallucis longus (61) can cause hallux valgus, and the bone can spread further due to force exerted by the flexor hallucis longus, making the cycle self-perpetuating. The flexor hallucis brevis, adductor hallucis (72), and abductor hallucis (71) become weak, allowing even further spread and deformity. A bunion, or swelling of the protective lubricating pad on the side of the big toe, can form and cause additional pain.

It is important not to wear high heels during childhood and adolescent developmental stages; if a young woman reaches age 20 with an abnormal bone angle of 10 degrees or less, she is unlikely to develop bunions later. Relief of trigger points may stop the progression or even reverse some of the bone and joint displacement of hallux valgus and subsequent bunions, though surgery may be necessary if the condition has progressed far enough.

Shin Splints and Tibial Periosteal Stress Syndromes

Anterior compartment syndrome is sometimes called anterior shin splints, which is easily confused with the generic term shin splints, used in the past to refer to any chronic pain in the front or middle of the lower leg associated with exercise. More recently, shin splints has come to refer specifically to irritation of the surface of the bone along the attachment of a muscle and is called periosteal irritation. In the front of the leg, periosteal irritation may develop when a runner first changes from a flat-footed to a toe-running style, begins training on a track or hill (especially downhill), or runs in a shoe that is either too rigid or too flexible. Trigger point self-help techniques will help resolve periosteal irritation.

Compartment Syndromes

A *muscle compartment* is a group of muscles within a particular part of the body, wrapped by strong, fibrous tissue called *fascia*. The fascia attaches the compartment to the bone, and each compartment has a blood and nerve supply. The lower leg contains four muscle compartments:

- *Superficial posterior compartment*, containing the soleus (59) and gastrocnemius (58) muscles;
- *Deep posterior compartment*, containing the flexor digitorum longus (61), flexor hallucis longus (61), popliteus (57), and tibialis posterior (60) muscles;
- *Anterior compartment*, containing the tibialis anterior (69), extensor hallucis longus (70), extensor digitorum longus (70), and peroneus tertius (64) muscles;
- *Lateral compartment*, containing the peroneus longus and peroneus brevis (64) muscles.

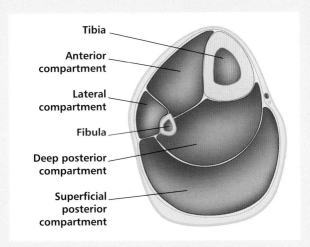

Compartment syndrome is where swelling within the muscle compartment causes increased pressure, which adversely affects blood and lymph circulation of the muscles inside. One of the causes of *anterior compartment syndrome* is tight, shortened calf muscles which overload weakened anterior compartment muscles. Acute causes of compartment syndrome may be an accident that crushes the leg, surgery, tight bandages or casts, burns, clotting, snakebites, or some medications.

Symptoms of compartment syndrome develop over time and are worse with activity, and pain persists for increasing amounts of time after exercise. The most noticeable symptoms are dull aching, tightness, pain, odd sensations, and diffuse tenderness over the entire belly of the involved muscles. It is important to see a health care provider *immediately*. If left untreated, compartment syndrome eventually causes scarring of the muscles and nerves and other permanent damage. Severe cases may even require amputation of the lower leg. A positive diagnosis is determined by measuring intramuscular pressure within the compartment.

Once a health care provider has successfully relieved pressure within the compartment, you should subsequently check for trigger points, since they were likely formed as a result of compartment syndrome.

Solutions

Orthotics Any condition affecting your leg and foot will probably improve immensely if you wear orthotic inserts in your shoes. See page 19, "Clothing."

Chair Make sure your chair is not compressing your thighs or causing problems in your calves. See page 15, "Ergonomics."

Sports Make sure you stretch and warm up prior to activities and stretch again afterward.

(For more information on these subjects and more conditions related to this region of the body, see *Trigger Point Therapy for Foot, Ankle, Knee & Leg Pain: A Self-Treatment Workbook* (DeLaune, 2010).)

Each muscle chapter in this section will contain additional solutions for these conditions and others affecting this part of the body.

56 Hamstrings Muscle Group

Biceps Femoris, Semitendinosus, and Semimembranosus

The *hamstring muscles* attach to the sit bone (ischial tuberosity) and the tibia and fibula bones below the knee. Their main functions are hip extension, which is bringing the leg back from midline, and knee flexion, which is bending your knee. These muscles are essential for walking, running, jumping, and bending forward.

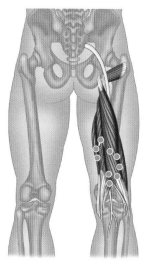

Rear view

Do not assume that just because your pain referral matches one of the pictures in this chapter that it is indeed coming from hamstring trigger points; trigger points in several other muscles have common referral patterns that overlap the referral patterns of the hamstring muscles. It is important to check the muscles listed under "Also Check," to make sure the referral is not from one or more of those muscles rather than the hamstrings.

Referred pain from trigger points in the hamstring muscles frequently gets diagnosed by both patients and practitioners as sciatic pain, because of the distribution pattern down the back of the leg. At least 80% of pain down the leg comes from trigger point referral from the hamstrings or gluteus minimus (62), not from "pinched nerves," herniated discs, or spinal stenosis in a lumbar vertebra (either a narrowing of the big hole in the vertebra that the spinal cord goes through, or a narrowing of the smaller holes the nerves travel out through). Since sciatica is usually assumed to be caused by compression of a nerve, pain referral from trigger points is probably more aptly called pseudo-sciatica.

If you have pain remaining after a laminectomy, check the hamstrings for trigger points.

Common Symptoms

- Pain referred over the back of the thigh, around the crease of the butt, over the back of the knee, and sometimes over the calf, worse with sitting due to pressure on the trigger points. Pain when walking, possibly even causing a limp, and pain when getting up from a chair, particularly if your legs have been crossed.
- Pain in the biceps femoris muscle can disrupt sleep.
- It may feel like the pain is only in the quadriceps femoris muscle group (65) on the front of the thigh, when in fact the problem is originating in the hamstrings and causing secondary trigger points to form in the quadriceps femoris group.
- There may be tingling and numbness when sitting in a chair that is too high, and restricted range of motion when bending forward to reach your toes.
- In above-knee amputees, phantom limb pain may come from trigger points in the hamstrings, particularly if the muscles were stretched to cover the bone.

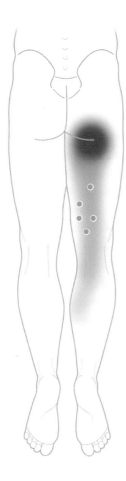

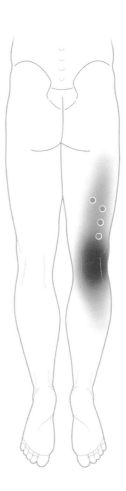

Causes and Perpetuation of Trigger Points, and Solutions

- Strain or partial tears of the hamstrings as a result of inadequate stretching before a sports activity, or auto accidents regardless of the direction of impact.
- Sitting in a chair where your feet do not touch the ground, children sitting in a high chair without a footrest, or sitting on a ski lift without a footrest.

Solutions

- Be sure to stretch prior to sports activities. If you swim, do not use the crawl stroke too much, but instead vary it with other strokes. If you bicycle, be sure your seat height is high enough so that your legs can straighten out as much as possible.
- If your chair is too high for you, buy or build a sloped footstool; you should be able to easily slip your fingers between your chair and thigh. Patio chairs can cause problems if there is a metal bar across the front and a sagging seat bottom. Make sure children in highchairs have footrests, and those at school have chairs or footrests of the proper height. When driving for long periods, use cruise control and take frequent breaks.

- Structural imbalances, such as a small hemipelvis (either the left or the right half of the pelvic bone) or short upper arms in relation to torso height that cause you to shift your weight forward.

Solutions

- See chapter 4, "Skeletal Asymmetries."

- Treatment of quadriceps femoris trigger points without also treating the hamstrings.

Solutions

- Check the quadriceps femoris muscle group (65) for trigger points and be sure to treat both.

Self-Help Techniques

Caution: Do not apply pressure to your legs if you have varicose veins in the area to be treated—it could release a clot that could go to your heart or brain! An acupuncturist or massage therapist should treat your legs, because they can avoid varicose veins. However, you may still do the stretches and exercises below.

In addition to treating the quadriceps femoris muscle group (65), you may need to treat the thoracolumbar paraspinal muscles (18), gluteus maximus (30), gluteus medius (31), and/or gluteus minimus (62) first, since these muscles can also restrict range of motion. You should also consider the piriformis (29), popliteus (57), gastrocnemius (58), and plantaris (59), since trigger points in those muscles can cause similar pain referral patterns, in addition to trigger points in the gluteus medius (31), gluteus minimus (posterior portion, 62), and vastus lateralis (65).

Tight hamstrings will tend to cause a flattened lumbar spine and a head-forward posture, resulting in problems in the quadratus lumborum (28), thoracolumbar paraspinal (18), iliopsoas (22), rectus abdominis (25), posterior neck (9), pectoralis minor (43), infraspinatus (35), subscapularis (37), teres minor (39), and supraspinatus (34) muscles. You should check these muscles for trigger points, particularly if you have upper-body symptoms that are only temporarily relieved. See chapter 7 for more information on head-forward posture.

Applying Pressure

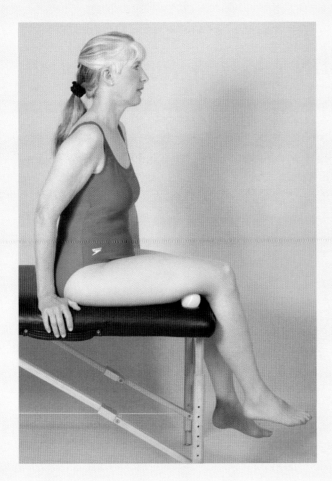

Pressure

Sit on a surface where your legs can dangle but are fully supported along the length of the thigh. Place a tennis ball under one thigh and use your hand to move the ball around to treat tender points. Repeat on the opposite thigh.

You may also treat the inner-thigh hamstrings by using your opposite hand to pinch the muscles between your thumb and fingers.

Stretches

In-Bathtub Stretch
See chapter 17.

Exercises

You may need to condition the gluteus maximus in order to inactivate hamstring trigger points. To condition the gluteus maximus, you must swim, hike uphill (this muscle is minimally used for normal walking), jump, or do some other vigorous activity while keeping your heart rate within your optimal range for aerobic respiration.

Also Check

Piriformis (29, piriformis and obturator internus). Gluteus medius (31). Gluteus minimus (62, posterior portion). Quadriceps femoris muscle group (65, vastus lateralis). Popliteus (57). Soleus and plantaris (59, plantaris). Gastrocnemius (58). Adductor muscles of the hip (67, adductor magnus). Iliopsoas (22).

Differential Diagnosis
If you are unable to relieve your symptoms with trigger point self-help techniques, you may need to see a health care provider to rule out osteoarthritis of the knee. Misalignment of the sacroiliac joint and L4 to L5 and L5 to S1 vertebrae can cause spasm and restriction of the hamstring muscles. See a chiropractor or osteopathic physician for evaluation and treatment.

57 Popliteus

The *popliteus* muscle is located behind the knee, attaching to the femur bone above and the tibia bone below. Its main function is to "unlock" the knee at the start of weight bearing.

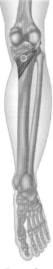

Rear view

Trigger points are usually found after trigger points in the gastrocnemius (58) or biceps femoris (56) have been inactivated, so be sure to work on those muscles first, if needed.

Common Symptoms

- Pain referred to the back of the knee when crouching, running, or walking, which is worse when going down stairs or downhill. Knee pain when straightening the leg.

- A slight decrease in range of motion, which will likely be unnoticeable.

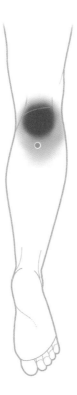

Causes and Perpetuation of Trigger Points, and Solutions

■ Sports that require you to twist, slide, and change direction suddenly, such as soccer, football, and baseball, or running or skiing downhill.

Solutions
■ If you do any of these sports activities, you may first need to condition this muscle gradually with the help of a physical therapist. Progressively add distance to your runs or hikes, rather than suddenly increasing the mileage. Avoid running or walking on side-slanted surfaces, or at least change directions periodically so you are running on the opposite slant. For example, return on the same side of the road instead of crossing and always facing traffic. Prior to an aggravating activity, take extra vitamin C and be sure to keep your legs warm.

■ Foot pronation, especially combined with the above activities.

Solutions
■ Do not wear high heels. Wear corrective orthotics to correct foot pronation problems. See chapters 2 and 4 for more information.

■ A trauma or strain that tears the posterior cruciate ligament in the knee.
■ Trigger points can develop in conjunction with a tear of the plantaris muscle (59).

Solutions
■ Work on the trigger points to the extent possible while the injury is healing and during recovery from the tear and/or surgery.

Self-Help Techniques

Applying Pressure

Caution: Do not apply pressure to your legs if you have varicose veins in the area to be treated—it could release a clot that could go to your heart or brain! An acupuncturist or massage therapist should treat your legs, because they can avoid the varicose veins. However, you may still do the stretches and exercises below.

Gastrocnemius Pressure
Do the gastrocnemius self-treatment first (see chapter 58), being careful to work close to the back crease of the knee.

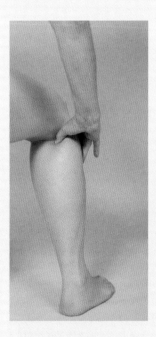 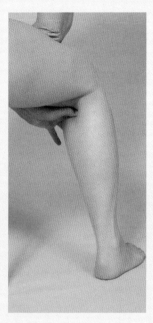

Popliteus Pressure
Sit in a chair and bend forward slightly, supporting yourself with one hand on your thigh. To work on the part of the muscle closest to the outside of your knee, use the thumb of the hand of the same side. To work on the part of the muscle closest to the inside of your knee (where the bulk of the muscle lies), use your thumb of the opposite hand. If you keep your thumb straight, it is easier to press through the overlying muscles into the trigger points in the popliteus. Be sure to get close to the crease of the knee to treat the entire muscle, but do not press right into the crease behind the knee—there are veins and nerves that are close to the surface. You may need the help of a massage therapist.

Also Check

Gastrocnemius (58). Hamstrings muscle group (56, biceps femoris).

Differential Diagnosis
If you are unable to relieve your symptoms with trigger point self-help techniques, you may need to see a health care provider to rule out a Baker's cyst, thrombosis of the popliteal vein, anteromedial and posterolateral instability of the knee, avulsion of the popliteus tendon, or a meniscus tear.

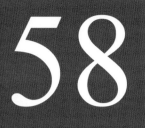

58 Gastrocnemius

The *gastrocnemius* muscle attaches to the femur bone, just above the knee. The Achilles tendon attaches both the gastrocnemius and the soleus muscles to the heel bone. The gastrocnemius works in conjunction with the other muscles on the back of the calf to control the forward rotation of the leg over the foot while walking, and it also helps stabilize the knee.

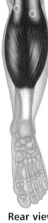

Rear view

Plantar fasciitis is caused by tension overload on the fascial attachment, or *plantar aponeurosis*, on the big bone in the heel (calcaneus), due to tightness in the gastrocnemius, soleus (59), abductor hallucis, flexor digitorum brevis, and/or abductor digiti minimi (71) muscles. The quadratus plantae (72) may also be involved. See chapter 55 for more information. Also see "Compartment Syndromes" in chapter 55, since the gastrocnemius muscle is located within the superficial posterior compartment. *If you have a compartment syndrome, it is important to see a health care provider immediately for treatment.*

If you have had a laminectomy in the lumbar area and still experience pain in the back of the leg, try searching for trigger points in the gastrocnemius muscle.

Common Symptoms

- Pain referred into the arch of the foot and over the back of the leg, back of the knee, and possibly back of the lower thigh.
- Pain when climbing steep slopes or over rocks, or walking on slanted surfaces.
- Difficulty straightening the leg completely when standing, and difficulty walking fast, with a tendency to walk with a flat-footed, stiff-legged gait.
- Calf cramps when sleeping.

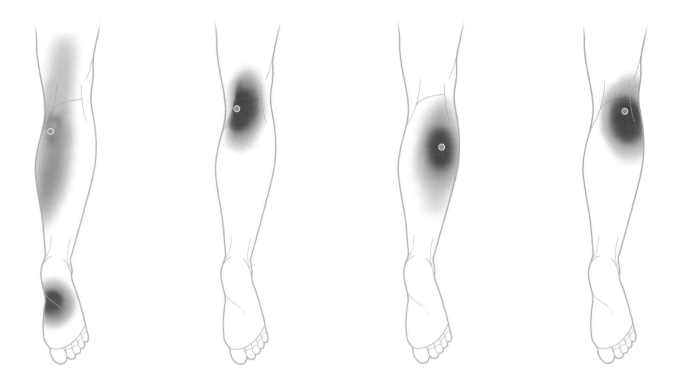

Causes and Perpetuation of Trigger Points, and Solutions

■ Sports activities such as walking, climbing, or running up steep slopes, over rocks, or on slanted surfaces, or riding a bicycle with the seat too low.

Solutions
■ Until the trigger points are inactivated, avoid walking up hills or on slanted surfaces. Stretch before and after athletic activities. Make sure your bike seat is not too low. If you swim, avoid the crawl stroke, since the kick causes you to point your toes.

■ Body positions that hold the muscle in a shortened or lengthened position for prolonged periods, such as standing while leaning forward for a long time, hooking your heel on a rung of a stool for an extended period, wearing high heels, driving a car with an accelerator pedal that is too horizontal, prolonged immobility with your toes pointed (such as when sleeping), or jobs that require a lot of squatting, for example working as a mechanic.

Solutions
■ Do not wear high heels. Avoid hooking your heels on the rung of a stool. Alternate standing and sitting positions, or if you must stand for long periods, stand more upright by correcting your posture (see chapter 7). Take breaks from squatting or use a low stool. Avoid wearing smooth leather shoes, particularly on a slippery floor. At night, place a pillow against the bottom of your feet to maintain a 90-degree angle between your feet and lower legs.
■ Use a car with an accelerator pedal that is not too stiff. If the accelerator pedal in your car is at a steep vertical angle, try attaching a wedge to the pedal with the big end at the bottom to reduce the angle of your foot. If it is nearly horizontal, experiment with attaching the big end of the wedge at the top. Using cruise control will help. Take breaks every 30 to 60 minutes.

■ Wearing socks, garters, or knee-high hose with an elastic band that is too tight, or wearing a cast.

■ Sitting in a reclining chair that places a lot of your leg weight on the calves, or sitting in a chair with a high front edge that impairs circulation or otherwise compresses the backs of your thighs.

Solutions

■ If your socks or hose leave a mark or indentation on your skin at the elastic band, the elastic is too tight and cutting off needed circulation. Buy socks and hose with a wider, looser band.

■ Sit in a chair at the proper height for you so that it is not restricting circulation in the back of your thighs or calves, and use a slanted footstool to elevate your lower legs if necessary. Using a rocking chair prevents prolonged immobility and increases circulation.

■ Muscle chilling, particularly if you have hypothyroidism.

Solutions

■ Sleep with a warm covering on your legs, such as knee-high pile socks or long-johns, an electric blanket, or a heating pad. During the day, keep your calves and body warm. Use a space heater near your legs if necessary. See chapter 4 for information on hypothyroidism.

■ Medical conditions such as viral infections or impaired circulation.

Solutions

■ Treat the underlying causes. See chapter 4 for information on treating viral infections. Talk to your health care provider regarding treatment of impaired circulation.

■ Calf cramps can be either a symptom of trigger points, or a cause and perpetuator of trigger points.

Solutions

■ Calf cramps are one of the most common symptoms of gastrocnemius trigger points and often occur when sleeping or sitting for too long with the toes pointed. When cramping occurs, rather than standing and walking immediately, instead gently flex the foot so the toes are moving toward your trunk, and then release. To reduce the tendency for your calves to cramp when sleeping, keep them warm at night by using a heating pad at bedtime, or use an electric blanket.

■ Calf cramps may also be brought on by dehydration, loss of/or inadequate intake of electrolytes (including potassium, calcium, magnesium, and salt), hypoparathyroidism, Parkinson's disease, and possibly diabetes. If you are experiencing calf cramps, try increasing your water intake and take a multimineral supplement. If you limit your salt intake severely and/or sweat heavily, try increasing your salt intake, unless otherwise directed by a health care provider. Doctors Travell and Simons (1992) found that taking 400 I.U. per day of vitamin E helped some patients tremendously. If you take a multivitamin be sure to count that amount of vitamin E toward the 400 I.U., and only take the larger dose for a maximum of two weeks, or for less if the cramps disappear sooner. Try vitamin B2 (riboflavin) if you have calf cramps during pregnancy. Some drugs, such as lithium, cimetidine, bumetanide, vincristine, and phenothiazines, can cause calf cramps, so you may need to talk to your health care provider to see if you can switch medications.

Self-Help Techniques

Check the gluteus minimus (posterior portion, 62) to ascertain whether trigger points there are causing and perpetuating satellite trigger points in the gastrocnemius. Also, check the tibialis anterior (69) and long extensors of the toes (70) for associated trigger points.

If the Achilles tendon feels tight, work on the gastrocnemius and soleus (59) muscle bellies to relax the tendon.

Applying Pressure

Caution: Do not apply pressure to your legs if you have varicose veins in the area to be treated—it could release a clot that could go to your heart or brain! An acupuncturist or massage therapist should treat your legs, because they can avoid the varicose veins. However, you may still do the stretches and exercises below.

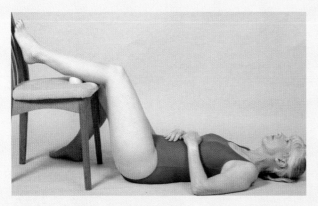

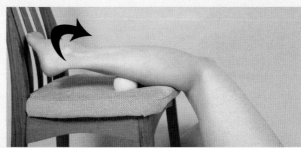

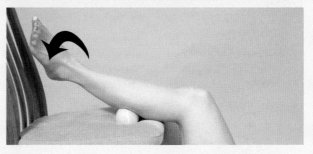

Gastrocnemius Pressure
Lie face-up with your butt pressed up close to a chair, coffee table, or other hard surface that is about the height you need to get a 90-degree angle bend at your knee. Place the ball on the hard surface and rest your calf on it, with gravity giving you the needed pressure. Be sure to work as much as you can from top to bottom, and rotate your leg side to side to get as much of the edges of the muscles as possible. You can move your leg over the ball, and you will need to move the ball with your hand at least once to treat all the points.

Then, sit up with your legs bent to one side, with one heel close to the pubic area and the other one out to the side. Hold a golf ball, tennis ball, or some other pressure device in the center of your palm and press it into tender points on your inner and outer lower legs to work the edges of the muscles.

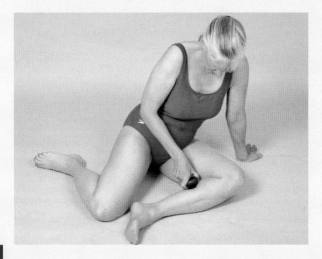

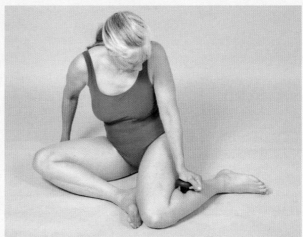

Stretches

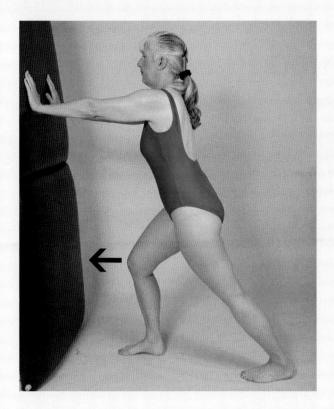

Gastrocnemius Stretch

Stand a short distance from a wall and place your hands on the wall at about head height. Place the leg to be stretched out behind you, with your knee straight, your heel on the floor, and your toes pointing straight forward. Let your hips move forward until you are getting a gentle stretch on the back of your lower leg. Look straight ahead so that your neck is not bent down.

Exercises

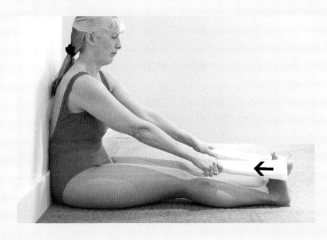

Seated Gastrocnemius Stretch

Sit with your back against a wall with your legs out straight. Put a thin, long towel around one foot and hold both ends of the towel with your hands. Gently press the ball of your foot against the towel for five seconds while you slowly inhale. As you exhale, release the pressure on your foot and use the towel to pull the ball of the foot toward you, giving you a gentle stretch on the back of the calf. Repeat three or four times with each foot.

Also Check

Soleus and plantaris (59, soleus). Hamstrings muscle group (56). Gluteus minimus (62, posterior portion). Tibialis anterior (69). Long extensors of the toes (70).

Differential Diagnosis

If the self-help techniques do not relieve the trigger points more than temporarily, you may need to see a health care provider to rule out damage to the nerve roots at the S1 level. You may also need to rule out a partial tear in the muscle ("tennis leg"), posterior compartment syndrome, thrombophlebitis, intermittent claudication, arteriosclerosis, or a Baker's cyst.

59 Soleus and Plantaris

The *soleus* muscle attaches to the tibia and fibula bones in the lower leg. The Achilles tendon attaches both the gastrocnemius and the soleus muscles to the heel bone. The soleus restrains the forward rotation of the tibia over the foot, contributes to knee stability, and provides ankle stability. The soleus muscle is known as the body's "second heart," due to its pumping action that returns blood from the lower leg to the heart. Flexing and extending the foot can greatly improve circulation in the legs.

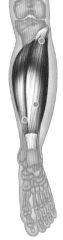

Soleus (rear view)

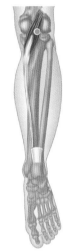

Plantaris (rear view)

The *plantaris* muscle is a thin, frail muscle that has considerable variations from person to person in structure and attachment locations, and may even be absent. It generally attaches to the femur above and turns into a thin tendon which passes in between the gastrocnemius and soleus muscles, to attach below to the heel bone. The bulk of the muscle fibers are found on the back of the leg, opposite the knee, in the popliteal space. The primary function of the plantaris is to point the foot and invert it toward the midline.

Achilles tendonitis may be due to trigger points causing shortening of the soleus and gastrocnemius (58) muscles. Pain will be diffuse and possibly burning in or around the Achilles tendon, and aggravated by activity. If the condition is severe, there may also be swelling, crackling sounds, or a tender nodule in the tendon. The cause is usually improper training or over-training. Corrective orthotics and shoes with a more flexible sole may help considerably.

Plantar fasciitis is caused by tension overload on the fascial attachment (plantar aponeurosis) on the big bone in the heel (calcaneus), due to tightness in the gastrocnemius (58), soleus, abductor hallucis, flexor digitorum brevis, and/or abductor digiti minimi (71) muscles. The quadratus plantae (72) may also be involved. See chapter 55 for more information. Also see "Compartment Syndromes" in chapter 55, since the soleus muscle is located in the superficial posterior compartment. *If you have a compartment syndrome, it is important to see a health care provider immediately for treatment.*

If you have heel pain, and a bone spur is found on the bottom of the big bone of the heel, do not assume the spur is the source of the pain. The other heel may have a spur that causes no pain, so trigger points may be the source of the pain, rather than the spur. An elevated serum uric acid level will cause a heel spur to become painful and is likely to aggravate trigger points in the soleus and other muscles.

The generic term shin splints has been used in the past to refer to any chronic pain in the front or middle of the lower leg associated with exercise. More recently, shin splints refers specifically to irritation of the surface of the bone along the attachment of a muscle and is called periosteal irritation, or in the case of the soleus muscle, soleus periostalgia syndrome. This is caused by repetitive exercise, such as running or aerobic dancing. At first, pain will be mild and occur later in the exercise, and will be relieved by rest. As the condition progresses, pain will be more intense, occur earlier in the exercise, and may not be relieved once the exercise has stopped. The surface of the bone, the periosteum, where the soleus attaches on the inside of the lower leg, can loosen and sometimes separate from the deeper part of the bone. A stress fracture can cause similar symptoms.

Common Symptoms

- Trigger points in either muscle can cause difficulty walking due to pain, especially uphill and up or down stairs.
- Trigger points in either muscle can cause an inability to flex the foot toward the knee, making it difficult to squat or kneel down to pick items up off the floor, which can subsequently lead to back pain if you are lifting by bending at the waist.

Soleus
- The most common trigger point in the soleus refers pain to the back and bottom of the heel and to the Achilles tendon. The second most common trigger point in the soleus is located close to the back of the knee and refers pain to the upper half of the back of the calf. An uncommon trigger point refers pain over the sacroiliac joint on the same side.

- Soleus trigger points may be the cause of "growing pains" in children.
- Trigger points and subsequent tightness of the soleus muscle can entrap the posterior tibial veins, posterior tibial artery, and tibial nerve, causing swelling of the foot and ankle and severe heel pain and tingling.

Plantaris
- Trigger points in the plantaris muscle refer pain behind the knee and to the upper half of the calf.
- Trigger points and subsequent tightness of the plantaris muscle can entrap the popliteal artery, which can cause calf pain.

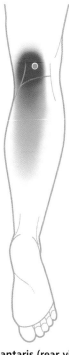

Plantaris (rear view)

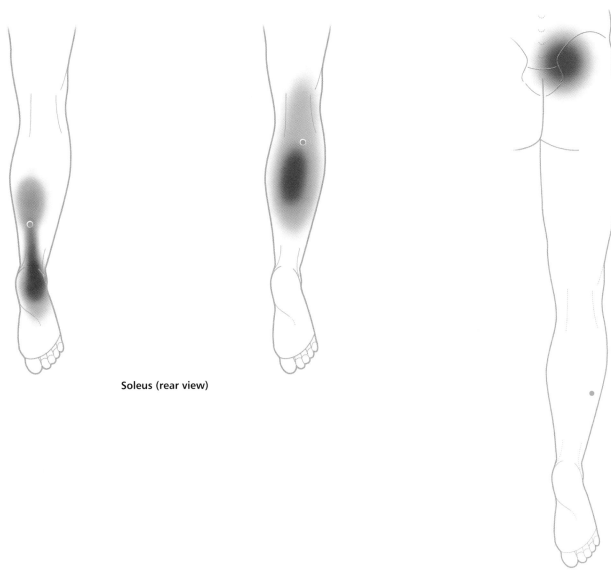

Soleus (rear view)

Soleus (rear view)

Causes and Perpetuation of Trigger Points, and Solutions

■ Sports activities such as running and jogging, or skiing and ice skating without the ankle support of stiffer boots. Walking, climbing, or running up steep slopes, over rocks, or on slanted surfaces, especially when you are not used to it.

Solutions
■ Stretch before and after athletic activities. Until the trigger points are inactivated, avoid walking up hills or on slanted surfaces. If you have pain when walking up stairs, try rotating your body to 45 degrees instead of facing forward, keep your body erect, and put your entire foot on the next step, rather than letting your heel hang off of the edge.

■ Wearing high heels, shoes with soles that are too stiff, or smooth-soled shoes on slippery surfaces.

Solutions
■ Do not wear high heels or smooth leather shoes, particularly on a slippery floor. If your shoes are so stiff they do not bend at the toes very well, you will need to find more pliable shoes. Proper shoes are so important to lasting relief of soleus trigger points that if you are unwilling to change your shoes, you can expect to need frequent treatment. See chapter 2, "Clothing," for more information.

■ Wearing socks, garters, or knee-high hose with an elastic band that is too tight.

Solutions

■ If your socks or hose leave a mark or indentation on your skin at the elastic band, the elastic is too tight and cutting off needed circulation. Buy socks and hose with a wider, looser band.

■ Sustained pressure against the calf, such as sitting in a reclining chair that places a lot of your leg weight on the calves. Sitting in a chair with a high front edge that impairs circulation or otherwise compresses the backs of the thighs, or sitting in a chair that is too high, so that you are not able to keep your feet flat on the ground.

Solutions

■ Sit in a chair at the proper height for you so that it is not restricting circulation in the back of your thighs, and use a slanted footstool to elevate the lower legs if necessary so that you can keep your feet flat. Using a rocking chair prevents prolonged immobility and increases circulation. Most recliner chairs or footrests place too much pressure on the calves. If you choose to use some kind of lower leg support, make sure you get something that supports the whole back of the lower leg and heels so that no one area takes all the weight of the leg.

■ Injuries such as a direct blow to the muscle, or a fall or near-fall.

Solutions

■ See chapter 4 for information on treating new injuries, then do the self-help techniques for the soleus muscle and the gastrocnemius muscle (58).

■ Referral from trigger points in the posterior portion of the gluteus minimus muscle.

Solutions

■ Check the gluteus minimus (62) for primary trigger points.

■ Prolonged immobility with your toes pointed, such as when sleeping or driving, or jobs that require a lot of squatting, such as working as a mechanic.
■ Chilling of the calf, especially combined with immobility.

Solutions

■ At night place a pillow against the bottom of your feet to maintain a 90-degree angle between your feet and lower legs. If you sleep on your back, try putting a small pillow under your knees. Wear knee-high fleece socks at night to prevent muscle chilling.
■ When driving for long periods, take frequent breaks and use cruise control.

■ One leg anatomically shorter than the other, since the short side bears more of the body weight.

Solutions

■ If you have one leg anatomically shorter than the other, you will need to see a specialist for compensating lifts. See chapter 4, "Spinal and Skeletal Factors," for more information.

Self-Help Techniques

Check the quadratus plantae (72), since it can also refer pain to the bottom of the heel. If you have trigger points in the soleus and also have knee pain, check the quadriceps femoris muscle group (65), since loss of function in the calf puts additional stress on the muscles of the front of the thigh.

If the Achilles tendon feels tight, work on the gastrocnemius (58) and soleus muscle bellies to relax the tendon.

Applying Pressure

Caution: Do not apply pressure to your legs if you have varicose veins in the area to be treated—it could release a clot that could go to your heart or brain! An acupuncturist or massage therapist should treat your legs, because they can avoid the varicose veins. However, you may still do the stretches and exercises below.

Gastrocnemius Pressure
The gastrocnemius pressure (see chapter 58) will also treat the underlying soleus muscle.

Stretches

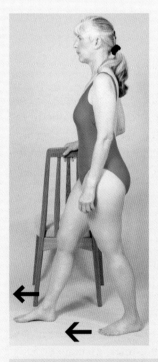
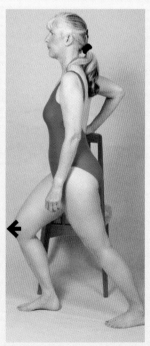

Soleus Stretch
Hold onto something for support and place one foot out in front of you, and one foot slightly behind you, with the toes of both feet pointing straight forward. Keeping your heel on the floor, bend the knee of the rear foot until you are getting a gentle stretch in the soleus muscle. Look straight ahead so that your neck is not bent down.

Also Check

Deep intrinsic foot muscles (72, quadratus plantae). Superficial intrinsic foot muscles (71, abductor hallucis). Gastrocnemius (58). Tibialis posterior (60). Long flexors of the toes (61). Tibialis anterior (69). Long extensors of the toes (70, extensor digitorum longus, extensor hallucis longus). Peroneal muscle group (64, peroneus tertius).

Differential Diagnosis
If you are unable to relieve your symptoms with trigger point self-help techniques, you may need to see a health care provider to rule out a rupture of a calf muscle, S1 nerve root irritation, thrombophlebitis, a ruptured popliteal cyst, or possibly a systemic viral infection. A ruptured muscle will cause sudden, intense pain at the time of an injury, followed by bruising that appears within one to two days. With thrombophlebitis there will be constant pain unaffected by activity level, as well as warmth and redness in the area.

60 Tibialis Posterior

The *tibialis posterior* muscle is located in between the bones of the lower leg, and its tendon attaches to several bones in the bottom of the foot. It helps distribute body weight evenly on the sole of the foot.

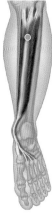

Rear view

Weakness or absence of this muscle causes severe overpronation, which means more of your weight is on the inside of the foot, and your foot and ankle roll in toward the midline. This leads to breakdown of one of the arches of the foot and then severe deformity. If a tight posterior tibialis is not treated, its tendon can become elongated or even rupture, accompanied by severe pain when walking and displacement of the bones of the foot. This condition requires diagnosis by an MRI. Any problems must be corrected within a few months to prevent irreversible damage.

The generic term shin splints, used in the past to refer to any chronic pain in the front or middle of the lower leg associated with exercise, now commonly refers specifically to irritation of the surface of the bone along the attachment of a muscle, and is called periosteal irritation. In the case of the tibialis posterior, shin splints usually develop in runners who are novices or in athletes who are poorly conditioned. At first, pain will be mild and occur later in the exercise, and will be relieved by rest. As the condition progresses, pain will be more intense, occur earlier in the exercise, and may not be relieved once the exercise has stopped. The surface of the bone, or periosteum, where the tibialis posterior attaches on the tibia, can loosen and sometimes separate from the deeper part of the bone. Also see "Compartment Syndromes" in chapter 55. *If you have a compartment syndrome, it is important to see a health care provider immediately for treatment.*

You will need the help of a professional to treat this muscle, but because tibialis posterior trigger points rarely occur alone, by treating the trigger points in other associated muscles, you can greatly speed your treatment and healing and help prevent permanent damage.

Common Symptoms

■ Pain referred primarily over the Achilles tendon, with spillover pain through the heel and the bottom of the foot and toes, and over the back of the calf.

■ Pain in the foot when running or walking, especially on uneven surfaces.

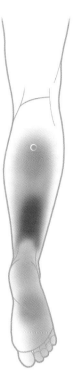

Causes and Perpetuation of Trigger Points, and Solutions

■ Running or jogging, especially on uneven ground or side-slanted surfaces, is the most common contributor to trigger point activation and perpetuation.

Solutions

■ Only walk or run on smooth, level surfaces until trigger points are inactivated. If you are unable to walk or run, try swimming and bicycling.

■ Shoes that are worn down on the inside or outside edges, or foot pronation.
■ A longer second toe, which causes an unstable ankle and foot rocking.

Solutions

■ Avoid high heels and shoes that do not fit properly. Wear good orthotics with arch support and a deep heel cup to prevent pronation. See chapter 2 for more information.

■ Systemic perpetuating factors such as hyperuricemia with or without symptoms of gout in the big toe, or polymyalgia rheumatica; both are diagnosed by a blood test. Obesity, hypertension, lupus, diabetes, peripheral neuropathy, smoking, and rheumatoid arthritis are also predisposing factors of problems with the tibialis posterior muscle and tendon.

Solutions

■ If you have been diagnosed with one of these conditions, you will need to treat the condition in order to get lasting relief from trigger points. You will probably need to periodically treat the trigger points when any flare-ups occur.

Self-Help Techniques

Applying Pressure

Caution: Do not apply pressure to your legs if you have varicose veins in the area to be treated—it could release a clot that could go to your heart or brain! An acupuncturist, physical therapist, or massage therapist should treat your legs, because they can avoid the varicose veins.

Gastrocnemius Pressure

The gastrocnemius pressure (see chapter 58) will help treat the tibialis posterior. The tibialis posterior is deep and next to the bone, so you may not be able to get to the whole muscle with self-help techniques. It is difficult to inject this muscle and not recommended. Ultrasound and stretching are effective, so you may need to see a physical therapist or other professional who can help with this.

Also Check

Long flexors of the toes (61, flexor digitorum longus, flexor hallucis longus). Peroneal muscle group (64, peroneus longus, peroneus brevis).

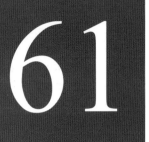

61 Long Flexors of the Toes

Flexor Digitorum Longus, Flexor Hallucis Longus

The *flexor hallucis longus* muscle attaches to the fibula bone and to the bottom of the bone in the big toe (great toe). The *flexor digitorum longus* muscle attaches to the tibia bone and the bottoms of the bones of each of the four lesser toes. These muscles help maintain equilibrium when your body weight is on the forefoot and help stabilize the foot and ankle while walking. Their primary action is flexing the end bone at the last joint on each of the toes, and assisting in flexing the other joints in the toes.

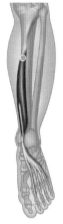
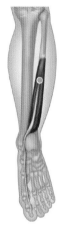

Flexor digitorum longus (rear view)   Flexor hallucis longus (rear view)

Hammer toes and claw toes can form when the long flexor muscles of the toes attempt to compensate for a flat foot caused by pronation. They can also form when the gastrocnemius (58) and soleus (59) muscles are weak, combined with a high arch and foot supination. This causes the outside and deeper rear calf muscles to try to compensate, but this is less common.

See the discussion of hallux valgus and bunions in chapter 55, since the flexor hallucis longus is involved in that condition. Relief of trigger points may stop the progression or even reverse some of the bone and joint spread and deformity of hallux valgus and subsequent bunions, though surgery may be necessary if the condition has progressed far enough.

The generic term shin splints, used in the past to refer to any chronic pain in the front or middle of the lower leg associated with exercise, now commonly refers specifically to irritation of the surface of the bone along the attachment of a muscle. This is called periosteal irritation, or in the case of these muscles, medial tibial stress syndrome. At first, pain will be mild and occur later in the activity, and will be relieved by rest. As this condition progresses, pain will be more intense, occur earlier during exercise, and may not be relieved once the exercise has stopped. The surface of the bone, or periosteum, where the flexor digitorum longus attaches on the inside of the lower leg, can loosen and sometimes separate from the deeper part of the bone. A stress fracture can cause similar symptoms.

The tendon of the flexor hallucis longus can rupture spontaneously if overloaded, without previous injury or disease, and must be repaired surgically.

Common Symptoms

■ Trigger points in the flexor digitorum longus refer pain primarily to the front half of the arch of the foot and into the ball of the foot. Sometimes pain is also referred into the second through fifth toes and, very occasionally, over the inside of the calf and ankle area.

■ Trigger points in the flexor hallucis longus refer pain to the bottom of the big toe and the ball of the foot adjacent to the big toe.

■ Probably pain with walking, and trigger points may occasionally cause painful cramping similar to gastrocnemius cramps.

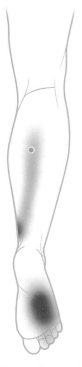

Flexor digitorum longus (rear view)

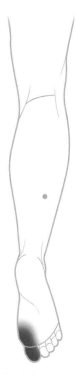

Flexor hallucis longus (rear view)

Causes and Perpetuation of Trigger Points, and Solutions

■ Walking, running, or jogging on uneven ground or sand, or on side-slanted surfaces.

Solutions
■ Until trigger points are inactivated, walk or run only on smooth surfaces, start with short distances, and increase mileage gradually. Try rowing, swimming, or bicycling instead.

■ Wearing shoes that are not very flexible or continuing to use shoes with worn soles and reduced cushioning.
■ Foot pronation, or having a second toe that is longer than the first toe, which causes an unstable ankle and foot rocking.
■ Weak gastrocnemius and soleus muscles combined with a high arch and foot supination.

Solutions
■ Do not wear high heels. Wear comfortable shoes with flexible soles and good shock absorption. Make sure that they do not cramp the toes and that the heels are not too loose. Replace worn shoes.

■ If your ankle is hypo-mobile (restricted movement), see a chiropractor or osteopathic physician to increase mobility. If it is hyper-mobile (moves too much), orthotics with good arch support and a deep heel cup, along with ankle-high shoes for support, will help stabilize the foot. You may need professional help to strengthen the gastrocnemius and soleus muscles.

Self-Help Techniques

Also check the tibialis posterior (60), superficial intrinsic foot muscles (71 – abductor digiti minimi, flexor digitorum brevis), and deep intrinsic foot muscles (72 – adductor hallucis, interossei, flexor hallucis brevis), since they have similar referral patterns.

Applying Pressure

Caution: Do not apply pressure to your legs if you have varicose veins in the area to be treated—it could release a clot that could go to your heart or brain! An acupuncturist or massage therapist should treat your legs, because they can avoid the varicose veins. However, you may still do the stretches and exercises below.

Gastrocnemius Pressure
The gastrocnemius pressure (see chapter 58) will also treat the long flexor muscles of the toes.

Stretches

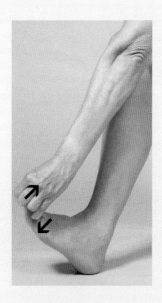

Long Flexors of the Toes Stretch
In a seated position, rest your heel on a stool or the floor with your ankle flexed toward your body. With your fingers, pull your toes toward you, and then slowly press your toes away from you, against your fingers. Relax, and then repeat.

Exercises

Walk in a swimming pool in waist-deep water, taking long strides.

Also Check

Tibialis posterior (60). Superficial intrinsic foot muscles (71). Deep intrinsic foot muscles (72, adductor hallucis, interossei, flexor hallucis brevis). Long extensors of the toes (70).

Differential Diagnosis
Pain on the inside of the ankle referred from trigger points in the flexor digitorum longus muscle can be easily mistaken for pain from tarsal tunnel syndrome. If you are not able to obtain relief with trigger point self-help techniques, you may need to see a health care provider for evaluation for other causes.

62 Gluteus Minimus

The *gluteus minimus* is the deepest of the gluteal muscles and attaches to the pelvis and the femur of the leg, crossing the hip joint. It helps keep the pelvis level when your weight is shifted to one leg, such as when walking.

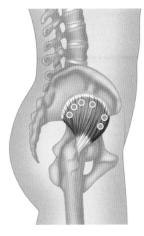

Referred pain from trigger points in the gluteus minimus muscle is frequently diagnosed by both patients and health care practitioners as sciatic pain because of the distribution pattern down the side and back of the leg. At least 80% of pain down the leg comes from trigger point referral from either the gluteus minimus or the hamstrings muscle group (56), and not from "pinched nerves," a herniated disc, or spinal stenosis in a lumbar vertebra (either a narrowing of the big hole in the vertebra that the spinal cord goes through, or a narrowing of the smaller holes the nerves travel out through). Since sciatica is usually assumed to be caused by compression of a nerve, referred pain from trigger points is probably more aptly called pseudo-sciatica.

If the pain feels deep in the hip joint, it is more likely coming from trigger points in the tensor fasciae latae muscle (63) instead of the gluteus minimus. If pain is over the sacrum (the bony triangle between the spine and the tailbone) or the sacroiliac joint (the joint where the sacrum and big pelvic bone meet), trigger points are more likely located in the gluteus medius muscle (31). If pain remains after a laminectomy surgery, check the gluteus minimus for trigger points.

Common Symptoms

- The anterior portion of the muscle refers pain down the side of the leg to the ankle, and possibly to a spot on the back of your buttocks, and may cause a limp when walking.
- The posterior portion of the muscle is partway between the side and the back, and refers pain over the gluteal area and down the back of the leg into the calf, and may also cause a limp when walking.
- Pain when running or hiking, or sleeping on the affected side, severe enough to wake you.
- Difficulty rising out of a chair after sitting for a while, and difficulty in finding a comfortable position standing, walking, or lying down.

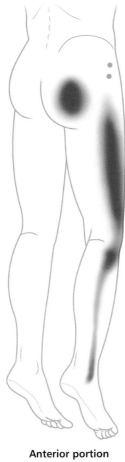

Anterior portion

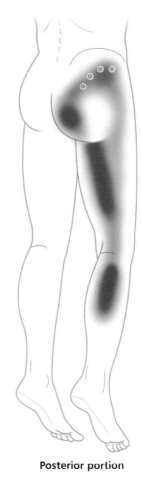

Posterior portion

Causes and Perpetuation of Trigger Points, and Solutions

■ Sudden or chronic overuse during sports activities, such as playing tennis, racquetball, or handball, or running too far or too fast, especially on rough ground.

Solutions
■ Runners and avid hikers often have gluteus minimus trigger points. If you have found trigger points with the self-help techniques, back off on your runs or hikes until the trigger points have improved dramatically. You can then slowly increase your mileage, staying out of the pain zone. I recommend doing both the ball self-treatment and ample stretching before and after a run or hike.

■ Postural problems, such as when sitting with a wallet in your back pocket, standing for long periods with your weight shifted to one side or with your feet too close together, walking with a limp from an injury, or sitting for too long, especially when driving.

Solutions
■ Do not carry a wallet in your back pocket. If you must stand for a long time, keep your feet apart and shift your weight frequently from one foot to the other. If you sit for long periods, move around the room every 15 to 20 minutes. Set a timer for 30 minutes and place it on the other side of the room to ensure that you will get up periodically to turn it off. Sleep with a pillow between your legs.

■ Direct injuries to the muscle, such as from a fall, or injections of medications, especially irritants.

Solutions

■ If you receive muscular injections, avoid the gluteus minimus. Injections into the gluteus medius and deltoid muscles are less prone to causing trigger points.

■ The sacroiliac joint out of alignment and/or a nerve root irritation.

Solutions

■ See a chiropractor or osteopathic physician to check the sacroiliac joint and lumbar vertebrae for alignment problems.

■ Obesity tends to overload the gluteus minimus muscles.

Solutions

■ If you are obese, do not over-exercise these muscles until trigger points have been inactivated and strength is built up gradually—see page 46, General Guidelines for Muscle Care. Walk with a wider stance.

■ Chilling of the muscle or the body as a whole.

Solutions

■ Keep your body and particularly the gluteus minimus muscles warm.

■ Structural inequalities, such as a small hemipelvis (either the left or the right half of the pelvic bone).

Solutions

■ If you have a small hemipelvis or other structural imbalance, see a specialist for compensating lifts and pads. See chapter 4 for more information.

Self-Help Techniques

Tightness in the opposite thoracolumbar paraspinal muscles can tilt and rotate the pelvis, causing pain in the hip joint and trigger points in the gluteal muscles. Be sure to work on the thoracolumbar paraspinal muscles (18) first, and the gluteal muscles (30 and 31) on both right and left sides.

If you only get temporary relief with the self-help techniques, check the quadratus lumborum (28), since trigger points in that muscle can cause and keep trigger points in the gluteus minimus activated.

Applying Pressure

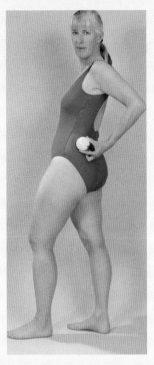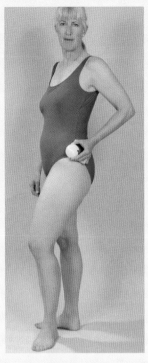

Gluteus Minimus Pressure

Be sure to work on the gluteus minimus muscles on both right and left sides of your body. Common trigger points in the gluteus minimus are found in the upper third of the back of your gluteal area, to over on the side between your hip joint and the top of your pelvis.

Lying face-up on a tennis ball, move the ball with your hand while searching for trigger points.

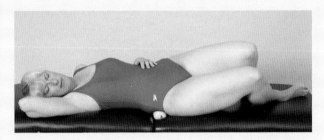

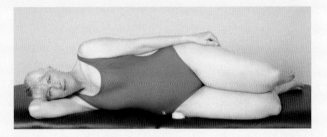

Start moving gradually out onto your side. By the time you work on the entire gluteus minimus muscle, you will be lying on your side. Many patients make the mistake of not getting far enough forward. If you are working over the seam of your pants, you are reaching all the points; otherwise, keep searching further forward.

Stretches

Gluteus Minimus Stretch Anterior Muscle Portion

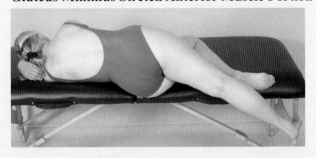

To stretch the anterior fibers of the gluteus minimus muscle, lie on your side on the edge of the bed with your back flush to the edge. Allow your top leg to drop behind you, off the edge. Allow gravity to give you a stretch. If you want more of a stretch, put the heel of your opposite leg on the side of your calf. Then move your heel closer to your knee for an even greater stretch.

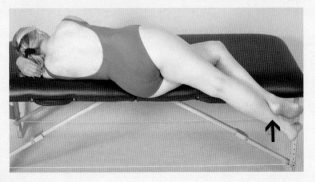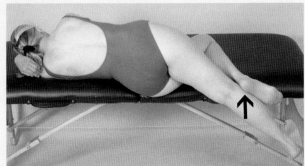

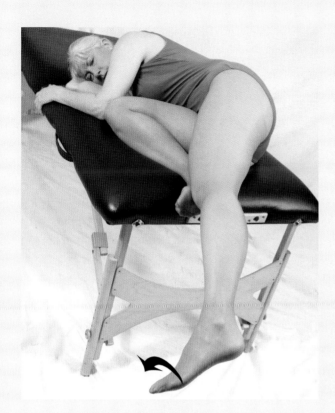

Gluteus Minimus Stretch Posterior Muscle Portion

To stretch the posterior fibers of the gluteus minimus muscle, lie on your side and position yourself at the foot of the bed with the top leg out over the end and slightly forward of the line of your trunk, with your toes slightly rotated toward the floor. Your bottom leg is bent at more than 90 degrees, so that it is still mostly on the bed. Let gravity give you a stretch.

Also Check

Piriformis (29). Gluteus medius (31). Tensor fasciae latae (63). Quadriceps femoris muscle group (65, vastus lateralis, satellite trigger points). Peroneal muscle group (64, peroneus longus). Quadratus lumborum (28). Gluteus maximus (30).

Differential Diagnosis

If the pain is very localized over the hip joint or perhaps from the buttocks down the side to the knee, it may be trochanteric bursitis, which is inflammation of a fluid-filled sack over the bone that allows the gluteus minimus tendon to glide over the bony prominence. The hip joint will be very tender to pressure, and applying pressure reproduces the symptoms. Gluteus minimus trigger points can also be misdiagnosed as bursitis, so it is always worth checking the surrounding muscles for trigger points and subsequent relief. Since, in every case of *true* bursitis that I have treated, the gluteus minimus muscle was also tight, I suspect tightness and trigger points are a causative factor for the bursitis. Acupuncture can treat bursitis: I lay the patient on their side and place four to five needles around the bursa and one in the center, which is called surround the dragon. I also needle points along the gall bladder meridian, in addition to any trigger points that are contributing to the irritation of the bursa.

I have found that if the pain is truly coming from a disc or a problem with a lumbar vertebra, the patient usually draws a referral pattern that starts as a thin line coming from a very specific spot on one side of a lumbar vertebra, and then continues into the gluteal area and down the leg. The pain is usually sharper and intense. If the pain referral starts in the gluteal area and not a discrete spot in the lumbar area, it is likely caused by trigger points in either the gluteus minimus or the piriformis muscles. If it does start next to a vertebra, you need to see a health care provider and have an MRI to be evaluated for disc problems and spinal stenosis. Acupuncture will help with disc problems, but will only help with the pain from spinal stenosis. It will not physically affect the spinal stenosis—that may require surgery. These surgeries usually have you back on your feet the day after the procedure.

63 Tensor Fasciae Latae

The *tensor fasciae latae* muscle attaches to the pelvic bone above, crosses the hip joint, and joins the iliotibial tract connective tissue, or iliotibial band, on the outer side of the thigh. It is used for both walking and standing by flexing and rotating the thigh, and moving the thigh out away from the midline, an action known as abduction. It also helps stabilize the knee.

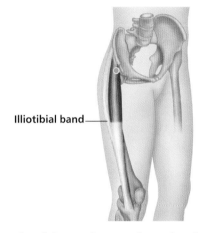

Illiotibial band

Referred pain must be differentiated from trigger point referral from the gluteus minimus (anterior fibers), gluteus medius, and vastus lateralis muscles. Pain may be misdiagnosed as trochanteric bursitis, so the term pseudo-trochanteric bursitis more aptly describes pain from trigger points.

Common Symptoms

■ Pain referred deep in the hip joint region, down the thigh on the side, and at the angle between the side and the front. Referred pain can also wrap around the front of the thigh and groin area.

■ Pain is more severe with movement, including walking rapidly.

■ An inability to sit for very long with the legs closer to the trunk at less than a 90-degree angle, and possibly an inability to lie on the affected side and/or the opposite side.

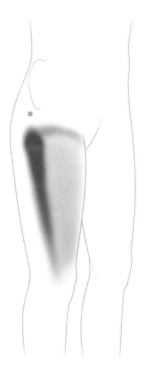

Causes and Perpetuation of Trigger Points, and Solutions

- Chronic overload such as running with an uncorrected foot pronation problem, having an anatomical leg-length inequality, or walking or running on side-slanted surfaces.
- In runners, poor conditioning and inadequate pre-stretching.
- Sudden trauma, such as jumping from a height.

Solutions

- Wear corrective orthotics to correct pronation problems—see chapter 2 for more information. If the soles of your shoes are worn, replace them.
- When a patient is examined face-up, it can appear that the affected leg is shorter than the other, so it is important for the diagnosing practitioner to release the tensor fasciae latae and determine if the bone of the leg is anatomically shorter than that of the unaffected leg before prescribing lifts.
- Avoid walking or jogging uphill until trigger points are inactivated. Avoid running or walking on side-slanted surfaces, or at least change directions periodically so you are running on the opposite slant. For example, return on the same side of the road instead of crossing and always facing traffic.

- Sitting or sleeping with the legs closer to the trunk at less than a 90-degree angle.

Solutions

- Avoid sitting in the cross-legged lotus position. When sleeping or sitting in a chair or car, maintain an angle of 90 degrees or greater between the torso and the thigh. A lumbar support will help with this, as will using cruise control and adding a thin pillow under the buttocks when driving.

Self-Help Techniques

Also check the gluteus minimus (62 – anterior portion) since the tensor fasciae latae is rarely involved alone, and because trigger points in the gluteus minimus can refer to the outside of the thigh and cause tightening of the iliotibial band. If your iliotibial band is tight, check both the tensor fasciae latae and the gluteus maximus (30) muscles, since this connective tissue helps attach both muscles to the leg. This condition is common in bowlegged runners whose feet pronate. Iliotibial tract friction syndrome causes diffuse pain and tenderness around the upper outside of the knee, which will probably be alleviated by using the self-help techniques for both of these muscles

Check the gluteus medius (31), rectus femoris (65), sartorius (66), iliopsoas (22), and quadratus lumborum (28), since trigger points in these muscles can cause similar referral patterns, and may also be involved in keeping trigger points in the tensor fasciae latae active. These muscles can also contain secondary trigger points caused by the tensor fasciae latae.

Applying Pressure

Thoracolumbar Paraspinal Pressure
As part of the tensor fasciae latae self-treatment, work on the thoracolumbar paraspinal muscles (18), because most of the time those muscles are also involved to some extent.

Tensor Fasciae Latae Pressure
Use a tennis ball on the bed. After working on the anterior portion of the gluteus minimus, move even further forward, so you are almost lying on your front—most people do not get far enough forward! The muscle goes from the pointy bony part of the front of your pelvis and is about five to eight inches long. If you put your hand in your front pocket, the muscle is under your hand.

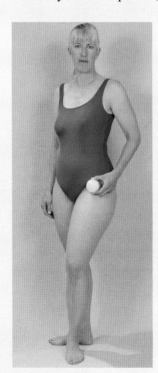
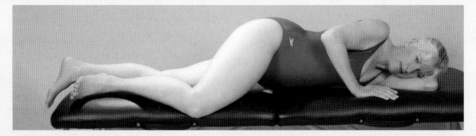

Stretches

Tensor Fasciae Latae Stretch
Position the front of your body flush with the edge of the bed, keeping your hips perpendicular. Hang your top leg off the bed in front of you, rotate your toes toward the ceiling, and let your leg dangle to allow gravity to give you the stretch.

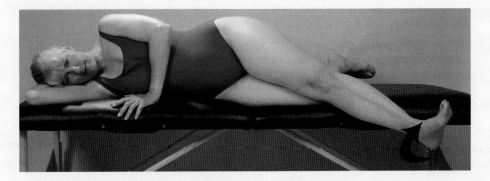

Quadriceps Side-Lying Stretch and Standing Stretches
The quadriceps femoris stretches (see chapter 65) also benefit the tensor fasciae latae.

Abdominal Stretch
See chapter 17. You may not be able to perform this stretch if you have back problems.

Thigh-Hip Extension Stretch
See chapter 22.

Also Check

Gluteus minimus (62, anterior portion). Gluteus medius (31). Gluteus maximus (30). Quadratus lumborum (28). Quadriceps femoris muscle group (65, vastus lateralis and rectus femoris). Iliopsoas (22). Sartorius (66).

> **Differential Diagnosis**
> If you are unable to relieve your symptoms with trigger point self-help techniques, you may need to see a health care provider to rule out an L4 nerve root irritation, arthritis of the sacroiliac joint, trochanteric bursitis, or peripheral nerve entrapment that causes meralgia paresthetica. See the gluteus minimus muscle (62) for information on bursitis, and the sartorius muscle (66) for information on meralgia paresthetica.

64 Peroneal Muscle Group

Peroneus Longus, Peroneus Brevis, Peroneus Tertius

The upper portions of the *peroneus longus*, *brevis*, and *tertius* muscles attach to the fibula, and their tendons attach to bones in the foot. These muscles stabilize and move the foot.

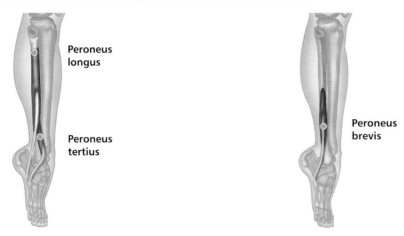

Peroneus longus

Peroneus tertius

Peroneus brevis

Because trigger points refer tenderness and pain in and around the ankle joint, pain referral can be misdiagnosed as arthritis or a chronic sprain. Weakness of any of the three peroneal muscles can contribute to "weak ankles," resulting in frequent ankle sprains and possibly ankle fractures. Sprains and fractures then further perpetuate trigger points, so treatment is critical to breaking this self-perpetuating cycle.

See "Compartment Syndromes" in chapter 55. If you have a compartment syndrome, it is important to see a health care provider immediately for treatment. Lateral compartment syndrome is likely to develop in runners who pronate and have abnormally mobile subtalar joints, or if the peroneus longus muscle ruptures. Once successfully treated, you should subsequently check for trigger points.

Common Symptoms

■ The peroneus longus and brevis refer pain and tenderness over and around the outside ankle bone, over a small area on the outside of the foot, and possibly over a small area over the outside of the lower leg. The peroneus tertius refers pain and tenderness more toward the front of the ankle and possibly behind the outside ankle bone and down toward and over the heel.

■ You may have weak ankles, which are easily broken or sprained over the outside, and you may have difficulty in-line or ice skating, unless the boots are very stiff.

■ If the deep peroneal nerve is entrapped, you may trip frequently due to an inability to lift your foot. Entrapment of the common peroneal nerve, superficial peroneal nerve, or deep peroneal nerve can cause pain and odd sensations, such as numbness on the front of the ankle and foot, accompanied by weakness of the ankle.

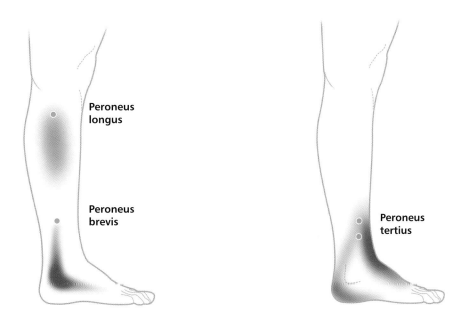

Causes and Perpetuation of Trigger Points, and Solutions

- ◼ Referred pain from trigger points in the anterior portion of the gluteus minimus muscle.
- ◼ Associated trigger points in the tibialis anterior and tibialis posterior muscles.

Solutions
- ◼ Be sure to also check the gluteus minimus (62 – anterior portion), tibialis anterior (69), and tibialis posterior (60) muscles for trigger points since they are often the cause of satellite peroneal muscle trigger points.

- ◼ Walking or running on side-slanted surfaces.

Solutions
- ◼ Walk or run on smooth, level surfaces until trigger points are relieved. Avoid slanted sidewalks, roads, or tracks.

- ◼ Sleeping with your toes pointed, or wearing high heels or shoes with a spike heel of any height.

Solutions
- ◼ At night, place a pillow against the bottom of your feet to maintain a 90-degree angle between your feet and lower legs. Do not wear spiked or high heels. Avoid shoes with pointed toes and inadequate room across the top of the toes. Your feet get wider as you get older, and shoes that may once have fit properly may now be too narrow. Any shoes that do not fit or are worn unevenly on the bottoms should be discarded. Buy shoes that have wide soles, such as athletic shoes, and get an orthotic insert with a deep heel cup and good arch support—most shoes made these days have minimal or no arch support. See chapter 2 for more information on footwear.

■ Wearing socks or knee-high hose with an elastic band that is too tight.

Solutions
■ If your socks or hose leave a mark or indentation on your skin from the elastic band, the elastic is too tight and cutting off needed circulation. Buy socks and hose with a wider, looser band.

■ Sprains or fractures in the lower leg, ankle, or foot, and/or immobilization with a cast.

Solutions
■ If you have pain remaining after a sprained or broken leg, ankle, or foot, try searching for trigger points in the peroneal muscles, since immobilization will cause trigger points.

■ Structural imbalances, such as a second toe longer than the first toe, or one leg anatomically shorter than the other.
■ Crossing one leg over the other can compress the common peroneal nerve.

Solutions
■ If your foot supinates due to a longer second toe (you will see excessive wear on the outside edge of the heel of your shoe), you will need to wear corrective orthotics. Crossing one leg over the other to compensate for a small hemipelvis (either the left or the right half of the pelvic bone) can compress the common peroneal nerve. If one leg is anatomically shorter than the other, you may have pain on only one side, even if you have a longer second toe on both sides. This is because your weight is shifted to the shorter side, causing a chronic overload of the muscles on that side. The leg may be "shorter" due to foot pronation and a low arch on the affected side, rather than a true unequal leg bone length. You will need to see a specialist for corrective orthotics or compensating lifts and pads for any of these conditions. See chapter 4 for more information.

Self-Help Techniques

Applying Pressure

Caution: Do not apply pressure to your legs if you have varicose veins in the area to be treated—it could release a clot that could go to your heart or brain! An acupuncturist or massage therapist should treat your legs, because they can avoid the varicose veins. However, you may still do the stretches below.

Gluteus Minimus Pressure
Check the gluteus minimus first (62, anterior portion), since the referred pain can cause satellite trigger points in the peroneal muscles.

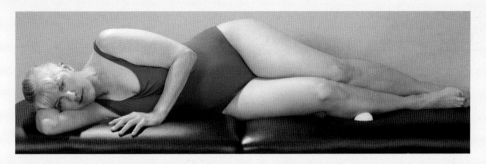

Peroneal Pressure
Lie on your side on the bed, with a tennis ball between the bed and the side of your lower leg, using gravity for pressure. You can move your leg over the ball to reposition it, but be sure to hold trigger points for eight seconds to one minute, following the general guidelines for self-help in chapter 5.

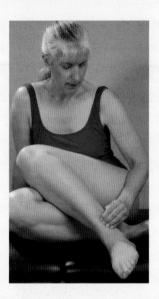

Then sit up with your leg out to the side on the bed and use the thumb of the same side to check for trigger points in the peroneus tertius, one to two inches above the outside ankle bone and closer toward the front of the leg.

Stretches

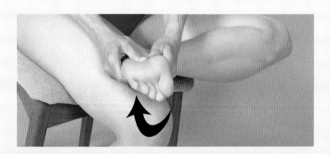

Peroneal Stretch
This stretch is most effective in a hot bath, but you may also sit in a chair. If you are stretching the left side, bring the left foot onto your right thigh. Rotate your foot so the bottom is toward the ceiling. You should feel the stretch on the outside of your lower leg.

Also Check

Gluteus minimus (62, anterior portion). Tibialis anterior (69). Tibialis posterior (60). Long extensors of the toes (70, extensor digitorum longus).

Differential Diagnosis
Trigger points in the peroneus longus can entrap the common peroneal nerve on the side of the leg just below the crease of the knee, and weaken both the anterior and the lateral compartment muscles. Loss of sensation from the entrapment is greatest in the triangular web between the first and second toes. If you are not able to relieve your symptoms with self-help techniques and are experiencing both the symptoms of common peroneal nerve entrapment and referred pain from peroneal trigger points, you need to see a health care provider to be evaluated for a ruptured disc in your back, some kind of cyst, or a rupture of the peroneus longus muscle.

65 Quadriceps Femoris Muscle Group

Rectus Femoris, Vastus Medialis, Vastus Intermedius, Vastus Lateralis

The *rectus femoris* muscle crosses both the hip and the knee joints, while the *vastus medialis, intermedius* and *lateralis* muscles only cross the knee joint. All four muscles come together to form a strong tendon which attaches to the kneecap, or patella, and the kneecap attaches to the tibia bone in the lower leg via the patellar ligament. The rectus femoris allows you to bend at the hip and all four muscles allow you to bend your knee.

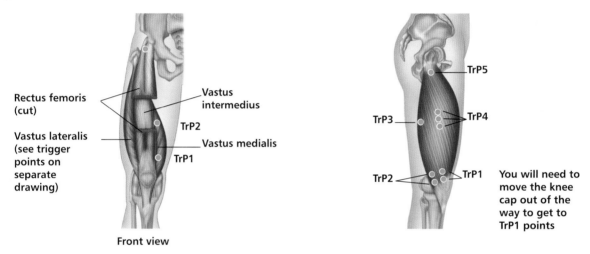

Rectus femoris (cut)

Vastus lateralis (see trigger points on separate drawing)

Vastus intermedius

TrP2

Vastus medialis

TrP1

Front view

TrP5

TrP3

TrP4

TrP2

TrP1

You will need to move the knee cap out of the way to get to TrP1 points

The vastus medialis and lateralis muscles are supposed to maintain normal positioning and tracking of the kneecap; however, tightness and trigger points in one or both muscles can pull the kneecap to one side or the other, causing structural damage between it and the underlying bones and joint. Trigger points in the quadriceps femoris muscle group are very common and frequently overlooked, mainly because they only minimally restrict range of motion, if at all. Doctors Travell and Simons nicknamed them the "Four-Faced Trouble Maker."

Pain from trigger points in the upper part of the vastus lateralis is commonly misdiagnosed as trochanteric bursitis. See the gluteus minimus muscle (62) for more information on bursitis.

Common Symptoms

- Pain referred on the thigh and knee, and possibly down the outside of the lower leg; see the pictures for all the trigger points and associated referral patterns.
- If you have weakness when extending your knee, you probably have either active or latent trigger points in the rectus femoris, vastus medialis, and/ or vastus intermedius muscles.

Rectus Femoris

- Pain referred deep in the knee, in and around the kneecap, and possibly on the front of the thigh at night in bed. Even though the pain is in the knee area, the most common trigger point is found just below the crease of the groin. Occasionally a trigger point will be found just above the knee and will refer pain deep into the knee joint.
- Going down stairs is more likely to be a problem than going up stairs.
- In above-knee amputees, phantom limb pain may come from trigger points in the rectus femoris, particularly if the muscle was stretched to cover the bone.

Vastus Medialis

- The trigger point closer to the knee refers pain to the front of the knee, and the trigger point about mid thigh refers pain over the inside of the knee and thigh.
- Toothache-like pain deep in the knee joint that can interrupt sleep and may be mistaken for inflammation of the knee.
- Trigger points only minimally restrict range of motion and may only affect leg function, rather than causing pain.
- Unexpected "buckling" of the knee produced by muscle weakness, which can lead to falls and injury. This will usually happen when walking on rough ground. If trigger points are found in both the vastus medialis and the rectus femoris, the hip may buckle.

Vastus Intermedius

- Intense pain at mid thigh, closer to the outside of the thigh. Pain is usually felt while moving and rarely when resting.
- Difficulty fully straightening the knee, which causes a limp when walking, especially after sitting for a while, and difficulty with climbing stairs.
- A buckling knee can be caused by a combination of trigger points in the vastus intermedius and the two heads of the gastrocnemius (58) below the crease at the back of the knee. This condition can also be caused by anterior subluxation of the lateral tibial plateau, which requires surgical correction. But since trigger points in the vastus medialis muscle are the more likely culprits, check that muscle first. Trigger points can also cause the kneecap to lock, though this is more commonly caused by trigger points in the vastus lateralis muscle.

Vastus Lateralis

- The vastus lateralis muscle develops multiple trigger points along the outside of the thigh, causing a variety of referral patterns along the outside of the thigh, knee, and possibly down into the calf. Trigger point referral can be misdiagnosed as trochanteric bursitis if pain is referred over the outside of the hip bone, or greater trochanter.
- Pain when walking and you may drag your foot on the affected side.
- Pain that disturbs your sleep when lying on the affected side.
- A "stuck patella" that can cause difficulty in straightening or bending the knee after getting up from a chair. If the kneecap is completely locked, the knee will be slightly bent and you cannot walk, and you are unable to sit without the leg supported in the locked position. Going up stairs is more likely to be a problem than going down them.

Ligamentous Trigger Point

- The lateral collateral ligament may refer pain to an area just above it on the outside of the knee.

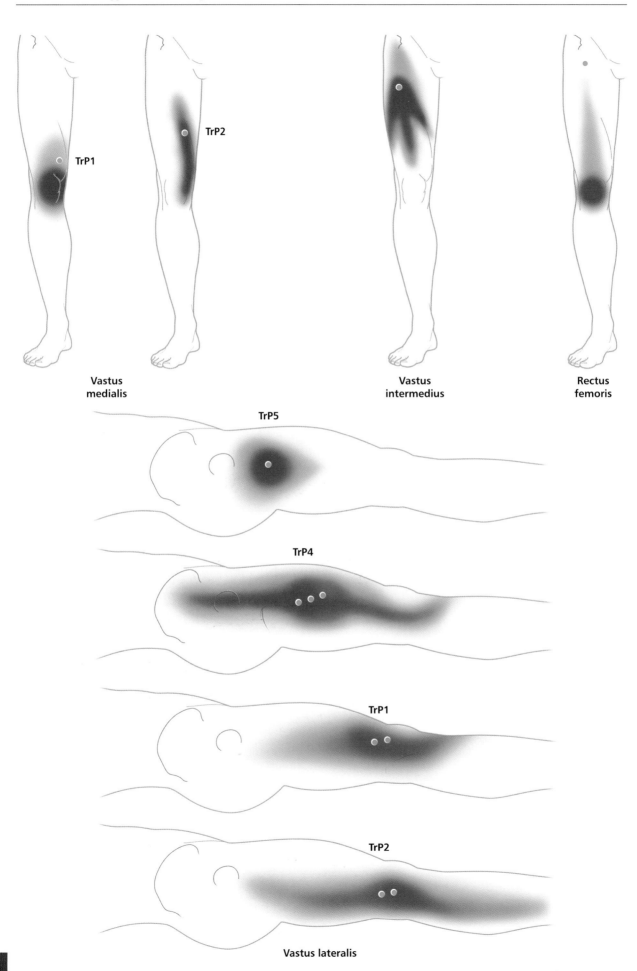

TrP1

TrP2

**Vastus
medialis**

**Vastus
intermedius**

**Rectus
femoris**

TrP5

TrP4

TrP1

TrP2

Vastus lateralis

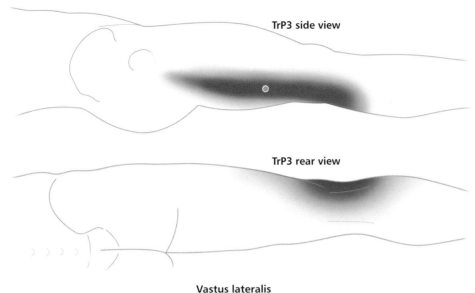

TrP3 side view

TrP3 rear view

Vastus lateralis

Causes and Perpetuation of Trigger Points, and Solutions

■ Injuries caused by stumbling (such as into a hole or off a kerb), sports, or a direct blow to the front of the thigh.
■ Overuse or improper conditioning exercises, such as deep knee bends, or knee extensions with a weight near the ankle.
■ Tightness in the hamstring muscles.
■ Active trigger points in the soleus muscle, which restrict the motion of the ankle and lead to overload of the quadriceps femoris muscle group.
■ Sitting with one foot under the buttocks.
■ Injections of drugs, such as insulin, into the thigh.
■ Any lengthy immobilization, such as wearing a leg cast.

Rectus Femoris
■ Sitting for a long time with a heavy weight on your lap.
■ Medical conditions such as a hip fracture and/or surgery, hip degenerative joint disease, or abnormal hip joint mechanics.

Vastus Medialis
■ Excessive foot pronation, possibly caused by flat feet.
■ Strenuous athletic activities such as jogging, skiing, football, basketball, and soccer.
■ A fall or a direct trauma to the knee joint and/or muscle.
■ Kneeling on a hard surface.

Vastus Intermedius
■ Trigger points develop secondary to trigger points in the other muscles of the quadriceps femoris group.

Vastus Lateralis
■ A sudden overload of the muscle or a direct trauma to the muscle, such as from sports accidents.
■ Sitting for a long time with your leg out straight.
■ Medical conditions such as hip degenerative joint disease or abnormal hip joint mechanics.

General Solutions

■ In the initial stages of treatment, you may wish to wear a neoprene knee brace, which will maintain warmth around the lower ends of the muscles and help remind you to be careful with the leg.

■ Wear corrective orthotics to solve foot pronation problems, and do not wear high heels. If one leg is anatomically shorter than the other, see a specialist to get a compensating lift.

■ Do not do deep knee bends or squats. See a physical therapist for a proper way to do knee extensions.

■ Avoid picking things up off the floor. Do not kneel for long periods of time; sit on a low stool and take frequent breaks. Avoid sitting in the same position for extended periods, especially with the thighs at less than a 90-degree angle to the trunk. Be sure to use a lumbar support. Do not sit with your legs extended straight out in front of you or with your foot under your buttocks. Sitting in a rocking chair helps keep the muscles mobilized. When getting out of a chair, use your arms to assist you in rising. When driving, use a lumbar support and a pillow or something similar under the buttocks to increase the angle between the torso and the thigh. Take frequent breaks.

■ If you have trigger points in the vastus medialis or vastus lateralis, sleep on the unaffected side with a pillow between your legs. Do not bring your thighs up toward your chest and do not straighten the legs out all the way either.

■ If you get intermuscular injections, ask your health care provider if another location would be acceptable.

■ It is important to identify and treat any lumbar vertebrae that are out of alignment or any hip alignment problems. See a chiropractor or osteopathic physician for evaluation and treatment.

Self-Help Techniques

Also check the gluteus minimus (62 – anterior portion) and the tensor fasciae latae (63) muscles, since they can have referral patterns similar to vastus lateralis trigger points. If pain is on the front or inside of the thigh, also check the adductor muscles of the hip (67 – adductors longus and/or brevis and gracilis). You will also need to check the hamstrings muscle group (56) and soleus muscle (59), since they can activate and perpetuate trigger points in the quadriceps femoris muscle group.

If you find trigger points in the rectus femoris, also check the other muscles of the group, as well as the iliopsoas (22) and sartorius (66) muscles. If you find trigger points in the vastus medialis, also check the rectus femoris, peroneus longus (64), adductor muscles of the hip (67), tensor fasciae latae (63), and gluteus medius (31). If you find trigger points in the vastus intermedius, also check the rectus femoris and vastus lateralis. If you find trigger points in the vastus lateralis, also check the gluteus minimus (62 – anterior portion).

Applying Pressure

Caution: Do not apply pressure to your legs if you have varicose veins in the area to be treated—it could release a clot that could go to your heart or brain! An acupuncturist or massage therapist should treat your legs, because they can avoid the varicose veins. However, you may still do the stretches and exercises below.

Hamstrings Pressure

Treat the hamstrings muscle group first (56), to avoid the cramping that can be caused by releasing the quadriceps femoris group. If you do not find trigger points in the hamstrings, you can probably skip this step in the future.

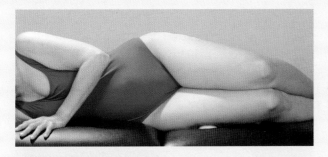

Vastus Lateralis Pressure

To treat the vastus lateralis muscle, start with the gluteus minimus (62 – anterior portion) and the tensor fasciae latae (63) self-help ball work. Then continue on down the side of your thigh, using your hand to move the tennis ball as you search for tender points. Be sure to work the whole length of the muscle.

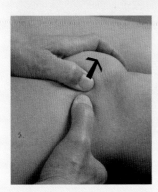

There may be some trigger points under the edge of the kneecap. Straighten out your leg, wrap your hands around your knee, and put both thumbs on the edge of the kneecap. Press the kneecap away from you while simultaneously pressing into trigger points in that area.

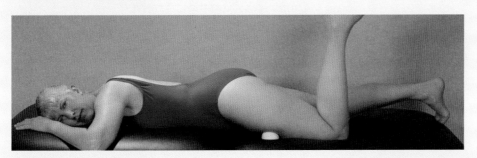

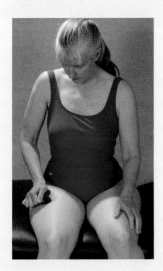

Rectus Femoris and Vastus Intermedius Pressure

To treat the rectus femoris and the underlying vastus intermedius, roll onto your stomach and, with your leg bent, move the tennis ball around, checking for tender points. Be sure to work the entire length of the muscles.

As an alternative, use a golf ball or other pressure device in the center of your palm and press into tender points. This is less effective than lying on the ball due to the thickness of the rectus femoris.

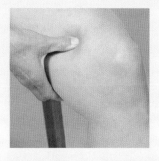

Vastus Medialis Pressure

To treat the vastus medialis, use your thumb, or a golf ball or other pressure device held in the center of the palm of your opposite hand, to press into tender points. It does not take a lot of pressure to treat these trigger points.

Stretches

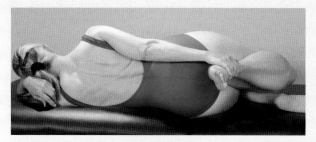

Quadriceps Side-Lying Stretch

Lying on your side on the bed, bend your bottom leg to almost a 90-degree angle to the trunk, so you can rest your top knee on the bottom foot. Grab the ankle of your upper leg and pull it up behind you, so you feel a stretch on the front of the thigh.

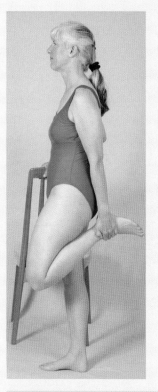
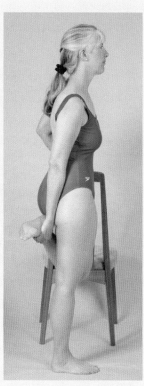

Quadriceps Standing Stretch

Hold onto a counter or other non-mobile piece of furniture for support. Grab your ankle using the hand of the same side and pull your leg up behind you. Then, with the opposite hand, grab the same ankle and pull your leg up behind you. The first part emphasizes the stretch of the vastus medialis, and the second part emphasizes the stretch of the vastus lateralis. Be sure to stretch both legs. This stretch is most effective when done in a warm swimming pool, holding onto the edge for balance.

Also Check

Hamstrings muscle group (56). Iliopsoas (22). Sartorius (66). Gluteus minimus (62, anterior portion). Tensor fasciae latae (63). Adductor muscles of the hip (67). Soleus and plantaris (59, soleus). Peroneal muscle group (64, peroneus longus). Gluteus medius (31).

Differential Diagnosis

There are many causes of knee pain, including ligament strains and tears, torn meniscuses, tendonitis, bursitis, kneecap fractures, and nerve entrapments. If you still have pain after inactivating trigger points, you will need to see an orthopedic doctor for evaluation. Even if other causes are found, trigger points are also likely involved, and treatment can help prepare you for surgery and help with recovery afterward.

66 Sartorius

The *sartorius* muscle crosses both the hip and the knee joints, and bends these joints in order to allow you to walk. It also rotates the thigh away from the body's midline, such as when placing your lower leg over the top of the opposite thigh. This muscle is very active during a variety of sports, especially those that require moving in several directions in rapid succession, such as basketball, tennis, and volleyball.

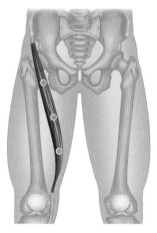

Trigger points in the lower part of the sartorius muscle refer pain in an area similar to the vastus medialis muscle (65), but pain from vastus medialis trigger points will feel deeper in the knee joint, rather than diffuse and superficial.

Common Symptoms

■ Referred pain that is superficial, sharp and tingling, felt at various points in the front of the thigh, and possibly superficial pain on the inside of the knee.

■ If the lateral femoral cutaneous nerve is entrapped, you may feel numbness, burning, or uncomfortable sensations in the front of your thigh, called meralgia paresthetica, which will be intensified by standing or walking.

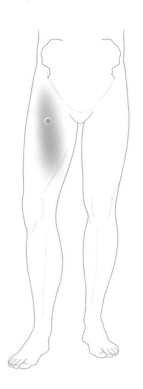
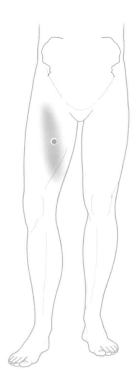
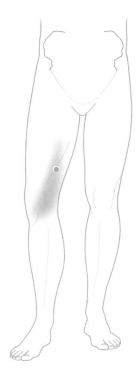

Causes and Perpetuation of Trigger Points, and Solutions

■ Excessive foot pronation.

Solutions
■ See chapter 2, "Footwear," to correct pronation.

■ Possibly a twisting fall.
■ Trigger points are usually found in conjunction with trigger points in the quadriceps femoris muscle group (65 – rectus femoris and vastus medialis), iliopsoas (22), pectineus (68), tensor fasciae latae (63), and adductor muscles of the hip (67).

Solutions
■ Do not sit cross-legged in the lotus position or with your ankle crossed over your opposite knee. Do not sleep with your knees drawn up tightly near your chest. Place a pillow between your legs.
■ If you have burning pain or odd sensations on the front of your thigh, try searching for trigger points below the pointy bony part of the front of your pelvis, and also work on the iliopsoas. Meralgia paresthetica (see above) may be caused by obesity, constricting garments or belts, one leg anatomically shorter than the other, or carrying a wallet in the front pants pocket. These causes will need to be addressed in order to obtain lasting relief.

Self-Help Techniques

Be sure to check for trigger points in the quadriceps femoris muscle group (65 - rectus femoris and vastus medialis), iliopsoas (22), pectineus (68), tensor fasciae latae (63), and adductor muscles of the hip (67), since the sartorius rarely develops trigger points on its own.

Applying Pressure

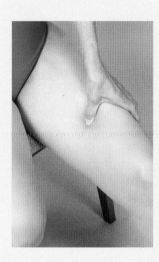

Sartorius Pressure
You may use the same pressure techniques as the vastus medialis and rectus femoris muscles (65), and you may also massage the muscle. Note how the muscle goes from the pointy part of the hip bone in front, crosses the front of the thigh, and then curves into your inner thigh as it approaches the knee. Be sure to work on all those areas so you will not miss any part of the muscle.

Also Check

Quadriceps femoris muscle group (65, rectus femoris and vastus medialis). Iliopsoas (22). Pectineus (68). Tensor fasciae latae (63). Adductor muscles of the hip (67).

67 Adductor Muscles of the Hip

Adductor Longus, Adductor Brevis, Adductor Magnus, and Gracilis

The *adductor longus*, *brevis*, and *magnus* muscles attach to the bottom of the pelvis on the upper end, cross the hip joint, and then attach along the femur below. The *gracilis* also attaches to the pelvis, but crosses both the hip and the knee joints, attaching to the tibia bone in the lower leg. The primary function of these muscles is to bring your leg toward the opposite leg, an action known as adduction.

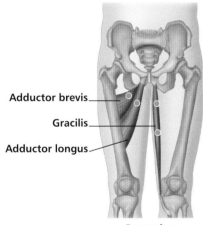

Adductor brevis

Gracilis

Adductor longus

Front view

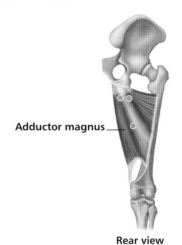

Adductor magnus

Rear view

Common Symptoms

Adductor Longus and Adductor Brevis
- Pain referred to the front of the thigh, over the front of the knee, and down the inside of the lower leg, and the pain feels deep. Pain is increased by standing and by sudden twists of the hip and may possibly only be felt during vigorous activity or muscle overload.
- Trigger points may cause stiffness of the knee, restricted range of motion in moving the thigh away from the midline of the body, and/or possibly restricted range of motion in rotating the thigh outward.

Adductor Magnus
- Pain on the front inside of the thigh, from the groin area down to the inside of the knee. Pain feels deep, possibly like it is shooting up into the pelvis and exploding like a firecracker. Pain may only occur during intercourse.
- The common trigger point high up between the legs may refer pain to the pubic bone, vagina, rectum, or possibly the bladder.
- You may have difficulty getting comfortable at night.

Gracilis
- Pain on the inside of the thigh that feels hot, stingy, and superficial. Pain may be constant at rest, and no change of position relieves it except for walking.

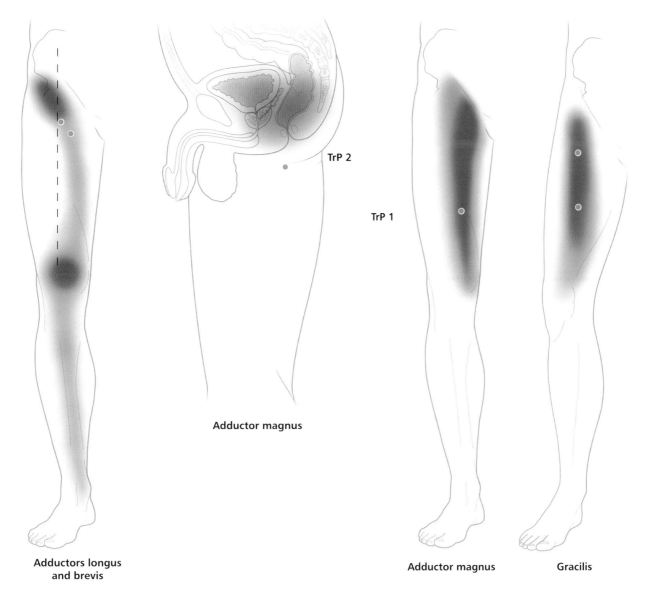

Adductor magnus

TrP 2

TrP 1

**Adductors longus
and brevis**

Adductor magnus

Gracilis

Causes and Perpetuation of Trigger Points, and Solutions

■ A sudden overload, for example trying to stop yourself from slipping on ice by attempting to keep your legs from spreading.

■ Activities such as horseback riding, running up or down hills, or long bike trips if you haven't trained for them. Skiing, most likely from snowplowing/wedge turns, or unexpectedly doing the "splits."

■ Sitting for long periods, especially when driving or with one leg crossed over the other knee.

Solutions

■ You may need to stop or modify activities until trigger points are relieved. When sleeping, put a pillow between your knees and try to keep your upper leg almost straight. Do not sit with your legs crossed, and if you must sit for long periods, stand and move around frequently.

■ Be sure to read chapter 4, particularly the sections on infections, nutritional problems, and organ dysfunction and disease.

Self-Help Techniques

If you get pain in the low back/upper gluteal area after working on the hip adductors, check the gluteus medius muscle (31) for trigger points. You may need to work on this muscle first in the future.

Apply moist heat to the upper front and inner thigh.

Applying Pressure

Parts of these muscles are more difficult to treat on yourself, so you will probably also need the help of a massage therapist, acupuncturist, or physical therapist to treat all the trigger points. Since the adductors magnus and brevis are so deep, it is hard to work on these muscles with massage alone. Ultrasound is an effective treatment.

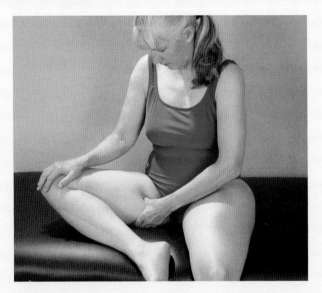

Hip Adductor Pressure
Sit with your legs bent to one side, with one heel close to the pubic area and the other one out to the side. Press a golf ball (or other pressure device in the center of your palm) into tender points on your inner thigh.

To access the upper portion of the adductor magnus, reach between your legs and find your sit bone with your fingers. Press the muscle attachment all around that area—it is easiest to use the hand of the opposite side. In addition to applying pressure to the adductor muscles, you may be able to lift and pinch part of this muscle group between the thumb and fingers of your opposite hand.

Stretches

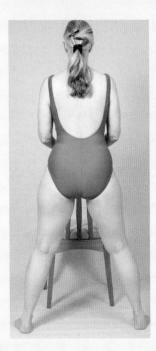
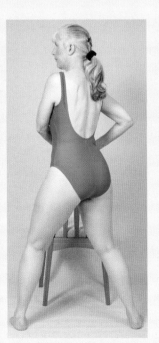
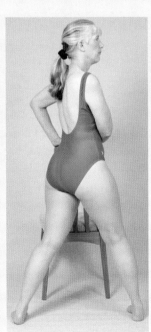

Hip Adductor Stretch
Hold onto a chair back, spread your legs apart almost as far as you can with your toes pointed straight forward, and gently rotate your pelvis away from the side you are stretching.

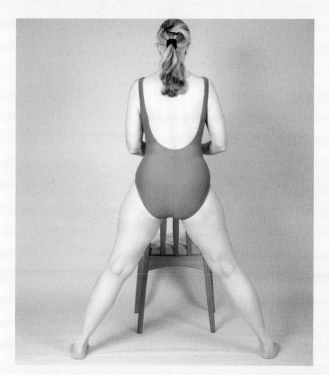

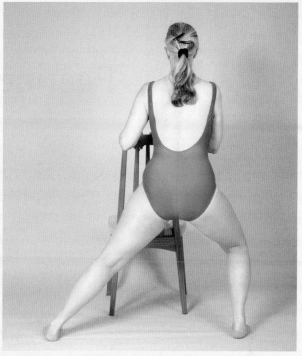

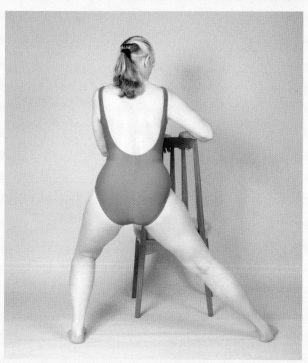

Pool Adductor Stretch

Hold onto a chair back, spread your legs apart almost as far as you can, and shift your weight to one side, allowing that knee to bend. The stretch is felt on the opposite inner thigh. It may be easier on your knees to do this stretch in a warm swimming pool in chest-deep water.

Also Check

Quadriceps femoris muscle group (65, vastus lateralis).

Differential Diagnosis

Three conditions may overload the hip adductors and cause chronic problems: pubic stress symphysitis, pubic stress fracture, and adductor insertion avulsion syndrome. If you are not able to relieve trigger points more than temporarily, you should see a health care provider to check for these conditions.

68 Pectineus

The *pectineus* muscle attaches to the pubic bone and to the femur bone of the thigh. It moves the leg toward the other leg and brings the knee toward the trunk (thigh flexion), and is used most when these two movements are combined.

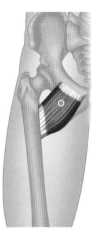

If pain remains after inactivating trigger points in the iliopsoas muscle (22) and adductor muscles of the hip (67), check the pectineus muscle.

Common Symptoms

- Deep aching pain just below the crease of the groin and possibly over the upper part of the thigh.
- Pain when sitting cross-legged or using your inner thighs to grip.

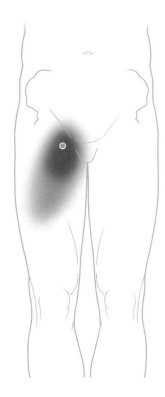

Causes and Perpetuation of Trigger Points, and Solutions

- Tripping or falling, or other sudden jerking trauma to the thigh.
- Horseback riding, or any other activity that requires you to grip strongly with your inner thighs.
- Sitting cross-legged or with the hips at less than a 90-degree angle to the torso.

Solutions

- Avoid strong gripping with your thighs until trigger points are inactivated. Do not sit in positions that aggravate trigger points. Sleep with a pillow between your legs.

- Trigger points can develop in association with conditions affecting the hip such as advanced osteoarthritis, with a fracture of the neck of the femur, or after surgery on the hip.
- One leg anatomically shorter than the other or a small hemipelvis (either the left or the right half of the pelvic bone).

Solutions

- See a specialist to correct any skeletal asymmetries. See a chiropractor or osteopathic doctor to check for lumbar vertebrae or sacroiliac joint alignment problems that may be causing a rotation of the pelvis.

Self-Help Techniques

Pain is rarely from trigger points in the pectineus muscle alone; be sure to check the adductor muscles of the hip (67) and the iliopsoas muscle (22) for trigger points.

Applying Pressure

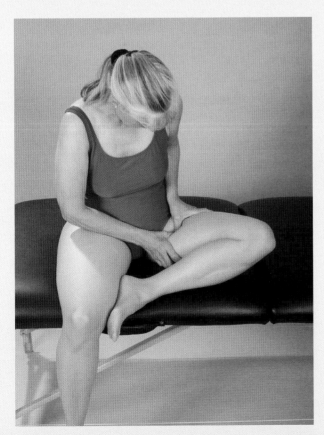

Pectineus Pressure
Sit with your knee rotated out to the side, if possible. Use one or both thumbs to apply pressure on the inner half of your thigh just below the crease of the groin. Be sure not to press too hard, since there are major nerves and arteries passing through that area.

Stretches

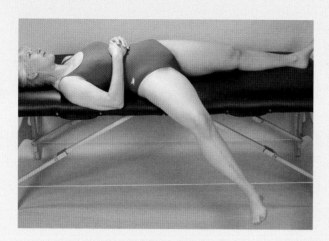

Pectineus Stretch

Position yourself on the edge of the bed, lying face-up, and hang your leg (including your thigh) at a 45-degree angle off the edge, allowing gravity to give you a stretch. If your foot touches the floor, you will need to find a higher surface to lie on.

Also Check

Adductor muscles of the hip (67). Iliopsoas (22).

Differential Diagnosis

If you are unable to relieve your symptoms with trigger point self-help techniques, you may need to see a health care provider to rule out obturator nerve entrapment, hip joint disease, pubic stress symphysitis (seen in runners and in contact sports such as ice hockey), which may occur concurrently with pectineus muscle trigger points.

69 Tibialis Anterior

The *tibialis anterior* muscle attaches to the tibia on the front of the lower leg and runs from the knee area down to its tendon attachments on some of the bones in the foot. It moves your toes up out of the way as you take each step when walking, running, hiking, etc. Trigger points in this muscle can be of particular concern because of the associated risks of falling due to balance problems and tripping.

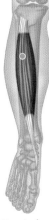

Front view

See "Compartment Syndromes" in chapter 55. If you have an anterior compartment syndrome, it is important to see a health care provider immediately for treatment. The most noticeable symptoms are tightness, dull aching, and diffuse tenderness over the entire belly of the tibialis anterior muscle, which is right next to the shin bone and runs from below the knee to about three-quarters of the way down the front of the leg. One of the causes of compartment syndrome is tight, shortened calf muscles which overload weakened anterior compartment muscles. This condition is sometimes called anterior shin splints, which is easily confused with the generic term shin splints used in the past to refer to any chronic pain in the front or middle of the lower leg associated with exercise. More recently, shin splints refers specifically to irritation of the surface of the bone along the attachment of a muscle and is called periosteal irritation.

Common Symptoms

- Pain referred over the front of the ankle and the top and side of the big toe. Possibly pain referred over the front of the lower leg and top of the foot.
- An inability to lift your toes out the way when walking, causing you to trip or fall.
- Ankle weakness or pain with motion.

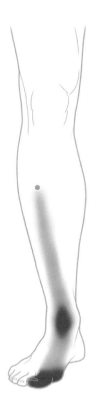

Causes and Perpetuation of Trigger Points, and Solutions

■ Direct trauma to the muscle, as in a direct blow or some other force severe enough to cause a sprained ankle or broken bone, or catching a toe on an object while walking.
■ Walking on rough ground or a slanted surface, or hiking in the spring after walking on level surfaces all winter.
■ A car accelerator pedal that is too horizontal or too vertical.

Solutions
■ Walk on smooth, level surfaces until trigger points are relieved. Then start adding short hills to strengthen the muscle. You can also start increasing the distance slowly, trying to stay within a range where the muscle does not get sore afterward.
■ If the accelerator pedal in your car is at a steep vertical angle, try attaching a wedge on the pedal with the big end at the bottom to reduce the angle of your foot. If it is nearly horizontal, experiment with attaching the big end of the wedge at the top. Using cruise control will help. Take breaks every 30 to 60 minutes.
■ At night, place a pillow against the bottom of your feet to maintain a 90-degree angle between your feet and lower legs.

■ Foot pronation.

Solutions
■ If your foot pronates you will need to get corrective orthotics. See chapter 2, "Footwear," for more information.

Self-Help Techniques

Trigger points in the tibialis anterior muscle usually occur in combination with trigger points in other leg muscles, and trigger points in other leg muscles also have similar referral patterns. Be sure to check the extensor hallucis longus and extensor digitorum longus (70), the extensor digitorum brevis and extensor hallucis brevis (71), the peroneus longus and tertius (64), the flexor hallucis longus (61), and the first interosseous (72) muscles.

Applying Pressure

Caution: Do not apply pressure to your legs if you have varicose veins in the area to be treated—it could release a clot that could go to your heart or brain! An acupuncturist or massage therapist should treat your legs, because they can avoid the varicose veins. However, you may still do the stretches below.

Gastrocnemius Pressure

It is essential to do self-help techniques on the calves first, since tightness in those muscles is likely the cause of trigger points in the tibialis anterior. If you release the tibialis anterior first, it could make the pain in the front of the leg much worse. See chapter 58.

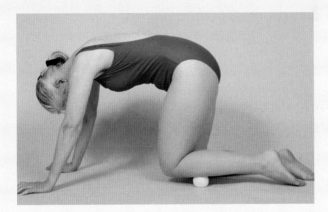

Tibialis Anterior Pressure

Even though most trigger points will be found in the upper third of the tibialis anterior, I like to work the entire length of the muscle. Get down on the floor on all-fours and place the tennis ball under the front of your lower leg. The weight of your leg should give you enough pressure. If you need more pressure, shift your weight toward the side you are working on. If you need less pressure, shift your weight away from the side you are working on. Be sure to keep your head relaxed and let it hang down.

Stretches

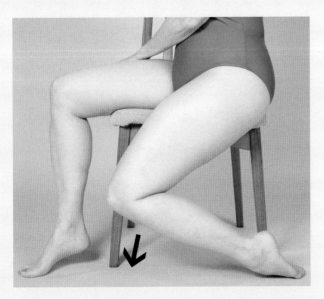

Tibialis Anterior Stretches

Sit sideways on the edge of a chair and drop your leg down so your toe is pointing behind you and the top of your foot is on the floor. Press your leg toward the floor until you get a gentle stretch. Adjust the position of your foot until you feel the stretch position that is best for you.

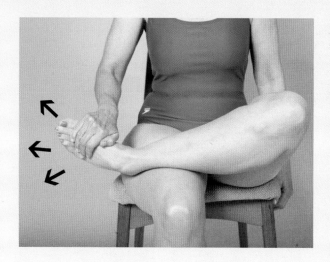

Cross your lower leg over the opposite thigh and pull the foot and toes back toward you with your hand, so you feel a stretch on the front of your leg. Moving your toes toward the ceiling or the floor will give you a slightly different stretch, so explore which angle works best for you.

Also Check

Long extensors of the toes (70, extensor hallucis longus, extensor digitorum longus). Superficial intrinsic foot muscles (71, extensor digitorum brevis, extensor hallucis brevis). Peroneal muscle group (64, peroneus tertius, peroneus longus). Long flexors of the toes (61, flexor hallucis longus). Deep intrinsic foot muscles (72, first interosseous).

Differential Diagnosis

If you are unable to relieve your symptoms with trigger point self-help techniques, you may need to see a health care provider to rule out a bunion, anterior compartment syndrome, and herniation of the tibialis anterior muscle. See a chiropractor or osteopathic physician to rule out an L5 vertebra or ankle bones out of alignment.

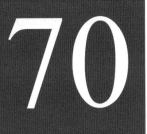

70 Long Extensors of the Toes

Extensor Hallucis Longus, Extensor Digitorum Longus

The *extensor hallucis longus* muscle attaches to the fibula bone and to the top of the bone in the big toe (great toe). The *extensor digitorum longus* attaches to both the tibia and the fibula bones in the lower leg, and to the tops of the bones of each of the four lesser toes. Both muscles prevent the forefoot from immediately slapping down upon heel-strike when walking, and they also help the foot clear the floor while the leg is swinging forward for the next step. They bring both the toes and the foot up toward the knees, an action known as dorsiflexion.

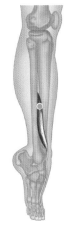
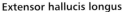

Extensor hallucis longus

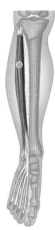

Extensor digitorum longus (front view)

Chronic tension of the long extensors of the toes can lead to hammer toe, claw toe, or mallet toe. Chronic tension in the flexor digitorum longus (61) and/or weakness in the lumbricals (72) can cause pain in the foot, leading you to lift your foot in a flat manner to avoid forefoot pressure, which overloads the extensor digitorum longus muscle. Wearing tight shoes can cause the lumbricals to atrophy or fail to develop normally during childhood, one possible initiator of the conditions mentioned above.

See "Compartment Syndromes" in chapter 55. If you have a compartment syndrome, it is important to see a health care provider immediately for treatment. One of the causes is tight, shortened calf muscles which overload weakened anterior compartment muscles. Once successfully treated, you should subsequently check for trigger points, since they were likely formed as a result of anterior compartment syndrome.

Pain from trigger points in the extensor digitorum longus muscle may be attributed to pain from the synovial joints in the bones of the foot, so be sure to check for trigger points if you have been given this diagnosis.

Common Symptoms

- Trigger points in the extensor digitorum longus refer pain mainly to the top of the foot and over the tops of the three middle toes, and sometimes over the front of the ankle and lower half of the front of the lower leg.
- Trigger points in the extensor hallucis longus refer pain over the top of the foot closest to the big toe, over the top of the big toe, and sometimes over the ankle and a little onto the front of the lower leg.
- When walking, the ball of the foot slaps down after heel-strike, or the foot will feel "weak."

- Trigger points can cause cramps at night in the front of the lower leg or when the toes are flexed toward the kneecaps for prolonged periods.
- Children and adolescents may experience "growing pains."
- The extensor digitorum longus can entrap the deep peroneal nerve and cause weakness in the muscles on the front of the lower leg and an inability to control the upward movement of the forefoot.

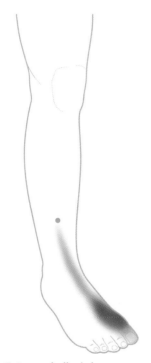

Extensor hallucis longus

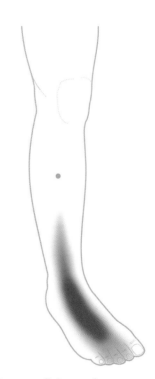

Extensor digitorum longus

Causes and Perpetuation of Trigger Points, and Solutions

- Injuries, such as tripping or falling, catching a toe on the ground when kicking a ball, a direct trauma to the muscle, or a stress fracture in one of the bones of the lower leg.
- Tight gastrocnemius (58) and/or soleus (59) muscles, which lead to a tight Achilles tendon, restricting foot movement.
- Lengthy immobilization of your foot either pointed or bent up toward your knee, such as when driving a car with an accelerator pedal that is too vertical or too horizontal, sitting in a chair with your feet tucked back a bit, wearing high heels, sleeping with your toes pointed, or wearing a cast or splint after a fracture or sprain.

Solutions

■ If the accelerator pedal in your car is at a steep vertical angle, try attaching a wedge on the pedal with the big end at the bottom to reduce the angle of your foot. If it is nearly horizontal, experiment with putting the big end of the wedge at the top. Using cruise control will help. Take breaks every 30 to 60 minutes.

■ Wear low heels or flat shoes with a wide base and buy some good orthotics. When sleeping, keep your feet at a 90-degree neutral angle, with the toes neither pointed nor bent up toward your knees—try putting a pillow against the bottom of your feet to maintain that position.

■ Keep your lower legs warm and covered. Avoid cold drafts and use a space heater near your legs if necessary. Protect your feet from cold floors.

■ If your ankle is hypo-mobile (restricted movement), see a chiropractor or osteopathic physician to increase mobility. If it is hyper-mobile (moves too much), orthotics with good arch support and a deep heel cup, along with ankle-high shoes for support, will help stabilize the foot.

■ Unaccustomed excessive walking, jogging, or running, especially on uneven ground.

Solutions

■ Until trigger points are inactivated, walk or run only on smooth surfaces, start with short distances, and increase mileage gradually. Try rowing, swimming, or bicycling instead.

■ Medical conditions, such as nutritional problems, L4 or L5 nerve root irritation, or anterior compartment syndrome (55).

Solutions

■ See chapter 3 to resolve nutritional problems. See a chiropractor or osteopathic physician if you have pain in your lumbar area and/or down your leg.

Self-Help Techniques

You may also need to check the peroneal muscle group (64), extensor digitorum brevis (71), and interossei (72), since trigger points in these muscles will also refer pain to the top of the foot, toes and ankle, and are easily confused with referral from trigger points in the extensor digitorum longus muscle. Also check the extensor hallucis brevis (71) and tibialis anterior (69), since trigger point referrals from these muscles are easily confused with those from the extensor hallucis longus muscle.

Applying Pressure

Caution: Do not apply pressure to your legs if you have varicose veins in the area to be treated—it could release a clot that could go to your heart or brain! An acupuncturist or massage therapist should treat your legs, because they can avoid the varicose veins. However, you may still do the stretches below.

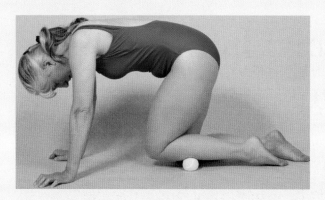

Long Extensors of the Toes Pressure

Get down on the floor on all-fours and place the tennis ball under the front of your lower leg. The weight of your leg should give you enough pressure. If you need more pressure, shift your weight toward the side you are working on. If you need less pressure, shift your weight away from the side you are working on. Try to bring your lower leg in toward your body's midline, so you are getting to the front outside angle of the lower leg.

You can also lie on your side with the tennis ball under your lower leg, again working toward the front outside angle of the lower leg.

Stretches

Tibialis Anterior Stretches
See chapter 69.

Also Check

Peroneal muscle group (64). Tibialis anterior (69).

Differential Diagnosis
Osteoarthritis or other conditions may cause inflammation, thinning, and possibly rupture of the extensor hallucis longus tendon, so you may need to see a health care provider for further examination and diagnosis.

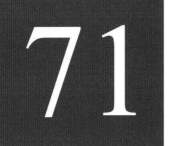

Superficial Intrinsic Foot Muscles

Extensor Digitorum Brevis, Extensor Hallucis Brevis, Abductor Hallucis, Flexor Digitorum Brevis, Abductor Digiti Minimi

The *extensors digitorum brevis* and *hallucis brevis* are on top of the foot, attaching to the top of the heel bone (calcaneus), and via tendons to the first through fourth toes. The *abductor hallucis*, *flexor digitorum brevis*, and *abductor digiti minimi* all attach to the bottom of the heel bone, and via tendons to each of the toes. As a group, the superficial intrinsic muscles of the foot control toe movement; they function as a unit to allow the flexibility to provide shock absorption and balance, as well as providing the rigidity and stability needed for walking.

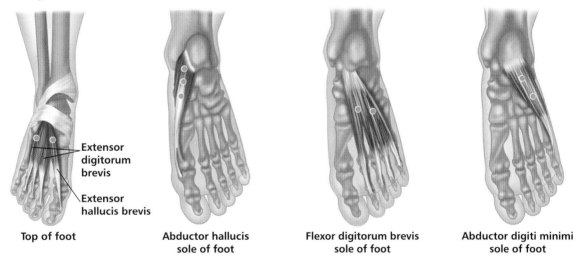

Extensor digitorum brevis

Extensor hallucis brevis

Top of foot   **Abductor hallucis sole of foot**   **Flexor digitorum brevis sole of foot**   **Abductor digiti minimi sole of foot**

Tightness and trigger points can lead to plantar fasciitis (see chapter 55), especially when combined with tightness in other muscles. Plantar fasciitis is caused by tension overload on the fascial attachment at the calcaneus (known as the plantar aponeurosis), due to tightness in the gastrocnemius (58), soleus (59), abductor hallucis, flexor digitorum brevis, and/or abductor digiti minimi muscles. The quadratus plantae (72) may also be involved.

Relief of trigger points may stop the progression or even reverse some of the spread of hallux valgus and subsequent bunions, though surgery may be necessary if the condition has progressed far enough. See the discussion on hallux valgus and bunions in chapter 55, and be sure to treat the abductor hallucis muscle for trigger points.

If you think you have an ankle sprain, but only feel pain in the foot and not the ankle area, it is likely caused by referral from trigger points in the muscles of the foot and not a sprain. If you have pain in your lower leg or ankle in addition to pain in your foot, symptoms are likely referred from trigger points in the leg or hip muscles.

Common Symptoms

- The extensor digitorum brevis and extensor hallucis brevis refer pain to the top of the foot, but slightly more toward the outside of the foot.
- The abductor hallucis refers pain and tenderness mainly to the side above the heel on the inside of the foot, with some spillover pain to the area above the arch and above the back of the heel.
- The abductor digiti minimi mainly refers pain to the ball of the foot behind the fifth toe, and possibly back a little further onto the sole of the foot.

- The flexor digitorum brevis refers pain and tenderness to the ball of the foot behind the second, third, and fourth toes, and people will usually indicate they have a "sore foot."
- A tendency to limp and an inability to walk very far due to pain, and possibly deep, aching pain even when you are not using your feet.
- The abductor hallucis can possibly cause tarsal tunnel syndrome by entrapping the posterior tibial nerve and its two branches—the medial and lateral plantar nerves—against the medial tarsal bones.

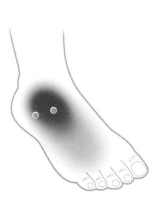

Extensor digitorum brevis, Extensor hallucis brevis top of foot

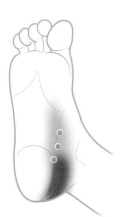

Abductor hallucis sole of foot

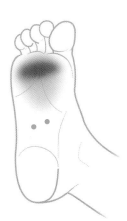

Flexor digitorum brevis sole of foot

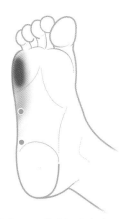

Abductor digiti minimi sole of foot

Causes and Perpetuation of Trigger Points, and Solutions

- Shoes that are too tight around the toes and ball of your foot, inflexible shoes (such as clogs), or foot pronation or supination.
- A second toe that is longer than the first toe can cause foot rocking, leading to trigger point formation in the abductor digiti minimi and abductor hallucis muscles.

Solutions

- Because of the deep, aching pain caused by trigger points in these muscles, you may have attempted to seek relief by trying many different kinds of shoes and inserts. Avoid high heels, shoes with narrow toes, and inflexible or slippery soles. Feet get wider and longer with age, so old shoes should be discarded. Pick a shoe with a wide base and cushioning, such as an athletic shoe. See the discussion of footwear in chapter 2.
- Orthotics may be uncomfortable if they press against trigger points, but after you have inactivated trigger points, wearing orthotics may be critical to obtaining lasting relief, especially if you have a longer second toe. Inactivating trigger points is crucial to eliminating pain.

- Repeatedly using your feet to pull yourself closer to your desk on a rolling chair.
- Walking or running on uneven ground or a side-slant.
- A fracture of the ankle or other bones of the foot, especially if a cast was used.
- Injuries by banging or stubbing your toes or falling.

Solutions

- Do not use your feet to move your chair around. Until trigger points are inactivated, walk or run only on smooth surfaces, start with short distances, and increase mileage gradually. Try rowing, swimming, or bicycling instead.

- Hypo-mobility or hyper-mobility of the joints of the foot.

Solutions

- If your ankle is hypo-mobile (restricted movement), see a chiropractor or osteopathic physician to increase mobility. If it is hyper-mobile (moves too much), orthotics with good arch support and a deep heel cup, along with ankle-high shoes for support, will help stabilize the foot.

- Gout, which is diagnosed by a blood test.

Solutions

- See chapter 4 for more information on gout and trigger points.

Self-Help Techniques

Check the extensor digitorum longus (70) and peroneus longus and brevis (64) muscles for trigger points, since their referral patterns are similar to those of the extensor hallucis brevis and extensor digitorum brevis. Also check the adductor hallucis (72), interossei (72), and flexor digitorum longus (61) muscles for trigger points, since their referral patterns are similar to those of the flexor digitorum brevis.

Applying Pressure

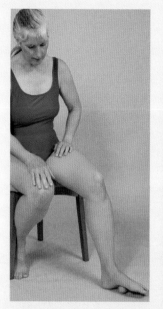
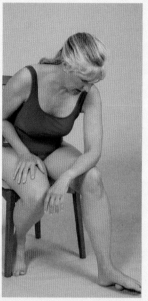
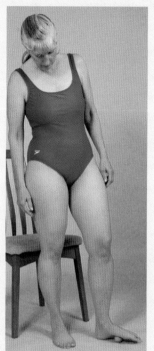

Plantar Foot Pressure
Sit in a chair and place your foot on top of a golf ball. You may roll it to different spots, holding pressure according to the general guidelines in chapter 5. Be sure to work into the edge of the arch and all the way out to the outside edge of the foot. As tenderness decreases, you can use your forearm to lean on your thigh to add pressure. If you need even more pressure, you can stand with your foot just resting on the ball, but do not shift any of your weight to that side so that you are actually standing on the ball.

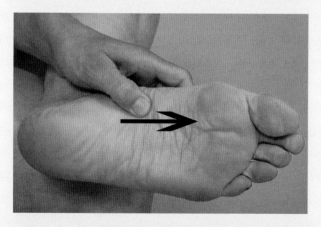

Then, sit and bring your foot across the opposite thigh, wrap your hands around your foot, and use one or both thumbs simultaneously to apply massage and pressure to the inside edge of your arch (the area that you cannot reach with the golf ball while your foot is on the floor).

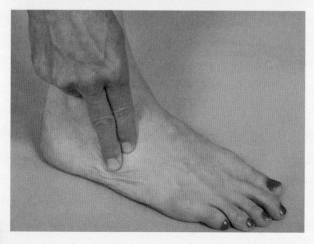

Dorsal Foot Pressure
To treat the extensors hallucis brevis and digitorum brevis, use your fingers or thumbs on the top of the foot, forward of the outside ankle bone.

Stretches

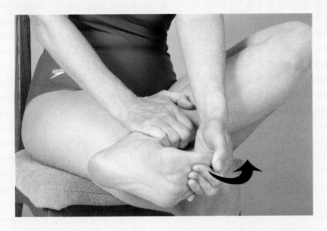

Toe Flexors Stretch
Put your foot over your opposite knee and use your opposite hand to stabilize your ankle. Use the hand of the same side you are treating to pull up on the toes, along with the entire foot. Doing this in warm water increases the benefits of the stretch.

Exercises

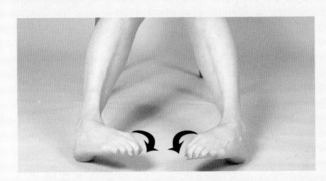 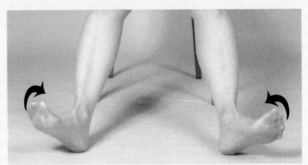

Active Toe Stretch
Sit with your legs stretched out and your heels on the floor. Point your toes while at the same time curling your toes and rotating your feet inward. Then transition to straighten your toes while bringing them up toward your knees and rotating your feet outward. This is a smooth movement. Repeat five times, pausing between each cycle.

Picking Up Marbles
Once trigger points have been inactivated for a few weeks, you can try picking up marbles with your toes to increase strength and coordination. Only do this for a couple of minutes at a time—reduce the length of time or stop entirely if soreness and pain increases.

Also Check

Long extensors of the toes (70, extensor digitorum longus). Peroneal muscle group (64, peroneus longus and peroneus brevis). Deep intrinsic foot muscles (72, quadratus plantae, adductor hallucis, flexor hallucis brevis, interossei). Long flexors of the toes (61, flexor digitorum longus). Gastrocnemius (58). Soleus and plantaris (59, soleus).

Differential Diagnosis
There are many structural problems, such as flat feet, congenital hypertrophy, an avulsion fracture, compartment syndromes, and bones that are out of alignment, that can cause foot pain. You may need to see a chiropractor, osteopathic physician, or other health care provider to be evaluated for causes of pain other than trigger points.

72 Deep Intrinsic Foot Muscles

Quadratus Plantae, Flexor Hallucis Brevis, Adductor Hallucis, and Interossei

The *quadratus plantae* is a muscle located deep in the bottom of the foot, attaching to the heel bone (calcaneus) and spanning the middle of the bottom of the foot. The *flexor hallucis brevis*, and *adductor hallucis* are also on the bottom of the foot, attaching to various bones in the foot and toes. The *interossei* are the deepest muscles in the foot and are located between the metatarsal bones. Like the superficial intrinsic foot muscles (71), the deep intrinsic foot muscles move the toes and function as a unit to allow the flexibility to provide shock absorption and balance, as well as providing the rigidity and stability needed for walking. The deep foot muscles probably help the toes adjust to variations in terrain and to dig in more effectively when walking on soft surfaces, such as sand.

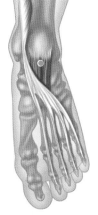 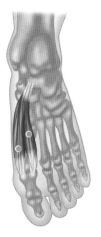 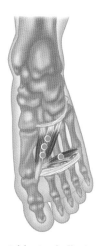 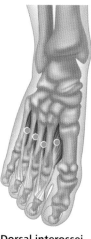 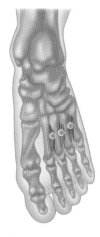

| Quadratus plantae
sole of foot | Flexor hallucis brevis
sole of foot | Adductor hallucis
sole of foot | Dorsal interossei
top of foot | Plantar interossei
sole of foot |

Muscular imbalances in the foot along with misaligned joints may lead to problems in the knee, hip, pelvis, and spine; therefore, treating trigger points in the feet and resolving the associated perpetuating factors may be crucial to resolving problems in other areas of the body.

See the discussion of hallux valgus and bunions in chapter 55, as the flexor hallucis brevis and adductor hallucis muscles are involved. Relief of trigger points may stop the progression or even reverse some of the spread of hallux valgus and subsequent bunions, though surgery may be necessary if the condition has progressed far enough.

The quadratus plantae muscle may be involved in causing plantar fasciitis. See chapter 55 for more information.

Common Symptoms

- The quadratus plantae refers pain and tenderness to the bottom of the heel.
- The adductor hallucis refers pain to the ball of the foot and is likely to cause a strange "fluffy" feeling of numbness and a sense of swelling of the skin over the ball of the foot.
- The flexor hallucis brevis refers pain and tenderness on the ball of the foot adjacent to the big toe and on the outside and top of the big toe, with spillover pain that may include most of the second toe.
- The interossei refer pain down the top of the toe closest to the affected muscle, and on the ball of the foot in a pattern closest to the affected muscle.

- Walking is limited due to pain.
- Numbness of the entire end of the foot accompanied by a feeling of swelling, mostly from trigger points in the flexor digiti minimi brevis, flexor hallucis brevis, or adductor hallucis muscles.
- The interosseous muscle between the first and second metatarsals (the bones attached to and behind the big toe and second toe) can cause tingling in the big toe that may also travel into the top of the foot and shin.
- Trigger points in any of the interossei muscles can cause hammer toes, which may disappear after inactivation of trigger points, particularly in younger patients.

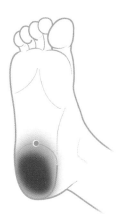
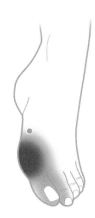
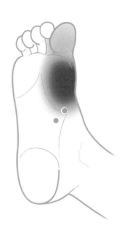
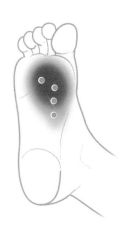

Quadratus plantae **Flexor hallucis brevis** **Adductor hallucis**

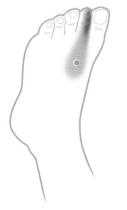
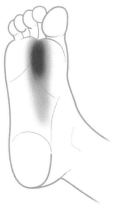

First dorsal interossei sample.
Referral corresponds to interossei
and will refer to adjoining toe

Causes and Perpetuation of Trigger Points, and Solutions

■ All of the causes and perpetuation of trigger points found in chapter 71, along with the solutions, also apply to the deep intrinsic foot muscles.
■ Chilling your feet in cold water or wearing wet socks in cold weather.

Solutions
■ Keep your feet warm and dry.

Self-Help Techniques

You may need to treat the extensor digitorum brevis (71) and/or extensor digitorum longus (70) first in order to prevent reactive cramping when you release the deep intrinsic foot muscles.

Trigger points in the deep intrinsic foot muscles are usually found in combination with trigger points in other muscles that refer pain to the foot, so be sure to check all the muscles listed for the foot in the pain guide found in chapter 6. Be sure to check the soleus (59), gastrocnemius (58), flexor digitorum longus (61), and abductor hallucis (71), since trigger points in those muscles can have somewhat similar referral patterns to the quadratus plantae. Check the gastrocnemius (58), flexor digitorum longus (61), and the flexor digitorum brevis (71) for trigger points, since their referral patterns can be confused with those of the adductor hallucis. Check the tibialis anterior (69), extensor hallucis longus (70), and flexor hallucis longus (61), since trigger point referral patterns could be confused with those of the flexor hallucis brevis.

Applying Pressure

Plantar Foot Pressure
See chapter 71.

Interossei Pressure
Buy a pencil eraser that fits on the end of a pencil. Using the tip of the eraser, press in between the bones of the foot on both the top and the bottom. As well as applying pressure, you can also move the eraser back and forth in the groove in between the long bones of the foot.

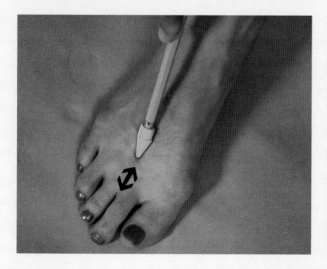
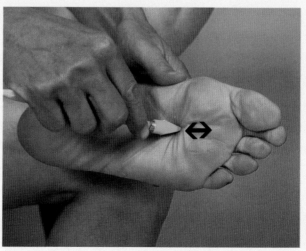

Stretches

The stretches and exercises are the same as in chapter 71.

Also Check

Soleus and plantaris (59, soleus). Gastrocnemius (58). Long flexors of the toes (61, flexor hallucis longus, flexor digitorum longus). Superficial intrinsic foot muscles (71, flexor digitorum brevis, abductor hallucis). Tibialis anterior (69). Long extensors of the toes (70, extensor hallucis longus).

Differential Diagnosis

If you are unable to relieve your symptoms with trigger point self-help techniques, you may need to see a health care provider to rule out stress fractures of the foot, structural deviations, or an injury to a sesamoid bone (the little bones on the ball of the foot at the base of the big toe) in the flexor hallucis brevis tendon.

Anyone with sore intrinsic foot muscles, particularly associated with inflammation of the big toe joints, should be tested for gout and subsequently managed, in order to obtain lasting relief with trigger point therapy.

References

Balch, J. F., & Balch, P. A.: 2000. *Prescription for Nutritional Healing: A Practical A-Z Reference to Drug-Free Remedies Using Vitamins, Minerals, Herbs, and Food Supplements.* New York: Avery.

DeLaune, V.: 2008. *Trigger Point Therapy for Headaches and Migraines: Your Self-Treatment Workbook for Pain Relief.* Oakland: New Harbinger Books.

DeLaune, V.: 2010. *Trigger Point Therapy for Foot, Ankle, Knee and Leg Pain: A Self-Treatment Workbook.* Oakland: New Harbinger Books.

Issbener, U., Reeh, P., and Steen, K.: 1996. Pain due to tissue acidosis: A mechanism for inflammatory and ischemic myalgia? *Neuroscience Letters*, 208:191–194.

Niel-Asher, S.: 2008. *The Concise Book of Trigger Points, second edition.* Chichester: Lotus Publishing.

Partanen, J., Ojala, T. A., and Arokoski, J. P. A.: 2009. Myofascial syndrome and pain: A neurophysiologic approach. *Pathophysiology*, doi:10.10266/j.pathophus.2009.05.001.

Shah, J. P, Danoff, J. V., Desai, M. J., Parikh, S., Nakamura, L. Y., Phillips, T. M., & Gerber, L. H.: 2008. Biochemicals associated with pain and inflammation are elevated in sites near to and remote from active myofascial trigger points. *Archives of Physical Medicine and Rehabilitation*, 89:16–23.

Simons, D. G., Travell, J. G., & Simons, L. S.: 1999. *Myofascial Pain and Dysfunction: The Trigger Point Manual. Vol. 1, The Upper Extremities, 2nd ed.* Baltimore, MD: Lippincott, Williams & Wilkins.

Simons, D. G., Travell, J. G., & Simons, L. S.: 1992. *Myofascial Pain and Dysfunction: The Trigger Point Manual. Vol. 2, The Lower Extremities.* Baltimore, MD: Lippincott, Williams & Wilkins.

Pronunciation of Muscle Names

MUSCLE NAME	PRONUNCIATION
Abductor Digiti Minimi	ab-DUK-ter DIJ-ih-tye MIN-ih-mye
Abductor Hallucis	ab-DUK-ter HAL-oos-is (or HAL-uh-kiss)
Adductor Brevis	ad-DUK-ter BREV-is
Adductor Hallucis	ad-DUK-ter HAL-ah-sis
Adductor Longus	ad-DUK-ter LONG-us
Adductor Magnus	ad-DUK-ter MAG-nus
Adductor Pollicis	ad-DUK-ter POL-ih-sis (or POL-ih-kiss)
Anconeus	an-KO-nee-us
Biceps Brachii	BYE-seps BRAY-kee-eye
Biceps Femoris	BYE-seps FEM-uh-ris
Brachialis	BRAY-kee-al-is
Brachioradialis	BRAY-kee-oh-ray-dee-AL-is
Buccinator	BUK-sih-NAY-tor
Bulbospongiosis	bul-boh-spun-jee-OH-ses
Coccygeus	KOK-si-jeez
Coracobrachialis	KOR-uh-ko-BRAY-kee-al-is
Deltoid	DEL-toyd
Diaphragm	DYE-ah-fram
Digastric	di-GAS-trik
Extensor Carpi Radialis Brevis	ek-STEN-ser KAR-pye ray-dee-AL-is BREV-is
Extensor Carpi Radialis Longus	ek-STEN-ser KAR-pye ray-dee-AL-is LONG-us
Extensor Carpi Ulnaris	ek-STEN-ser KAR-pye ul-NAIR-is
Extensor Digitorum	ek-STEN-ser dij-i-TOH-rum
Extensor Digitorum Brevis	ek-STEN-ser dij-i-TOH-rum BREV-is
Extensor Digitorum Longus	ek-STEN-ser dij-i-TOH-rum LONG-us
Extensor Hallucis Brevis	ek-STEN-ser HAL-ah-sis BREV-is
Extensor Hallucis Longus	ek-STEN-ser HAL-ah-sis LONG-us
Extensor Indicis	ek-STEN-ser IN-di-kis
External Abdominal Oblique	eks-TER-nal ....oh-BLEEK
Flexor Carpi Radialis	FLEK-ser KAR-pye ray-dee-AL-is
Flexor Carpi Ulnaris	FLEK-ser KAR-pye ul-NAIR-is
Flexor Digiti Minimi Brevis	FLEK-ser DIJ-ih-tye MIN-ih-mye BREV-is
Flexor Digitorum Brevis	FLEK-ser dij-i-TOH-rum BREV-is
Flexor Digitorum Longus	FLEK-ser dij-i-TOH-rum LONG-us
Flexor Digitorum Profundus	FLEK-ser dij-i-TOH-rum pro-FUN-dis
Flexor Digitorum Superficialis	FLEK-ser dij-i-TOH-rum soo-per-fish-ee-AL-is
Flexor Hallucis Brevis	FLEK-ser HAL-oos-is (or HAL-uh-kiss) BREV-is
Flexor Hallucis Longus	FLEK-ser HAL-oos-is (or HAL-uh-kiss) LONG-us
Flexor Pollicis Longus	FLEK-ser POL-li-sis LONG-us
Frontalis	fron-TAL-is

MUSCLE NAME	PRONUNCIATION
Gastrocnemius	GAS-trok-NEE-mee-us
Gemellus	jem-EL-us
Gluteus Maximus	GLOO-tee-us MAK-sim-us
Gluteus Medius	GLOO-tee-us MEE-dee-us
Gluteus Minimus	GLOO-tee-us MIN-ih-mus
Gracilis	GRASS-ih-lis
Iliocostalis Lumborum	ILL-ee-oh-KOS-tal-is lum-BOR-um
Iliocostalis Thoracis	ILL-ee-oh-KOS-tal-is tho-RAS-is
Iliopsoas	ILL-ee-oh-SOH-is
Infraspinatus	IN-frah-spy-nah-tus
Intercostals	in-ter-KOS-tals
Interossei (Foot)	in-ter-OSS-ee
Interosseous (Hand)	in-ter-OSS-ee-us
Ischiocavernosus	is-kee-oh-KAV-er-no-sus
Lateral Pterygoid	...TER-i-goid
Latissimus Dorsi	lat-ISS-im-is DOR-sye
Levator Ani	leh-VAY-tor A-nye
Levator Scapula (e)	leh-VAY-tor SCAP-yoo-lee
Longissimus Capitis	lon-JIS-i-mus KAP-i-tis
Longissimus Thoracis	lon-JIS-i-mus tho-RAS-is
Masseter	mah-SEE-ter
Medial Pterygoid	...TER-i-goid
Multifidi (dus)	mul-TIF-i-dus
Obturator Externus	OB-tu-RA-tor ex-TER-nus
Occipitalis	ok-sip-i-TAL-is
Opponens Pollicis	oh-POH-nenz POL-i-sis (or POL-i-kiss)
Orbicularis Oculi	or-bik-yoo-LAIR-is OK-yoo-lye
Palmaris Longus	PAL-mar-is LONG-us
Pectineus	pek-tin-EE-us
Pectoralis Major	pek-toh-RAL-is MA-jer
Pectoralis Minor	pek-toh-RAL-is MYE-ner
Peroneus Brevis	per-oh-NEE-us BREV-is
Peroneus Longus	per-oh-NEE-us LONG-us
Peroneus Tertius	per-oh-NEE-us TER-shee-us
Piriformis	peer-uh-FOR-miss
Plantaris	plan-TEHR-iss
Platysma	pluh-TIZ-MUH
Popliteus	POP-lih-TEE-us
Pronator Teres	PRO-nay-ter TAIR-eez
Pyramidalis	PIR-ah-mid-ah-liss

MUSCLE NAME	PRONUNCIATION
Quadratus Lumborum	quad-DRAT-us lum-BOR-um
Quadratus Plantae	quad-DRAT-us PLAN-tee
Rectus Abdominis	REK-tus ab-DOM-i-nis
Rectus Femoris	REK-tus FEM-uh-ris (or fem-OR-is)
Rhomboid	ROM-boyd
Sartorius	sar-TOR-ee-us
Scalene	SKAY-leenz
Serratus Anterior	ser-RAY-tus an-TEER-ee-or
Semimembranosus	sem-ee-mem-brah-NO-sis
Semispinalis Capitis	sem-ee-spy-NAY-lis KAP-i-tis
Semitendinosus	sem-ee-ten-din-OH-sis
Soleus	SOH-lee-us
Sphincter Ani	SFINGK-ter A-nye
Splenius Capitis	SPLEH-nee-us KAP-i-tis
Splenius Cervicis	SPLEH-nee-us SUR-vuh-sis
Sternalis	stern-AH-liss
Sternocleidomastoid	STERN-oh-KLYE-doh-MAS-toyd
Subclavius	sub-CLAY-vee-us
Suboccipital	sub-ahk-SIH-pih-tul
Subscapularis	sub-SKAP-yoo-lar-is
Supinator	SOO-pin-ayt-er
Supraspinatus	SOO-prah-spy-nah-tus
Temporalis	tem-poh-RAL-is
Tensor Fasciae Latae	TEN-sor FASH-ee (or FASH-ee-ay) LAT-tee
Teres Major	TER-eez MA-jer
Teres Minor	TER-eez MYE-ner
Tibialis Anterior	tib-ee-AL-is
Transverse Perineum	...per-uh-NEE-uhm
Trapezius	trah-PEE-zee-us
Triceps Brachii	TRY-seps BRAY-kee-eye
Vastus Intermedius	VAS-tus in-ter- MEE-dee-us
Vastus Lateralis	VAS-tus lat-er-AL-is
Vastus Medialis	VAS-tus mee-dee-AL-is
Zygomaticus	zye-goh-MAT-ik-us

General Index

Index of Muscles